Musculoskeletal Disorders in Primary Care

RCGP Curriculum for
General Practice Series

# Musculoskeletal Disorders in Primary Care

*A guide for GPs*

*Edited by*
Louise Warburton

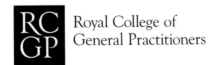

The Royal College of General Practitioners was founded in 1952 with this object:

*'To encourage, foster and maintain the highest possible standards in general practice and for that purpose to take or join with others in taking steps consistent with the charitable nature of that object which may assist towards the same.'*

Among its responsibilities under its Royal Charter the College is entitled to:

*'Diffuse information on all matters affecting general practice and issue such publications as may assist the object of the College.'*

**British Library Cataloguing-in-Publication Data**
A catalogue record for this book is available from the British Library

© Royal College of General Practitioners 2012

Published by the Royal College of General Practitioners 2011
1 Bow Churchyard, London EC4M 9DQ

**Disclaimer**
This publication is intended for the use of medical practitioners in the UK and not for patients. The authors, editors and publisher have taken care to ensure that the information contained in this book is correct to the best of their knowledge, at the time of publication. Whilst efforts have been made to ensure the accuracy of the information presented, particularly that related to the prescription of drugs, the authors, editors and publisher cannot accept liability for information that is subsequently shown to be wrong. Readers are advised to check that the information, especially that related to drug usage, complies with information contained in the *British National Formulary*, or equivalent, or manufacturers' datasheets, and that it complies with the latest legislation and standards of practice.

Designed and typeset at the Typographic Design Unit
Printed by Hobbs the Printers Ltd
Indexed by Susan Leech

ISBN: 978-0-85084-333-0

# Contents

List of contributors    *vii*
Preface    *xvii*
List of abbreviations    *xix*


**Introduction** | *Louise Warburton*    1

**Chapter 1** | *John Tanner*
The management of acute back and neck pain    9

**Chapter 2** | *Steve Longworth*
Chronic back and neck pain    35

**Chapter 3** | *Krysia Dziedzic and Lindsay M. Bearne*
The principles of physiotherapy    65

**Chapter 4** | *Caroline Anne Mitchell and Ade Adebajo*
Primary care diagnosis and management of shoulder disorders    85

**Chapter 5** | *Martyn B. Speight and Jon Greenwell*
Hip and knee problems    109

**Chapter 6** | *Anthony Redmond and Anne-Maree Keenan*
Foot problems    133

**Chapter 7** | *Adrian Dunbar and Daniel Wardleworth*
Tendonopathy    169

**Chapter 8** | *Claire Y. J. Wenham and Philip G. Conaghan*
Osteoarthritis    185

**Chapter 9** | *Pam Brown*
Osteoporosis and metabolic bone disease    213

**Chapter 10** | *Peter Glennon*
Fibromyalgia and allied syndromes    239

**Chapter 11** | *Elspeth Wise*
Acute arthropathies   263

**Chapter 12** | *Peter Lanyon*
Rheumatoid arthritis: ongoing management   283

**Chapter 13** | *Philip S. Helliwell and Laura C. Coates*
Spondyloarthropathy   307

**Chapter 14** | *Graham Davenport*
Connective tissue diseases   335

**Chapter 15** | *Jean Oliver*
Hypermobility   357

**Chapter 16** | *David Walker*
Polymyalgia rheumatica and giant cell arteritis   371

**Chapter 17** | *Helen Foster*
Musculoskeletal problems in children and adolescents   381

**Chapter 18** | *Alastair Wass and Brian Fitzsimons*
Pre-hospital emergency care and the management of burns   409

**Chapter 19** | *Edward Roddy and Michael Doherty*
Gout   439

**Chapter 20** | *Nerys Williams*
Musculoskeletal disorders and working-age health   453

Colour figures   473

Index   489

# Contributors

**Dr Louise Warburton** MRCGP DFFP DRCOG DM-SMed has been a GP for 20 years and GPwSI in musculoskeletal medicine and rheumatology for six years. Prior to that she was a rheumatology clinical assistant for eight years. She currently works with the Telford community rheumatology service and musculoskeletal interface service. She is President of the Primary Care Rheumatology Society and has been a Medical Editor of *Hands On* for Arthritis Research UK. Dr Warburton is a specialist GP on the Guidelines Development Group for NICE in the preparation of guidelines for *Rheumatoid Arthritis* (CG79) and is author of articles for a variety of GP magazines and other publications in the medical field. She is a member of the MSK specialist collection for www.evidence.nhs.uk.

**Dr Ade Adebajo** is a Consultant Rheumatologist in South Yorkshire. His academic interest is in the field of health services research and educational research in the field of rheumatology. He has a particular interest in the interface between primary and secondary care rheumatology. In addition to his clinical commitments, Dr Adebajo is Associate Director of Teaching for the University of Sheffield Medical School. He also leads an active and vibrant research group. He has published and lectured extensively and sits on a number of international committees. He is a tutor on the twice-yearly South Yorkshire GP Registrar course and regular gives talks to GPs on rheumatological conditions. Dr Adebajo is Associate Editor for a major rheumatology journal and sits on the editorial board of several international journals. He has also edited and contributed to several books. He has written widely on shoulder problems and has conducted various research studies on this topic. Dr Adebajo is a Board Member of the Arthritis and Musculoskeletal Alliance (ARMA), the umbrella body for all patient and professional groups dealing with musculoskeletal conditions in the UK. Dr Adebajo is a member of the Cochrane Collaboration. He is a Fellow and Examiner of the Royal College of Physicians (United Kingdom). He is the Regional Adviser for the North of England for the Royal College of Physicians and Surgeons of Glasgow. He is a recent External Examiner for the University of London MBChB Examinations and a Fellow of the American College of Physicians. He is an External Adviser for Postgraduate Courses and in particular the musculoskeletal course at the University of Bradford. He also teaches at Sheffield Hallam University and the Liverpool School of Tropical Medicine. He has been a Temporary Adviser to the World Health Organization on two occasions and is an Associate Editor of NHS Evidence. He is a Lead Clinical Tutor for one of the European League against Rheumatism (EULAR) online course modules and has also contributed to the Royal College of General Practitioners online learning programme. His academic appointments include a professorial chair in the United States.

**Dr Lindsay M. Bearne** qualified as a physiotherapist from King's College London, specialising in musculoskeletal and rheumatological physiotherapy. She has worked clinically in the NHS, private hospitals and in private practice. After obtaining an MSc in Sports Science from Loughborough University in 1992 and a PhD from Kings' College London in 2000, Dr Bearne worked in research and academia developing an interest in the consequences and rehabilitation of chronic musculoskeletal conditions, specifically inflammatory arthritis. In 2002, Lindsay was appointed a lecturer in Physiotherapy at King's College London where she teaches medical, nursing and allied health professionals, and supervises undergraduate and postgraduate research projects. She has published original research and contributed to books, national guidelines and information pamphlets aimed at patients and practitioners. She continues to work in clinical practice and liaises with patient self-help groups such as the National Rheumatoid Arthritis Society. Lindsay is currently a Trustee and Research Officer of the British Health Professionals in Rheumatology. At King's College London, Lindsay is a member of an interdisciplinary health and social care research division that undertakes programmes of research to improve the quality of services and health and social outcomes relating to individual clinical and social needs, service delivery and organisation, and the wider social and policy context of care.

**Dr Pam Brown** MRCGP s an Edinburgh graduate who has been a GP in Swansea, South Wales, for more than a quarter of a century, most recently in an inner-city practice. She was a founder member of the Primary Care Rheumatology Society (PCR) and has worked closely with both the PCR and the National Osteoporosis Society throughout their respective 25-year histories. She was an author and tutor on the Diploma in Primary Care Rheumatology at the University of Bath until 2010, and is now involved in the development of the Musculoskeletal Module of the University of Bath's MSc in Primary Care. Pam is a member of the Welsh Osteoporosis Advisory Group and clinical assistant in the metabolic bone clinic, and is currently helping develop a fracture liaison service in Swansea. Pam recently joined Public Health Wales as a Primary Medical Care Adviser, and is a GP appraiser. Pam writes regularly for the GP journals on her three passions – osteoporosis, obesity and diabetes.

**Dr Laura Coates** MBChB PhD MRCP Dip Epi qualified in 2003 from the University of Liverpool and is currently working as a rheumatology trainee in the Yorkshire Deanery. She has recently completed her PhD entitled 'Improving the outcome of psoriatic arthritis'. She is a member of the Group for Research and Assessment of Psoriasis and Psoriatic Arthritis (GRAPPA) and the psoriatic arthritis and MRI imaging groups of the Outcome Measures in Rheumatology Clinical Trials (OMERACT) Network.

**Prof. Philip Conaghan** MB BS PhD FRCP FRACP holds the Chair of Musculoskeletal Medicine at the University of Leeds, and is a Consultant Rheumatologist for the Leeds Teaching Hospitals NHS Trust. He is a Senior Investigator for the UK National Institute for Health Research (NIHR) and is Deputy Director of the NIHR Leeds Musculoskeletal Biomedical Research Unit. His research incorporates a spectrum from translational and proof-of-concept work through to large clinical trials. His major research interest is understanding pharmacotherapeutic response in rheumatoid arthritis, psoriatic arthritis and osteoarthritis, with a special focus on the roles of imaging. He has just completed his term as Chair of the EULAR Standing Committee on Imaging, and is lead for the Imaging and Biomarker stream of OMERACT. He chairs a Working Group of the OARSI FDA Osteoarthritis Initiative, is Chair of the Arthritis Research UK's national Osteoarthritis Clinical Studies Group and was previously Chair of the UK National Institute for Health and Clinical Excellence (NICE) Osteoarthritis Clinical Guidelines group. He has authored over 200 publications as peer-reviewed papers, review articles and book chapters.

**Dr Graham Davenport** FRCGP is a single-handed rural GP and, having been taught by Frank Dudley Hart at Westminster Hospital, has maintained his interest in rheumatology through the Primary Care Rheumatology Society (PCR) of which he is a past-President. Dr Davenport completed an MSc in rheumatology in 1999, with his thesis on 'How to reduce the gastro-intestinal complications of non-steroidal anti-inflammatory drugs in primary care' and has been involved in postgraduate education for GPs as a lecturer, trainer, course organiser and appraiser. He has a particular interest in osteoporosis and is involved in the development of osteoporosis guidelines. He ran a successful Train the Trainers Osteoporosis Conference in London in 2010. He represents the RCGP on the Health Professional Partner Forum of the National Osteoporosis Society, the Executive Committee of the National Hip Fracture Database and the steering group of the National Audit of Falls and Bone Health in Older People. He is also the RCGP's Clinical Champion for Osteoporosis (Musculoskeletal Medicine). Dr Davenport is involved in several research and audit studies, and is currently organising a primary care-based research study into the management of carpal tunnel syndrome. He has chaired a working party to develop guidelines for the early management of inflammatory arthropathy (the 'S-factor'), which has been released recently, and he is running a series of musculoskeletal educational days for GPs and registrars under the auspices of the RCGP and the PCR.

**Prof. Michael Doherty** is Head of Department and Director of Clinical & Epidemiological Research at the Arthritis Research UK Pain Centre, the University of Nottingham.

**Dr Adrian Dunbar** has worked as a GP for 22 years whilst acquiring an interest in musculoskeletal medicine and education for primary care. For the last 6 years he has worked as a GP with a Special Interest in musculoskeletal medicine and chronic pain management. He is also an Associate Postgraduate Dean at the Department of Postgraduate General Practice Education, Yorkshire and Humber Deanery, University of Leeds.

**Prof. Krysia Dziedzic** qualified as a physiotherapist at Manchester Royal Infirmary in 1982. Her clinical career was undertaken in Withington, Sevenoaks, Medway and Rochester Hospitals and at the Staffordshire Rheumatology Centre, the Haywood, Burslem. She completed her PhD at Keele University in 1997 and became a Senior Research Fellow and a Keele and West Midlands Physiotherapy Clinical Trialist, a post focusing on enhancing evidence based physiotherapy practice through randomised, controlled clinical trials. In 2000 she was appointed Arthritis Research UK Senior Lecturer in Physiotherapy. Prof. Dziedzic works as part of an interdisciplinary research team at Keele that was awarded Arthritis Research UK funding as the Arthritis Research UK Primary Care Centre in 2008 and was recognised in 2009–10 by the award of a prestigious Queen's Anniversary Award to Keele University. She was awarded a personal chair by Keele University in 2010, as Arthritis Research UK Professor of Musculoskeletal Therapies. Prof. Dziedzic had been president of the British Health Professionals in Rheumatology and was co-author of the ARMA Standards of Care for Osteoarthritis and the NICE recommendations for the management of osteoarthritis. She is a member of the Keele research team collaborating with Graham Davenport and the Primary Care Rheumatology Society to develop a randomised, controlled trial in primary care for carpal tunnel syndrome.

**Dr Brian Fitzsimons** graduated from the University of Aberdeen in 1987 and obtained his MRCGP in 1991. Initially he spent nearly five years as an associate GP between Scourie/Kinlochbervie and Durness Practices, before moving to partnership in Lochinver for nearly six years. Family illness led to a move to Tain in 2001. He is a very active BASICS GP and MIO for NHS Highland. He has been a trainer with the British Red Cross in the Highlands for five years, and became a BASICS UK Instructor in April 2010.

**Prof. Helen Foster** FRCP FRCPCH DCH Cert Med Ed is Professor of Paediatric Rheumatology at Newcastle University and Honorary Consultant, Newcastle Hospitals NHS Trust.

**Dr Peter Glennon** MA MMEDSc FRCGP DCH DRCOG DipIMC is a full-time GP, trainer and senior partner at Browning Street Surgery, Stafford. He is a former clinical assistant and GPwSI in rheumatology and a former editor of *Synovium*, a newssheet produced by Arthritis Research UK.

**Dr Jon Greenwell** qualified in general practice in 2006. Since then he has also undertaken training in sports and exercise medicine. He currently shares his time between working for NHS Bradford and Airedale as a GP with a Special Interest in musculoskeletal medicine and working in elite sport, as team physician to Leeds Carnegie and Leeds Rhinos rugby teams, and as medical officer to the British swimming team. Dr Greenwell developed and teaches on the Postgraduate Diploma in Musculoskeletal Medicine with Rheumatology at the University of Bradford, aimed at developing GP skills and training further GPwSIs.

**Dr Philip S. Helliwell** qualified in 1972 at the University of Oxford after an initial degree in psychology and physiology. Dr Helliwell received specialist training in nuclear medicine before spending five years in primary care. He was appointed as a consultant rheumatologist in 1990, and to an academic post in 1996. His current research programme includes clinical subgroups and diagnostic criteria for psoriatic arthritis, and clinical and biomechanical studies of the foot/ankle in musculoskeletal disorders.

**Dr Anne-Maree Keenan** is Assistant Director of the NIHR Leeds Musculoskeletal Biomedical Research Unit (LMBRU). After qualifying as a podiatrist in Melbourne, Australia, Dr Keenan worked in public and private sector positions, before taking on a full time teaching and academic role, initially at

LaTrobe University, then at the University of Western Sydney before moving to Leeds in 2002. Her research interests are in osteoarthritis, plantarfasciitis and the efficacy of foot orthoses, where she has published over 45 papers. She has methodological expertise in clinical trials, observational studies and patient-centred outcome measures. Dr Keenan is the Leeds Teaching Hospital's Trust Research lead for Musculoskeletal Disease and is the LMBRU's patient and public involvement lead.

**Dr Peter Lanyon** DM FRCP MRCGP DRCOG graduated from the University of Birmingham in 1986, and initially trained in general practice, where the large community burden of musculoskeletal disorders amongst the working population sparked his interest in rheumatology. He therefore decided to leave general practice to obtain further training in this area, and has been a Consultant Rheumatologist at Nottingham University Hospital since 1999. He is the RCP Regional Specialty Adviser for Rheumatology in the East Midlands, and a member of the BSR Clinical Affairs Committee. He has been actively involved in GP education for the last 20 years as a member of the PCR Society Steering Committee, and is a past author and tutor for the University of Bath Diploma in Primary Care Rheumatology.

**Dr Stephen Longworth** MSc FRCGP DM-SMed DPCR qualified 30 years ago and has been a full-time GP in Leicester for 25 years. He has also worked in the Shoulder Clinic of the Department of Orthopaedic Surgery at Leicester General Hospital, and currently works there in the Spine Clinic for one session per week as a Specialist Doctor. Dr Longworth was the first GP with a Special Interest in Musculoskeletal Medicine in Leicester and co-authored a paper in the BJGP about the effectiveness of this approach to managing musculoskeletal problems. He has a master's degree in Sport and Exercise Medicine and diplomas in Musculoskeletal Medicine and Primary Care Rheumatology. He was a GP Trainer for 10 years, is currently an Appraiser and undergraduate Tutor, and has been a Visiting Professor in the Department of Clinical Skills at St George's University Medical School in the Caribbean. He is a past President of the Primary Care Rheumatology Society and was a Tutor and Examiner for the Diploma in Primary Care Rheumatology at the University of Bath. He is co-author of the bestselling book *Injection Techniques in Orthopaedic and Sports Medicine*, which has been translated into French, Greek and Chinese. The 4th edition will be published in 2011 under the new title *Injection Techniques in Musculoskeletal Medicine: a practical manual for clinicians in primary and secondary care*. Dr Longworth also co-authored the chapter on clinical assessment in *The ABC of Spinal Disorders* from BMJ Books and has written articles about musculoskeletal topics for *Update, Prescriber, GP* and others. He has been a guest expert on Radio 4 medical programmes *Case Notes* and *Check Up* on the topics of back and shoulder pain. In 2001 he made an educational video on 'Shoulder Pain in Primary Care' with the Video Education Unit at the University Hospitals of Leicester NHS Trust. He has been published twice in *Nature* (in their science fiction story feature 'Nature Futures').

**Dr Caroline Anne Mitchell** MBChB MD FRCGP DRCOG PGCertMEd has been a GP in Sheffield since 1990 and a part-time Senior Clinical Lecturer at the University of Sheffield (Academic Unit of Primary Care) since 1993. She has had an interest in musculoskeletal disorders, specifically shoulder pain, having co-authored articles on the topic for the *British Medical Journal*, the Arthritis Research Campaign, the *ABC of Rheumatology* and also an e-learning module for the RCGP. Her MD was an RCT evaluation comparing physiotherapy interventions for total knee replacement and she continues to have an academic interest in evidence-based primary care interventions for knee osteoarthritis. Most recently she has been a member of the content development and steering groups for the NHS Choices patient shared-decision aid for knee arthritis. She currently represents the RCGP on the Standing Committee for Rehabilitation Medicine at the Royal College of Physicians.

**Jean Oliver** is a physiotherapist working in Cambridge.

**Dr Anthony Redmond** PhD is a Senior Lecturer in the Section of Musculoskeletal Disease at the University of Leeds Institute for Molecular Medicine and an Honorary Professor in Clinical Biomechanics at Staffordshire University. He heads the Leeds foot and ankle studies group 'FASTER', and contributes to a portfolio of work in rheumatology and orthopaedics across the Leeds NIHR Musculoskeletal Biomedical Research Unit and the Institute for Medical and Biological Engineering. Studies cover the basic science of the lower limb in rheumatic diseases; clinical trials in osteoarthritis, rheumatoid arthritis, soft-tissue rheumatism, ankylosing spondylitis and hypermobility syndrome, as well as translational studies in bioengineering and joint-replacement technologies. Dr Redmond contributed to the NICE guidelines for osteoarthritis and rheumatoid arthritis and was lead author of the ARMA/PRCA National Standards of Care for foot problems in musculoskeletal diseases. He has authored more than a dozen books and book chapters and published more than 50 journal articles in the fields of biomechanics and musculoskeletal and neuromuscular medicine. Anthony is currently Chair of the Arthritis and Musculoskeletal Alliance (ARMA), the umbrella body for the UK musculoskeletal community.

**Dr Edward Roddy** graduated from the University of Nottingham in 1997 and subsequently undertook training in general medicine in Nottingham and Western Australia. On his return to the UK in 2001, he embarked upon specialist training in rheumatology in the East Midlands. During this period, he undertook his doctoral thesis under the supervision of Prof. Michael Doherty at the University of Nottingham, researching the epidemiology and treatment of gout in primary care. He came to Keele University in 2007 as a Clinical Lecturer in Rheumatology at the Arthritis Research UK Primary Care Centre and Honorary Consultant Rheumatologist at the Haywood Hospital. He is a fellow of the Royal College of Physicians.

**Dr Martyn B. Speight** MB ChB Dip Sports Med DMS-Med FFSEM MLCOM is a musculoskeletal and sports physician, as well as a registered osteopath. Dr Speight has been a full-time practitioner of musculoskeletal (MSK)/sports and exercise medicine (SEM) for the last 12 years. Prior to this he worked in all areas of the NHS dealing with MSK problems (orthopaedics, rheumatology, GP and A&E medicine) before deciding to specialise. He has a very eclectic/holistic approach to MSK problems, drawing on many different modalities/management strategies, including osteopathic techniques. His clinical work is based in Otley and Leeds, currently in private practice, working in close liaison with multidisciplinary teams including all related disciplines across the spectrum of MSK/SEM. He is a tutor and faculty member at the London College of Osteopathic Medicine. He has a very keen interest in the development of MSK as a specialty subject, and as such has regular commitments to BIMM's teaching programme as well as lecturing at various venues. His main areas of clinical interest are lower-limb problems in athletes/sportspeople and lumbar pelvic pain syndromes. His past experience with elite sports has been in tennis players, whilst at present he has regular involvement with both Super League rugby league players and Guinness Premiership rugby union players, as well as full-time endurance athletes.

**Dr John Tanner** BSc FFSEM DM-SMed DSMSA qualified in 1977 and trained first as a GP before specialising in orthopaedic and sports medicine. He ran a sports injury clinic in Milton Keynes for seven years, a medical osteopathic practice in Bermuda for four years and on return to the UK developed the Oving Clinic as a multidisciplinary practice in West Sussex. He has been running a practice in Guildford for the last four years and does procedures at Mount Alvernia Hospital. He also worked as an Associate Specialist at Odstock Rehabilitation in the Pain Management team for ten years and for two years in orthopaedics at Worthing. He has authored three books, *Better Back*, *Your Guide to Back Pain* and *The BMA Guide to Back Care*. He pioneered the use of extracorporeal shockwave therapy in tendinopathy in the UK, and has a special interest in chronic musculoskeletal and spinal pain, interventional pain relief techniques and psychological management. He is an Instructor for the International Spinal Intervention Society and sits on its European Faculty. He has set up a new course for postgraduate training for doctors in Musculoskeletal Medicine, teaching regularly throughout the UK. He works at BUPA Health and Wellbeing as Co-Clinical Lead at the Barbican and takes referrals from GPs and colleagues covering a wide range of problems.

**Dr David Walker** MA MD FRCP is a Consultant Rheumatologist at Freeman Hospital, Newcastle Upon Tyne Hospitals NHS Trust. His research interest is in education, including primary care. He is on the Arthritis Research UK Education Strategy Committee and regularly attends the Primary Care Rheumatology Society.

**Dr Daniel Wardleworth** MBChB MRCGP is a GP at the Haworth Medical Practice, Keighley. He has a special interest in musculoskeletal conditions.

**Alastair Wass** FRCS FCEM qualified from St Thomas' Hospital in 1987 and subsequently passed FRCS in 1992. Thereafter he undertook higher specialist Accident & Emergency training in Yorkshire, based in York, Leeds and Wakefield. He was appointed to his consultant post in 1996 and has remained at the Mid Yorkshire Hospitals (Pinderfields & Pontefract) ever since. He has been heavily involved with training of emergency medicine trainees as Regional Training Programme Director, Chair of the Yorkshire Deanery Speciality Training Committee and a former member of the College of Emergency Medicine (CEM) Training Standards Committee. He is an examiner for the fellowship examination for the CEM and an active Advanced Trauma Life Support Course director/instructor. He also sits on one of the CEM Article 14 assessment panels and is the current Vice-Chair of the Yorkshire & Humber CEM Regional Board. More recently, he has become involved with the National Clinical Advisory Team, looking into strategic issues surrounding rationalisation of emergency medicine services.

**Dr Claire Y.J. Wenham** is a Clinical Research Fellow within the NIHR Leeds Musculoskeletal Biomedical Research Unit at Chapel Allerton Hospital, Leeds. She is currently taking time out of her specialty registrar training to undertake an MD, studying targeted treatments for osteoarthritis using imaging-detected pathology and has a particular interest in the role of synovitis in osteoarthritis.

**Dr Nerys Williams** is a Consultant Occupational Physician based in the West Midlands who is currently working for the Department for Work and Pensions. She also works part time in an upper-limb clinic in the NHS. Her interests include obesity and disability assessment.

**Dr Elspeth Wise** is a salaried GP in Washington, Tyne and Wear. She was a holder of an Arthritis Research Campaign Educational Fellowship and recently completed her MD thesis looking at trainee GPs' musculoskeletal education. She has a continuing interest in primary care musculoskeletal education and lectures at the BMJ Musculoskeletal Masterclasses and on the University of Bradford Diploma of Musculoskeletal Medicine with Rheumatology. She currently works for one session a week in the Rheumatology Department of the Freeman Hospital, Newcastle upon Tyne.

# Preface

Musculoskeletal disorders make up approximately 20% of all consultations in primary care. GPs are therefore required to have knowledge of everything from a fractured toe to systemic lupus erythematosus!

Traditionally, teaching for undergraduates in musculoskeletal disorders has been brief and does not cover many of the common conditions very well.

This volume is an attempt to remedy this situation.

I have drawn together a group of experts in musculoskeletal medicine and rheumatology, and they have produced a textbook that is aimed at the primary care physician. We have considered common presentations of these disorders, their treatment, current guidelines on management and when to refer onwards to specialist care. Osteoporosis, inflammatory arthritis, burns and minor injuries are just some of the topics covered.

We have also addressed each disease with reference to the domains of primary care management in RCGP curriculum statement 15.9, *Rheumatology and Conditions of the Musculoskeletal System* (Including Trauma). Case histories are included in each chapter to make the information more relevant for primary care.

I hope that the book is user friendly and will dispel some of the myths about treatments for musculoskeletal problems. I also hope that in our 'brave new world' of GP commissioning, this book will support doctors in their quest to commission the best musculoskeletal care for our patients.

My thanks go to all the authors for their excellent contributions and to Dr Rodger Charlton for his comments.

Louise Warburton

# Abbreviations

ACL    anterior cruciate ligament
ACR    American College of Rheumatology
ACS    acute coronary syndrome
ADL    Activities of Daily Living
ANA    antinuclear antibody
APS    antiphospholipid syndrome
ARC    Arthritis Research Council
ARMA   Arthritis and Musculoskeletal Alliance
ASIS   anterior superior iliac spine

BASDAI    Bath Ankylosing Spondylitis Disease Activity Index
BASICS    British Association for Immediate Care
BNF       *British National Formulary*
BSR       British Society for Rheumatology

CAM      complementary and alternative medicines
CBT      cognitive behavioural therapy
CCP      cyclic citrullinated peptide
CEM      College of Emergency Medicine
CFS      chronic fatigue syndrome
CK       creatine kinase
CNB      chemical, nuclear, biological
COT      consultation observation tool
COX-2    cyclo-oxygenase-2
CREST    calcinosis, Raynaud's, oesophageal dysmotility,
         sclerodactyly and telangiectasia
CRP      C-reactive protein
CRPS     complex regional pain syndrome
CSAG     Clinical Standards Advisory Group
CT       computerised tomography
CTDs     connective tissue diseases
CVD      cardiovascular disease

DDA      Disability Discrimination Act
DEN      doctor's educational need
DES      Directed Enhanced Service
DIP      distal interphalangeal
DMARDs   disease-modifying antirheumatic drugs

DRESS   drug rash with eosinophilia and systemic symptoms
DVT   deep-vein thrombosis
DXA   dual-energy X-ray absorptiometry

EMDC   Emergency Medical Dispatch Centre
EMEA   European Medicines Agency
EMG   electromyography
ENAs   extractable nuclear antigens
EPP   Expert Patient Programme
ESR   erythrocyte sedimentation rate
EULAR   European League Against Rheumatism

FAI   femero-acetabular impingement
FBC   full blood count
FMS   fibromyalgia syndrome
FSD   functional somatic disorder

GCA   giant cell arteritis
GI   gastrointestinal
GPwSI   General Practitioner with a Special Interest
GTN   glyceryl trinitrate

HAV   hallux abducto valgus
HIV   human immunodeficiency virus
HM   hypermobility
HMS   hypermobility syndrome
HRT   hormone-replacement therapy
HRUS   high-resolution ultrasound
HSE   Health and Safety Executive

IASP   International Association for the Study of Pain
IBD   inflammatory bowel disease
IBS   irritable bowel syndrome
ICATS   Independent Care and Treatment Service
ICE   ideas, concerns and expectations
ICF   International Classification of Functioning
IFT   interferential therapy
IHD   ischaemic heart disease
IMB   intermetatarsal bursitis

JHS  joint hypermobility syndrome
JIA  juvenile idiopathic arthritis

LBP  low-back pain
LDL  low-density lipoprotein
LLLT  low-level laser therapy
LMAs  laryngeal mask airways

MDT  multidisciplinary team
ME  myalgic encephalomyelitis
MRI  magnetic resonance imaging
MSF  Musculoskeletal Services Framework
MS  monosodium urate
MSK  muskuloskeletal
MTP  metatarsophalangeal
MUA  manipulation under anaesthesia
MUPS  medically unexplained physical symptoms

NAI  non-accidental injury
NICE  National Institute for Health and Clinical Excellence
NNO  number needed to offend
NNT  number needed to treat
NOGG  National Osteoporosis Guideline Group
NREM  non-rapid eye movement
NPSA  National Patient Safety Agency
NRAS  National Rheumatoid Arthritis Society
NSAIDs  non-steroidal anti-inflammatory drugs

OA  osteoarthritis
OARSI  Osteoarthritis Research Society International
OHP  occupational health physician

PBC  practice-based commissioning
PCL  posterior cruciate ligament
PCT  Primary Care Trust
PEME  pulsed electromagnetic energy
PIP  proximal interphalangeal
PMH  previous medical history
PMR  polymyalgia rheumatica
PPE  personal protective equipment
PPI  proton pump inhibitor

PRICE   protection, rest, ice therapy, compression and elevation
PSA   prostate-specific antigen
PSIS   posterior superior iliac spine
PTH   parathyroid hormone
PUN   patient's unmet need
PV   plasma viscosity

QoF   Quality and Outcomes Framework

RA   rheumatoid arthritis
RCT   randomised controlled trial
REMS   Regional Examination of the Musculoskeletal System
RF   rheumatoid factor
RICE   rest, ice, compression and elevation
RIMA   reversible inhibitor of monoamine oxidase type-A
RTA   road traffic accident
RTC   road traffic collision

SARA   sexually acquired reactive arthritis
SERMs   selective oestrogen receptor modulators
SFOA   synovial fluid signs of OA
SLE   systemic lupus erythematosus
SLR   straight-leg raise
SNRI   serotonin-norepinephrine reuptake inhibitor
SS   symptom severity
SS   systemic sclerosis
SSRI   selective serotonin reuptake inhibitor
STAT   Society of Teachers of the Alexander Technique
SWD   short-wave diathermy

TBSA   total body surface area
TCAD   tricyclic antidepressant
TENS   Transcutaneous Electrical Nerve Stimulation
THA   total hip arthroplasty
TKA   total knee joint arthroplasty
TNF   tumour necrosis factor
TPD   tibialis posterior dysfunction
TSH   thyroid-stimulating hormone
TSS   toxic shock syndrome

UC   ulcerative colitis
ULT   urate-lowering therapy
URTI   upper respiratory tract infection

VAS   visual analogue score
VZIG   varicella-zoster immune globulin

WAD   whiplash-associated disorders
WHO   World Health Organization
WPI   widespread pain index
WRULD   work-related upper-limb disorder
WRULS   work-related upper-limb syndrome

# Introduction

*Louise Warburton*

## Prevalence of musculoskeletal conditions

Musculoskeletal (MSK) conditions make up 15–20% of GP consultations. At present it is estimated that around 17.3 million people in the UK, which is over one third of the adult population, have back pain. Up to 8.5 million people have joint pain, over 4.4 million have moderate to severe osteoarthritis and over 650,000 have inflammatory arthritis.[1] Prevalence is shown on Table 1.

Table 1 ○ *Musculoskeletal disease prevalence rates (per 100,000 person years at risk)*

| Disease | All ages (>16) | (95% CI) |
|---|---|---|
| All MSK events | 13,275 | (13,215, 13,336) |
| Soft-tissue rheumatism and chronic widespread pain | 4068 | (4034, 4104) |
| Back pain | 3747 | (3715, 3779) |
| Osteoarthritis | 1724 | (1702, 1746) |
| Rheumatoid arthritis | 215 | (207, 223) |
| Polymyalgia rheumatica | 165 | (159, 172) |
| Osteoporosis | 135 | (129, 141) |
| Ankylosing spondylitis | 37 | (34, 40) |
| Systemic lupus erythematosus (SLE) | 13 | (12, 15) |
| Scleroderma | 6 | (5, 7) |
| Gout | 6 | (4, 7) |

*Source*: Royal College of General Practitioners. *Rheumatology and Conditions of the Musculoskeletal System (Including Trauma).*[2]

## Costs to the individual and society

The vast number of individuals involved means that MSK conditions have huge resource implications. The total cost of back pain alone to the economy has been estimated at between 1% and 2% of gross national product, and the NHS/community care services spend over £1 billion on services for back pain.[1] In 1999–2000, £2148 billion was spent on Incapacity Benefit payments to people with arthritis and related conditions.

MSK conditions are not only common and costly to the economy but they also have major impacts on patients' lives. In the *Health Survey for England* of 2001, diseases of the MSK system were the most common cause of disability (40%).[3]

It therefore follows that all GPs and all registrars will be exposed to patients suffering from MSK disorders. The challenge for primary care is to diagnose these conditions and treat them appropriately, preventing them from becoming chronic and incurring costs to the individual and society.

## Aims of this book

This book is aimed at offering GP registrars a core text of knowledge. It is also aimed at GPs who wish to refresh or supplement their knowledge of MSK disorders. It is written with the RCGP curriculum statement in mind;[2] this statement covers trauma, burns, mechanical problems, osteoarthritis and inflammatory arthritis.

### *RCGP core competences and assessing musculoskeletal conditions*

The MSK system is fundamental to our daily lives: it is responsible for our mobility and it features in our every waking, and sometimes even sleeping, moment. It is therefore high in the patient's conscious experience and any small malfunction will be quickly recognised. Many pathologies or conditions of the MSK system will cause PAIN and a large number of consultations about the MSK system will be about pain. Because pain produces an emotional response, the consultations will also be about emotions.

Such consultations can therefore be demanding on the practitioner. Not only will the practitioner have to make an assessment and diagnosis of the problem, but also he or she will have to acknowledge the emotional status of the patient, or the consultation will be dysfunctional. This of course is part of taking a holistic approach to the patient, as described in the core competences of being a GP. These are listed below:

1 ▷ **Primary care management** ▶ manage a whole range of
   unselected patients, often with multiple conditions, as part
   of a multidisciplinary team and act as the patient's advocate
   within the healthcare system.
2 ▷ **Person-centred care** ▶ effective doctor–patient relationship
   with respect for patient's autonomy; aim to work in partnership
   and provide continuity of care over time.
3 ▷ **Specific problem-solving skills** ▶ use history, examination
   and appropriate investigations, along with knowledge of prevalence
   and incidence of disease within the community population, to
   manage conditions effectively.
4 ▷ **A comprehensive approach** ▶ promote health and manage
   multiple pathology and chronic diseases. Offer appropriate
   management options from prevention and treatment to
   rehabilitation and palliation.
5 ▷ **Community orientation** ▶ balance needs of individual patient
   with needs of community as a whole in a healthcare system with
   finite resources.
6 ▷ **A holistic approach** ▶ take into account the patient's psychological, social and spiritual beliefs.

To illustrate some of these points, we can consider the case of Ethel, who
consulted with her GP because of a painful and swollen knee. Ethel was
75 years of age and her GP noted the fact that the knee was causing Ethel
difficulties with mobility and was disturbing her sleep. He examined the
knee and found that it was indeed swollen. He noted from her past history
that Ethel had rheumatoid arthritis (RA) but was only on paracetamol. He
decided to refer Ethel to the visiting General Practitioner with a Special
Interest (GPwSI) in Rheumatology, who visited the practice every fortnight
as part of the practice-based commissioning musculoskeletal service.

The GPwSI assessed Ethel using the core competences of general practice:

**PRIMARY CARE MANAGEMENT**

*CLINICAL MANAGEMENT*

The GPwSI took a clinical history and found that Ethel had suffered from
RA for 30 years and had been under the care of the local rheumatology unit.
She had been attending for annual review. She had never had any disease-
modifying therapy (disease-modifying antirheumatic drugs, DMARDs),
partly because of her fears about these therapies and partly because she had
been lost to follow-up at various points in the past. She had also been seeing

junior members of the team at each visit, who were not as experienced as the consultant.

Ethel has severe joint disease with ulnar deviation of her fingers, loss of hand function, fixed flexion deformities of her elbows and a large knee effusion on the left. She had marked quadriceps wasting of the left thigh. She was also very thin and showed all the signs of well-established RA. She could hardly walk.

The GPwSI looked at the co-morbidities of RA that Ethel most certainly had – osteoporosis and cardiovascular disease – and considered how to diagnose and manage these.

### WORKING WITH COLLEAGUES AND TEAMS

The GPwSI reviewed Ethel's notes and the last few clinic letters. He decided that he would involve other members of the multidisciplinary team (MDT) and referred Ethel to the practice physiotherapist. He also referred her to the practice social worker to discuss her current care package (which was none) and the possibilities of extra support for Ethel and her husband.

He also arranged a bone density scan to screen for osteoporosis and blood tests to check disease activity (ESR and CRP, haemoglobin) and fasting lipids.

### PRIMARY CARE ADMINISTRATION AND IMT

All the recent clinic letters were scanned into Ethel's records for ease of access. The GPwSI noted that Ethel had not had her annual influenza vaccination, despite an invitation, and had never had a pneumovax. He was able to offer these to Ethel that day. She agreed to have them once the reasons were explained.

Ethel's RA problem had been filed under past problems in her GP computer record, so the GPwSI reactivated the problem as a current condition. This was so it was more obvious to other members of the MDT using her records.

### PERSON-CENTRED CARE

### COMMUNICATION AND CONSULTATION SKILLS

The GPwSI explored Ethel's health beliefs about her RA and what she thought about her swollen knee. He allowed her to talk about her fears of DMARDs, which would be used to treat her RA, and why she had never agreed to take them. He also asked about Ethel's support at home (husband) and what his health was like. Did Ethel have any children or relatives nearby?

4

## SPECIFIC PROBLEM-SOLVING SKILLS

### *DATA-GATHERING AND INTERPRETATION*

A full examination revealed the extent of Ethel's RA and the degree of joint damage that had happened over the years. The GPwSI made a functional assessment of Ethel's mobility; she used a walking stick but was prone to falls.

### *MAKING A DECISION*

It was clear that Ethel was not being treated in an optimal fashion. There were many pathologies that needed addressing. Blood tests had revealed high inflammatory markers and a normochromic and normocytic anaemia, again a sign of high disease activity.

Ethel needed treatment for osteoporosis.

## A COMPREHENSIVE APPROACH

### *MANAGING MEDICAL COMPLEXITY AND PROMOTING HEALTH*

Ethel's case was certainly complex; she had unmet health needs but also some fears and mistrust of the medical establishment. The GPwSI had to take all these factors into account when formulating a treatment plan. He decided to consider Ethel's health holistically and invited her husband to attend at the next consultation so that his views could be taken into account.

## COMMUNITY ORIENTATION

Ethel and her husband lived in a housing estate five miles from the local hospital. They found it difficult to get to appointments there, as Ethel could not get on and off the bus very easily and could only walk about 400 metres. They did not possess a car.

The GPwSI therefore decided that she would be best managed at the GP practice and any hospital appointments (such as the bone density scan) could be arranged with hospital transport. Conversely, Ethel was well known in the community, and friends and neighbours helped her on a daily basis with shopping.

## A HOLISTIC APPROACH

After all these factors were taken into account, Ethel's health and care had been assessed and treated holistically. The GPwSI did not offer Ethel DMARDs until he had seen her several times and established a rapport with her and her husband. She would now trust him and was less fearful of the side effects of the medication. A social worker visited them and arranged some help with Ethel's self-care such as bathing.

Ethel attended some physiotherapy sessions at the practice and, on the recommendation of the physiotherapist, was then referred to the hospital Falls Clinic so that she could have an occupational therapy assessment and be provided with a proper walking aid.

The GPwSI also aspirated and injected Ethel's left knee with 40 mg of methylprednisolone, and this produced an immediate benefit.

### *Using the framework*

Each MSK condition presented in the chapters of this book can be assessed and treated using this framework. The framework provides the GP or GP registrar with a 'toolkit' that can be used for each patient seen in the course of his or her work.

As GPs, we are uniquely placed to treat our patients holistically, and patients do not always have to travel to specialist care appointments within hospital settings. Through practice-based commissioning, there are often local networks of primary care expertise where patients with MSK problems can be assessed, in a similar way to Ethel.

### Audit and quality of treatment

At the time of writing, MSK disorders are not part of the Quality and Outcomes Framework (QoF) for general practice in the UK. Despite their prevalence and importance in terms of disease impact for the individual and society because of days of work lost, there is no special incentive to look at these conditions and audit them within general practice. MSK conditions therefore currently sit far back in the consciousness of the average GP.

It is to be hoped that this situation will be remedied in the future. Until then, we must all strive to educate ourselves and our peers about the importance of these conditions in society, and hope that they become an important part of the practice agenda.

We must continue to audit our performance. Revalidation will probably place practice and individual audit high on the agenda, and MSK conditions would be ideal for a novel audit that falls outside the QoF.

*Further resources*

There is an abundance of guidance for the care of MSK conditions available. The following resources can be accessed online:

▷ the Arthritis and Musculoskeletal Alliance (ARMA) has produced standards of care for patients with MSK conditions and provides an excellent resource and basis for practice audit (**www.arma.uk.net**)
▷ the British Society for Rheumatology has several useful guidelines, including two on RA and guidelines on the side effects and monitoring of DMARDs (**www.rheumatology.org.uk**)
▷ the National Institute for Health and Clinical Excellence (NICE) has recently produced guidelines on osteoarthritis and RA (**www.nice.org.uk**)
▷ the Primary Care Rheumatology Society offers educational resources and guidance (**www.pcrsociety.org**)
▷ Arthritis Research UK provides physician and patient literature (**www.arthritisresearchuk.org**)
▷ NHS Evidence Specialist Collections (**www.evidence.nhs.uk**), NHS Evidence (**www.library.nhs.uk/musculoskeletal**) and Athens (also at **www.evidence.nhs.uk**) – registration required
▷ the British Institute of Musculoskeletal Medicine (BIMM) offers educational resources for non-inflammatory MSK conditions (**www.bimm.org.uk**)
▷ the National Osteoporosis Society has its own guidelines for osteoporosis (**www.nos.org.uk**).

## Conclusion

I hope that those who use this book find that it enriches their lives and practice. My aims have been to present MSK conditions in a straightforward way that is focused on primary care. Treating patients with arthritis is very rewarding. My own professional life has been focused on these patients and it has brought me many benefits.

Finally I would like to thank all the experts who have contributed to this book. This book could not have produced without their hard work and dedication.

**References**

1 • Arthritis and Musculoskeletal Alliance. *Standards of Care for People with Back Pain, Inflammatory Arthritis and Osteoarthritis* London: ARMA, 2004.

2 • Royal College of General Practitioners. *Rheumatology and Conditions of the Musculoskeletal System (Including Trauma)* (curriculum statement 15.9) London: RCGP, 2007, www.rcgp-curriculum.org.uk/PDF/curr_15_9_Rheumatology_and_musculoskeletal_ problems.pdf [accessed October 2011].

3 • Bajekal M, Prescott A. *Health Survey for England 2001: disability* London: The Stationery Office, 2003.

# The management of acute back and neck pain

*John Tanner*

## 1

## Introduction

Back and neck pain are common reasons for consulting the primary care doctor. In population surveys the point prevalence for back pain in the population is between 20–30% at any one time. Further, approximately 20% of the adult population will have experienced symptoms from their neck within the last 12 months. It is estimated that in the West approximately 70% of the population will experience some significant back pain at some time in their lives; it can therefore be said that spinal pain can be regarded as a natural condition of mankind. However, its impact on healthcare resources and economic costs in Western industrialised society is significant.

In 1994 the Clinical Standards Advisory Group (CSAG) on back pain[1] reported on the impact on sickness absence and claims for incapacity benefit. It was noted that, although the incidence and prevalence of back pain was thought not to have increased over the preceding decades, the costs of payments for disability were rising exponentially, which was believed to be related to the disability benefits system. This report also highlighted the need to reorganise services and improve education of the management of back pain at all levels.

The diagnosis and management of back and neck pain have not changed significantly (except perhaps lesser use of X-rays and greater use of MRI scans) over the last 15 years because it is only recently that services are being reorganised to enable implementation of these guidelines.[2] The main thrust of this report has been to divert referrals from secondary care to an intermediate level of service based in the community – Independent Care and Treatment Service (ICATS) – which is staffed by a multidisciplinary team including a doctor with a special interest in musculoskeletal medicine, a specialist or extended-scope physiotherapist, podiatry, and ideally facilities for functional rehabilitation. To complement this there has also been a move to transfer some aspects of the pain service into the community.

The surgical management of disc prolapse and radicular pain has shifted towards microdiscectomy, enabling quicker recovery and reduced postoperative morbidity. The increased use of minimally invasive techniques such as the X stop for decompression of a stenosed spinal canal has been a significant advance. The X stop is a mechanical device that is placed between the spinous processes in the lumbar spine. It can be expanded once inserted, and helps to open up the spinal canal and nerve root foraminae.

It is too early to know whether these changes in service delivery have made any difference to clinical outcomes. However, there are already several reports from audits of these musculoskeletal services that show reduced access times, high patient satisfaction and significant cost savings.[3]

During this time legislation has changed in such a way as to make certification for stress at work an acceptable reason for prolonged sickness absence. As a result, in the last 10 years sickness absence due to chronic back pain has plateaued. However, this may simply reflect a change in the way illness is labelled rather than a real change in the natural history of chronic back pain.

During the same period there have been two widely quoted studies, one in Victoria, South Australia,[4] and the other in the Glasgow region,[5] which have shown the benefit of a media campaign to change beliefs about back pain in relation to how acute episodes of back pain are managed. The main benefits have been reduced work absence and reduced use of healthcare resources. At the same time, however, there has been a perceptible increase in patients' expectations of the ability of modern medicine to cure back pain, together with a media-fuelled rise in health anxiety. There is greater awareness of back pain and its sequelae, which continue to produce high demand on healthcare resources.

Musculoskeletal disorders account for approximately 25% of all consultations in primary care. Back pain accounts for 3–7% of all GP consultations and is the third most commonly reported symptom after headache and tiredness.[6]

Before discussing triage diagnosis and management it is important to understand how our conceptual model of back pain as a disease needs revising.

GPs are well aware that up to 30% of all consultations are about 'medically unexplained symptoms'. Previously, the tendency was for doctors to attempt to classify symptoms into a recognised pattern, syndrome or disease entity, and dismiss those that could not be categorised or search for functional or psychosomatic reasons to explain them. If the patient persisted with his or her symptoms then a psychiatric referral may have been made. There are now well-thought-out management guidelines that help GPs handle uncertainty and manage these patients more appropriately.[7]

Understanding neck and back pain requires a good grasp of these new principles. Most experienced clinicians who have been managing patients with spinal pain for many years will openly admit that they do not know what precisely is wrong in 70% of cases. In other words, an exact tissue diagnosis cannot be made on the basis of history and physical examination alone. These are the tools that the GP has to rely on.

In the past, medicine has been preoccupied with a disease model and therefore the causes of back pain have often erroneously been attributed to osteoarthritis or degenerative disc disease, simply because it has been identified on an X-ray or a scan. Similarly, congenital abnormalities such as spina bifida occulta and minor anatomical derangements such as spondylolysis and spondylolisthesis have too readily been identified as the main aetiology.

Back pain often begins in childhood or adolescence, where the prevalence may be as high as 15%. It remains at this level until the peak incidence of more severe back pain between the ages of 40 and 55, following which severe, disabling back pain tends to decrease towards the end of life.

The natural history is for the spine to shorten and stiffen with ageing, with impairment of posture and osteoporotic changes. There is also the development of the characteristic changes of spondylosis, which is the remodelling of vertebrae as an adaptation to gravitational stress and the metabolic processes of osteoarthrosis.

The intervertebral disc is a specialised structure composed of a fibrous ring, the annulus fibrosis, and a pulpy matrix, the nucleus pulposus contained between the end plates of the vertebra that are lined with hyaline cartilage (see Figure 1.1 on p. 473). The disc has a high water content, approximately 90% at birth, which diminishes progressively with age to about 70%. This dehydration of the disc tends to increase the stiffness of the functional segmental unit and possibly render it more vulnerable to injury since its capacity to absorb loading is reduced.

The lower lumbar segments, particularly L3/4, L4/5 and L5/S1, and the lower cervical spine segments C5–T1, are most prone to degenerative changes. Population surveys of radiological evidence of degeneration, and its association with the presence of symptoms, have consistently shown a very low correlation, i.e. structural abnormalities related to ageing and degeneration do not indicate the source of pain.[8] Epidemiologically, back pain peaks in the middle decades whereas ageing and degenerative changes will tend to progress throughout life. With an increasingly aged population, however, a small rise in the incidence of chronic back pain related to the secondary effects of degenerative change on spinal canal width, which causes spinal stenosis, has been observed.

One result of the predilection for doctors to label symptoms with the name of a disease such as spondylosis or osteoarthritis, which is merely a description of changes seen on X-ray, is the instillation of fear and anxiety in the patient's mind. This is called a *nocebo effect* (the opposite of placebo – likely to induce real or imagined harm) and doctors should avoid falling into this pitfall. Patients are already quite anxious enough about their pain and its meaning.

The absence of identifiable disease tends to lead to the common categorisation of back pain as either 'simple back pain' when referring to an acute episode or 'non-specific/mechanical back pain' when chronic. However, the reader of this book and the more serious-minded practitioner should be encouraged to search for specific signs of 'dysfunction' on a general, regional and spinal segmental level, which may point the way to the most appropriate treatment. Dysfunction implies the presence of pain and/or disordered motion in the absence of demonstrable pathology. When applied to the spinal segment it is defined by the World Health Organization (WHO) (ICD 739) as the impaired or altered physiological function of related components within the somatic system.

For a greater understanding of the meaning of the term 'dysfunction' refer to Chapter 9 of *The Back Pain Revolution* by Gordon Waddell.[9] This was proposed as a revolution in our understanding of back pain when published. However, it was well described and researched in osteopathic literature as early as the mid-1950s.

Understanding and recognising dysfunction enables the practitioner to make a positive diagnosis leading to specific management. To see how musculoskeletal dysfunction is assessed and treated, the GP should observe a physiotherapist or osteopath at work. *Unfortunately, chiropractic teaching still embodies the outmoded concept of 'subluxed vertebra', which rarely occurs except in traumatic cases.*

The third important area in relation to this subject is to understand the interaction between the mind and body in relation to musculoskeletal pain. Much research over the last 20 years has focused on the psychological factors that predict the slide from acute to chronic back pain and the psychological factors associated with a poor prognosis. These are called the *yellow flags*. Students are referred to the work of Burton, Main, Watson and many others who have highlighted the importance of psychosocial factors such as fear-avoidance behaviour, anxiety and depression.[10] People with painful physical symptoms and anxiety often exhibit an increased perception of bodily discomfort, and by focusing on these symptoms and their significance become acutely aware of this 'dis-ease' in their body.

Professor of anthropology and London GP, the late Cecil Helman made a similar point in the 1980s:

*Illness is what the patient feels when he goes to the doctor and disease is what he has on the way home from the doctor's office. Disease, then, is something an organ has; illness is something a man has. Illness refers to the subjective response of the patient to being unwell; how he, and those around him, perceive the origin and significance of this event; how it affects his behaviour or relationships with other people; and the steps he takes to remedy this situation. It includes not only his experience of ill-health, but the meaning he gives to that experience. Even responses to physical symptoms, such as pain, can be influenced by social and cultural factors; these factors can in turn affect the presentation of the symptoms and the behaviour of the patient and his family.*

Furthermore, Helman goes on to say that, 'Illness can occur in the absence of disease.'[11]

Patients who present with high levels of anxiety and depression, i.e. distress, are the ones who are most at risk of becoming chronic.

To summarise, the role of the practitioner is to identify serious pathology or *red flags*. These only account for a small percentage of back and neck pain presentations (approximately 1%, although this may rise to 5% in the over-65-year-olds).

Second, he or she is advised to make a thorough search for signs of *dysfunction* when performing clinical history and examination. This is in order to make a positive diagnosis and enable appropriate advice and explanation of the pain to be given and to indicate treatment.

Third, he or she must be aware of the impact of distress and the *yellow flags* on the presentation, recovery and final outcome of the patient's episode. Attention to disease, dysfunction and distress provides a holistic appraisal that hopefully will lead to improved communication and satisfying consultations with these patients.

Fourth, the GP will manage most 'simple' back pain in the community, promoting the maintenance of *activity*. This is opposed to the traditional concept of rest as a treatment, utilising simple analgesics and the skills of physical therapists in manual therapy, acupuncture, and a structured activation approach within the cognitive milieu of 'hurt does not mean harm'.

The CSAG guidelines for low-back pain (LBP) are reproduced as Figure 1.2 (see overleaf).

Figure 1.2 ○ *CSAG guidelines for low-back pain*

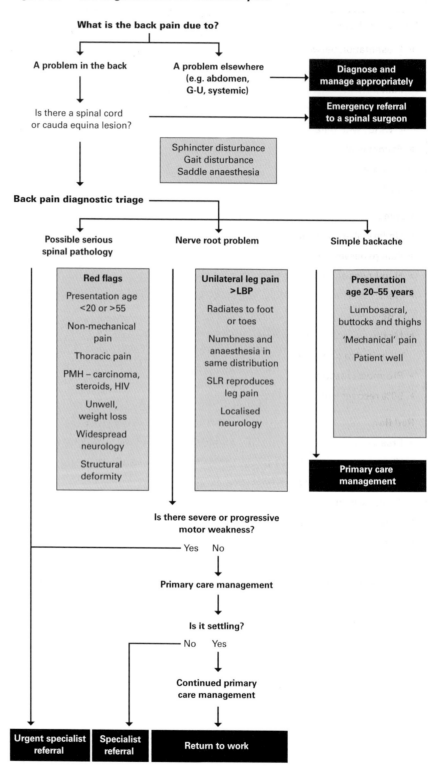

14

*Source*: Clinical Standards Advisory Group. *Back Pain*.[1]

Box 1.1 ○ *Diagnostic triage including red flags*

### Simple backache

- ▶ Presentation between ages 20 and 55.
- ▶ Lumbosacral region, buttocks and thighs.
- ▶ Pain 'mechanical' in nature.
  - ▷ Varies with physical activity.
  - ▷ Varies with time.
- ▶ Patient well.
- ▶ Prognosis good.
- ▶ 90% recover from acute attack in 6 weeks.

### Nerve root pain

- ▶ Unilateral leg pain worse than low-back pain.
- ▶ Pain generally radiates to foot or toes.
- ▶ Numbness and paraesthesia in the same distribution.
- ▶ Nerve irritation signs.
  - ▷ Reduced straight-leg raise (SLR), which reproduces leg pain.
- ▶ Motor, sensory or reflex change.
  - ▷ Limited to one nerve root.
- ▶ Prognosis reasonable.
- ▶ 50% recover from acute attack within 6 weeks.

### Red flags for possible serious spinal pathology

- ▶ Presentation under the age of 20 or onset over the age of 55.
- ▶ Violent trauma, e.g. fall from a height, RTA.
- ▶ Constant, progressive, non-mechanical pain.
- ▶ Thoracic pain.
- ▶ Previous medical history (PMH) – carcinoma.
- ▶ Systemic steroids.
- ▶ Drug abuse, HIV.
- ▶ Systemically unwell.
- ▶ Weight loss.
- ▶ Persisting severe restriction of lumbar flexion.
- ▶ Widespread neurological signs and symptoms.
- ▶ Structural deformity.

*Continued overleaf*

**Cauda equina syndrome / widespread neurological disorder**

► Difficulty with micturition.

► Loss of anal sphincter tone or faecal incontinence.

► Saddle anaesthesia about the anus, perineum or genitals.

► Widespread (> one nerve root) or progressive motor weakness in the legs or gait disturbance.

► Sensory level.

**Inflammatory disorders (ankylosing spondylitis and related disorders)**

► Gradual onset before age 40.

► Marked morning stiffness.

► Persisting limitation of spinal movements in all directions.

► Peripheral joint involvement.

► Iritis, skin rashes (psoriasis), colitis, urethral discharge.

► Family history.

The next stage in the early management of back or neck pain is the vital importance of communicating the doctor's findings to the patient, giving advice and education or deciding on referral pathways. The patient's initial contact with the first healthcare provider with first-time low-back pain and his or her experience of this sets the scene for the future, especially in regard to recurrences. The doctor will use his or her skills in communication and in person-centred care to inform the patient about the diagnosis and management. Using knowledge of colleagues, he or she will be able to refer onwards to a suitable practitioner, such as a physiotherapist. This initial consultation will allow the doctor to use all the six core competences of consultation and, in doing this, provide a satisfactory outcome for the patient.

## Importance of physical examination

The above are skills generic to the well-trained GP and are essential in the management of patients with spinal pain. Establishing a rapport with the patient, listening carefully and giving the patient time, and conducting a comprehensive physical examination will go a long way to meeting these expectations. You will see from the CSAG guidelines (see Figure 1.2 on p. 14) that, after initial triage of patients into simple back pain, nerve root pain or possible serious pathology, most often the GP is called upon to explain there is 'nothing seriously wrong', 'to stay as active as possible' and to expect natural recovery within a few weeks. Conveying this message to a patient in pain requires all the consultation skills that a doctor possesses and which he or she develops in training and work. It also calls for a holistic approach to the care of the patient.

The GP needs to have a reasonable understanding of concepts of musculoskeletal dysfunction in order to explain what is meant by simple mechanical back pain and how the spine may be appearing to function perfectly well and free of pain one moment, and be immobilising the patient a few hours later. The use of a model showing the structures in the spine including the vertebrae, discs and nerves, and a chart showing the muscles, is very helpful in initial education.

An appreciation of the patient's commitments at work and at home is also vital and is again part of the holistic approach to the consultation. Wherever possible it is important for the patient to continue working. Patients who stop working take longer to recover and lose fitness and self-esteem.

## Therapeutics in primary care management

Use paracetamol with codeine preparations for acute simple back pain, ascending the analgesic ladder (WHO). Supplement with NSAIDs in the absence of contraindications, and prescribe tramadol for moderate to severe pain. Muscle relaxants are only required in the presence of muscle spasms that cannot be diagnosed without proper examination.

Escalate the ladder rapidly to strong opiates for severe radicular pain. A low dose of tricyclics such as amitriptyline 10–25 mg may be required to control the pain. If it cannot be controlled there needs to be *a fast-track pain relief service for epidural or nerve root block with steroid.*

## Referrals and the musculoskeletal team

Most Primary Care Trusts now employ an ICATS team to assess patients with back pain. The composition of this team and the development of the service may vary from region to region, but it is expected that there will be guidelines on referral pathways that have been worked out locally and should be abided by as far as possible. This is again part of the competences of the GP (working with colleagues and teams), to be aware of local referral networks and the competences of specialists and their teams. Direct referral to physiotherapy is available in some areas and even patient self-referral.

Children under the age of 16 with worrying or serious back pain will obviously be referred directly to the relevant paediatric department since they will not come under the adult services provision.

## Physical examination

It is strongly recommended that if a patient is not improving or worsening within 10–14 days of the initial presentation and appropriate triage that he or she is examined more comprehensively at review along the lines outlined below. (This is taken from an information leaflet from the British Institute of Musculoskeletal Medicine entitled *The Ten Minute Back Examination*.)[12]

### Observation

1 ▷ Observe the patient's expression, demeanour, body language (illness communication) as he or she enters the room.

2 ▷ Watch the patient's gait (limp, ataxia, etc.). Watching a patient walk can give information about his or her diagnosis. An 'antalgic' gait can occur when patients shift their centre of gravity to avoid loading acutely painful limb joints or an inflamed nerve root. An ataxic gait can be caused by alcohol intoxication, cerebellar disease, or loss of descending column function. A Trendelenburg gait, swaying the trunk over the affected limb on weight bearing, can occur in gluteal-muscle weakness or unstable hip pathologies. A high-stepping gait occurs in loss of proprioception in the feet and a foot drop in L4 root deficit. Loss of hip extension in osteoarthritis (OA) may shorten the stride on the affected side and produce a limp, while loss of internal rotation will cause the foot to turn out.

#### STANDING

An essential examination consists of the following:

1 ▷ Inspection (symmetry, posture): look at the patient from the front, back and side. Note lateral lists or obligatory stoop.

2 ▷ Ask the patient to perform a voluntary trunk motion in flexion, extension and side bending (limitation, site of pain produced, pattern) and conduct a modified Schober's test (lumbar intervertebral motion). When asking the patient to perform voluntary motion, observe asymmetrical range of motion by comparing side bending, while observing for aberrant movements such as 'catches'. Warn the patient to tell you if pain is felt and where. A form of Schober's test can be used to evaluate lumbar flexion: while the patient is at full forward bend, place your outstretched thumb and index in the midline to span the

patient's lumbosacral area, with your thumb at the level of the posterior superior iliac spine (PSIS) and your index as high as you can reach on the spine. The span between these digits will be about 15 cm. Ask the patient to extend up to a neutral erect position. The span between your thumb and index should decrease by around 5 cm. Less than 3 cm will indicate significantly decreased lumbar spinal flexion.

Optional examination when history or examination thus far suggests further assessment.

**3** ▷ Supported squat (hip and knee joints; quads and gluteal strength) and one leg standing with rise onto toes (gluteus medius and calf strength; ataxia): the patient gets support by resting hands on yours. Difficulty with rising onto the toe may indicate calf weakness associated with the S1 nerve root deficit, while unsteadiness may indicate ataxia. Repeated rises may be required to elicit lesser degrees of weakness.

**4** ▷ Palpate the landmarks – iliac crests, posterior superior iliac spine (PSIS) and anterior superior iliac spine (ASIS) (pelvic tilt, torsion or asymmetry) and erector spinae tone. This will help you confirm what you found visually on postural evaluation. A lateral tilt shown by all pelvic landmarks is the most reliable sign for a true short leg.

**SITTING**

**1** ▷ Inspection (symmetry, posture): a pelvis that is tilted laterally when standing but levels when the patient is seated is typical of a true leg length difference. It is also a good time to observe the patient's seated posture.

**2** ▷ Slump test (dural irritability): this is used to apply stress to the dural coverings of nerve roots within the vertebral canal to determine whether they cause pain. The test is performed with the patient in a seated position. In order: the back is slumped, the knee extended, the trunk leans forward and the foot dorsiflexed. If pain is produced in low back or legs, progression through the sequence is halted and forward bending of the neck onto the chest is added to test the effect of this movement on the pain. Provided no movement of back or legs takes place, pain below the waist that is accentuated and relieved by flexion and extension of the neck can be assumed to originate around inflamed dural investments of nerve roots, most likely in association with a herniated lumbar disc.

Figure 1.3 ○ *The slump test*

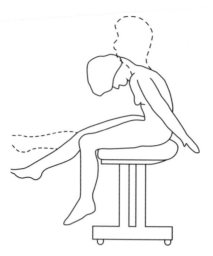

Source: Copyright © BIMM.
Reproduced by permission.

**SUPINE LYING**

An essential examination consists of the following:

**1** ▷ SLR and site of pain produced (quantify non-specific restriction): a limited SLR may have many causes as it is not as specific as the slump test, and can indicate knee, hamstring, pelvic and spinal problems as well as lumbar disc herniation. The latter diagnosis is more likely if pain is produced below the knee. The SLR is useful to quantify and chart a patient's response to treatment.

Hip flexion, rotations at 90° of flexion and abduction (hip joint pathology): stress along femur at 90° hip flexion and slight adduction to elicit pain (sacroiliac joint pain). Carry out knee flexion, extension, valgus and varus stresses at 30° flexion, rotation at 90° and additional tests if indicated (knee joint pathology). Unrecognised hip and knee problems may confuse diagnosis and will need to be taken into account in a treatment plan.

If history or examination, thus far, suggests further assessment, the optional examination is as follows:

**2** ▷ Apparent leg length at the ankle (short leg; lumbopelvic asymmetry): ask the patient to raise his or her buttocks off the table and then settle back down while the legs are stretched out straight. Compare the position of the medial malleoli and check the level of the tibial tuberosities to distinguish lower-leg differences. Also palpate the height of the ASIS.

Differences in 'apparent leg length' may be due to asymmetrical position of the lumbar spine or pelvis.

3 ▷ Abdominal palpation for masses and pulses (aneurysm, malignancy, hepatomegaly, arterial occlusion): these tests would be useful to rule out some of the red-flag situations associated with lower-back pain. Trauma, weight loss, systemic features of infection, a history of malignancy and long-term corticosteroid use may stimulate increased vigilance. Acute cauda equina syndrome will mainly be diagnosed by symptoms such as anaesthesia/paraesthesia in the saddle area (numbness when wiping with toilet paper), an onset of bowel or bladder dysfunction, increasing neurological deficit in one or both legs, and sometimes erectile or sexual dysfunction. Pain is quite variable. Any of these symptoms should trigger tests of perineal sensation and anal tone. Especially if the patient is older than 50 or younger than 10, a search for hepatomegaly, para-aortic lymphadenopathy, dilated aorta, bruits or loss of femoral pulses, may yield crucial diagnostic findings.

4 ▷ Tests of muscle strength: isometric strength of hip flexion L2, knee extension L3, foot extension L4, hallux extension L5, foot eversion S1 (motor deficit; muscle or tendon abnormality); sensation (sensory loss); reflexes including Babinski (L & UMN deficits). The patient has been a passive player in the examination up until muscle testing. It is a good idea to let the patient know that he or she is about to do something active to avoid confusion and ensure prompt co-operation. In older people, hamstrings often go into distressing cramp when their strength is tested: S1 and S2 roots can be tested equally well by buttock clench, foot plantar flexion and eversion.

Loss of muscle strength in a particular myotome may indicate a disc prolapse in the lumbar segment above this level, especially if the patient also has back pain.

### Time required for examining the back

For further assessment of the back, the author appreciates that there will not be time in a 10-minute consultation to perform such a thorough back assessment. However, specialist GPs will be able to perform all of this examination in a 20-minute appointment.

21

**PRONE LYING**

**1** ▷ Tenderness 1" from midline at each spinal level (pain generator near segmental muscles or facet joints): tenderness in this location may indicate pain generated in the underlying muscle or zygoapophyseal joint, or be allodynia reflecting central sensitisation caused by nociceptive inputs from segmentally related sources.

**2** ▷ Anterior springing at each segmental level (pathological change in vertebrae and spinal joint, e.g. osteomalacia, neoplasia, infection): this should be done carefully as it can be quite pain provoking. It is especially important if your history has led you to think about red flags such as osteomalacia, compression fractures, neoplasms and infection. Some disc lesions also may give a positive result. Applying a tuning fork to the sensitive level or percussing a level of positive springing may help to confirm your working diagnosis.

**3** ▷ Buttock clench (weakness of gluteal muscles): feel for symmetry of tone and palpate for atrophy, which would indicate S1 deficit or gluteal-muscle problems.

**4** ▷ Hip extension and rotations at zero flexion (hip joint pathology): have one hand over the joint to localise motion to the hip and monitor for limitation and end feel. Limited extension may indicate psoas or anterior hip joint problems.

**5** ▷ Prone knee flexion (femoral nerve root sleeve irritability): with the patient prone and hip extended, flex the knee towards the buttock to perform the 'femoral nerve stretch'. This is another dural test to check for lesions involving the L2, L3 and L4 nerve root, but like SLR is non-specific as other structures may provoke pain in this position.

**LATERAL LYING ON LEAST PAINFUL SIDE, THEN REPEATED ON THE OTHER SIDE**

**1** ▷ Erector spinae muscle pliability and tenderness in upper, middle and lower lumbar areas (abnormal muscle function and pain sensitivity due to primary or secondary dysfunction): feel for areas where the normal level of pliability is reduced and the muscle feels stiffer and may be tender, as may be tighter strands felt within the muscle and spanning many segments. Abnormal function of muscles may be the only sign associated with a persistent impairment in non-specific back pain.

2 ▷ Rotation provocation test of L5–T9 spinous processes (painful motion barrier in rotation at specific segmental level): pain generated as the spinal joint reaches a barrier to further passive torsion may locate the segmental source more accurately than other signs. This is a difficult technique to master without formal demonstration.

3 ▷ Contour of spinous processes palpated to elicit a shelf, a sign of spondylolisthesis. Stress applied in direction of abnormal shift to elicit pain (symptomatic spondylolisthesis).

---

### Interpretation

The presence of spinal nerve root/dural problems associated with disc herniation may be determined from the history, most commonly painfully limited forward bending, reduced SLR, a positive slump test, and in severe cases neurological deficits.

Lumbar root entrapment causes pain referred to the leg often with temporary or persisting neurological deficits but SLR, slump and forward bending typically do not provoke the leg pain. However, backward bending and/or ipsilateral side bending often will.

In the above situations, single nerve root deficits may be found. When multiple root function is impaired further investigation is usually indicated to exclude other pathology.

In dysfunction of a spinal joint, locally paraspinal tenderness and decreased pliability of muscles are found. The slump and SLR tests are typically negative while torsional stress applied to painful segments provokes pain. Forward bending and side bending, usually particularly to one side, are most likely to be limited by pain.

Postural pain on standing is usually produced in backward bending or when an excessive lumbar lordosis buckles during axial loading through the shoulders.

---

Box 1.2 ○ *Case study 1*

A 37-year-old man who is a regular runner and cyclist attends your surgery two weeks after the acute onset of low-back pain whilst gardening. Initially he could hardly stand and could not go to work. He consulted an osteopath after three days, who treated him gently with manual therapy and advised him to rest and to consider giving up running. (He had had a couple of milder episodes in the last two years.)

He had improved and gone back to work. He had also recently returned to the osteopath and was treated by manipulation but only two days ago sneezed and 'gone back to square one'.

His pain is low down in the left lumbar region radiating into the buttock, and his back feels 'crooked'. It is worse bending and sitting for more than ten minutes, after which he can hardly straighten up.

He wants to know what is wrong, whether he needs a scan or other investigation, if he is getting the right treatment, and if he should be back at work. He is also concerned about having to give up running, which he finds 'a great stress buster'.

He has a sedentary job, commutes to work 10 km by cycling and has a wife and one-year-old boy.

---

Your examination finds a tall, slim man with his trunk listing to the left. He can perform a full squat from standing with his back straight. Active flexion increases this appearance and is limited by pain. His slump test is positive on the left, straight leg raising 40° on left, 80° on right; power, sensation and reflexes are normal. He has a full range of hip motion, negative sacroiliac stress tests, and negative anterior spring test of the lumbar segments.

▷ What is the likely diagnosis?
▷ Does he need any further investigation?
▷ Would you alter or add anything to his current treatment from the osteopath?
▷ Do you think he should stay at work?
▷ Should he stop running in the long term for fear of damaging his back?

---

## Management of neck pain

Neck pain is almost as common in the community as back pain, with an estimated prevalence of 25% of the adult population in the last year, though it is rarely as disabling.[13] Nevertheless, it accounts for considerable morbidity when chronic. This may happen following 'whiplash injury' in motor vehicle accidents, or in the elderly with severe degenerative disease of the joints.

Most episodes are short lived and best managed in primary care. One way to guide management of neck pain is by age of presentation rather than by pathology, as shown below.

### Child under five years

Infants with acute wryneck should be referred to paediatric orthopaedics for possible atlantoaxial rotatory subluxation or congenital torticollis.

### Child between ten and 16

Patients in this group who present with acute wryneck/torticollis (neck side bent in one direction and rotated in the other) have an acute segmental dysfunction. They should be managed with analgesics, a soft collar at night only, and an active range of motion exercises. If not resolved in the expected ten days, refer to physical therapy for manual therapy.

### Young adult, 20–40 years

Acute torticollis occasionally progresses to full-blown disc syndrome with root irritation or compression. Management is above.

Neck pain after trauma may occur at any age. A large study on A&E patients from the USA [14] indicates that if there is no midline tenderness over the cervical spine, normal alertness, no intoxication, no focal neurological deficit, and no other distracting painful injury, plain X-rays can be omitted and bony injury would be missed in only 1% of cases (Hoffman's criteria).

Neck pain following a road traffic accident is a common reason for attendance in primary care for a number of reasons. Acceleration–deceleration injury involving the soft tissues, spinal joints and discs, nerves and central nervous system is collectively termed 'whiplash associated disorders' (WAD). *Patients intending to make a claim will want detailed documentation of the mechanics of the accident, initial symptoms and signs, and treatment instituted. It is in the interest of the GP to ensure that this is carefully documented for if a lawyer requests details.*

Obviously WAD can occur at any age; pain and stiffness develop between one hour and two days (depending on severity), classically following a rear-end collision. It should be classified and treated according to the Quebec Task Force guidelines:[15]

▷ **grade I** ▶ pain and stiffness, no physical signs – manage symptoms with simple analgesics, advice on active range of motion exercises and posture. No collar

▷ **grade 2** ▶ neck complaints, physical signs, i.e. restricted motion – as above and refer early for mobilisation/manipulation. Acupuncture works well for persisting muscle tension. Avoid prolonged passive treatment courses

▷ **grade 3** ▶ neck complaints plus neurological signs – moderate or strong analgesics, a collar at night may help, refer to musculoskeletal team

▷ **grade 4** ▶ neck complaints, fracture/ dislocation – should be managed through A&E to neurosurgery.

If symptoms of mechanical pain persist beyond three months, refer to a specialist for diagnostic work-up for facet arthropathy, present in over 50% of cases.[16]

Bony injury is sometimes missed on plain X-ray, even in high-velocity accidents, so consider referral for CT scanning if Hoffman's criteria are met.[14]

Treat actively and screen for development of psychosocial factors and post-traumatic stress disorder, which may develop over the first three months and portend a worse prognosis. Discouragement from litigation will lead to a better outcome, but angry and hurting patients can rarely be dissuaded. Paradoxically, settlement of claims, often delayed for up to two years or more, does not lead to a cure.

Disc prolapse may present as an acute torticollis picture and progress to a full-blown disc herniation, with radicular pain down the arm in a more or less dermatomal distribution with paraesthesiae in the hand and fingers. Often the worst pain is in the posterior cervicoscapular region but referred pain from dural irritation may be felt in the upper pectoral area also. This pain is severe and debilitating, requiring strong analgesia. Start at level 2 but be prepared to go quickly to level 3 on the analgesic ladder. Adding low-dose tricyclics is helpful together with postural advice for upright and sleeping positions.

*An X-ray or MRI scan do not add to management at this stage.*

Consider early referral for epidural or nerve root block with steroid if pain is not adequately controlled.

The natural history is for this to resolve over 6–8 weeks; very few require surgery. Full recovery of nerve deficit may take 6–9 months. Cord compression rarely results from disc prolapse in the neck.

Postural pain is caused by sustained static posture. For example, long hours on a computer, at a workstation or a similar activity may lead to chronic muscle tension in the head, neck and shoulders.

Alternatively, the forearm and wrist posture for repeated keystroke or

26

mouse work can lead to diffuse arm pain or 'repetitive strain symptoms' (the term 'injury' is no longer used).

This is managed by recommending a workstation assessment, liaising with the occupational health department at the workplace or other key personnel, observing posture in your surgery and giving quick, simple advice along the Alexander principle lines[17] for video of techniques,[18] and recommending regular exercise and stretches to break the monotony of prolonged computer work. Brief manual therapy may be recommended in the acute crisis to avoid work absence.

---

## Red flags

There are four red flags:

1 ▷ To recognise the first is simple enough. The patient with known inflammatory disease, commonly rheumatoid arthritis, after some years may *develop axial neck pain*, fine crepitus, a sense of fatigue in maintaining posture and occasionally frank instability. Even without these symptoms up to one third of patients will have synovitis and other changes such as pannus and erosions in the upper cervical region on MRI.

2 ▷ The second is *progressive weakness, sensory disturbance in the upper limbs* causing loss of dexterity, sometimes accompanied by weakness and incoordination of the lower limbs and mild neck pain. Neurological examination and reduced range of motion in the cervical spine secondary to spondylosis reveal the suspected diagnosis of cervical myelopathy. A neurosurgical opinion should be sought.

3 ▷ The third is more difficult because it may simply present as neck pain with restricted motion that *progresses relentlessly* and only involves nerve roots and spinal cord late in the picture. All the red flags described in the back pain triage apply, particularly a past history of cancer in one of the common primaries that metastasise to bone. X-rays and ESR or CRP together with a bone profile may be sufficient to clinch the diagnosis.

4 ▷ The fourth red flag is the patient who presents with *radicular pain in the arm or cervicoscapular pain that progresses to involve the lower trunk of the brachial plexus*. He or she may be a smoker or present with other constitutional symptoms. This will alert the GP to order a chest X-ray with

apical views as well as a pathology screen, which may reveal the primary (pancoast) tumour in the lung apex.

---

## Physical examination

**Posture** ▶ note the asymmetric posture of acute wryneck, forward head or chin poke position of the hurried, driven type (a typical type A personality). This is the consequence of dorsal kyphosis, deafness, or antalgic position due to large disc prolapse.

**Muscle wasting** ▶ chronic asymmetric posture may cause this, amyotrophy of the scapular muscles (C6 segment), deltoid wasting (C5 or disuse), and small muscles of the hand (T1 root compression may be a red flag), trapezius upper fibres in accessory nerve palsy or post radiotherapy.

**Active range of movements** ▶ symmetrical restriction suggests spondylosis of ageing or inflammatory disease. Painful, asymmetric restriction indicates local joint dysfunction, facet joint pain or disc prolapse.

Screen the scapular movements for co-ordination, fluency and power on resisted shoulder shrug. Screen the arm and shoulder if pain or radicular symptoms radiate distal to the point of the shoulder.

**Specific test** ▶ foraminal closing test (combined rotation and extension) provokes radicular pain or sensory symptoms in upper limb in root entrapment.

**Neurological tests** ▶ for power, sensation, reflexes including Babinski, if there are any symptoms in upper or lower limbs.

**Passive testing** ▶ performed when patient upright as a gentle assessment of the 'feel' at end of range.

**Palpation** ▶ soft tissues of the neck and shoulder for tone, trigger points, posterior joints for tenderness.

---

**Box 1.3** ○ *Case study 2*

---

A 40-year-old woman presents with a history of right neck and shoulder pain of three months' duration with tingling in the ring and little fingers. She says she took her children for a rollercoaster ride and developed neck pain and stiffness soon after that. She is a single parent and works in an office.

She is suffering constant pain, worse after a day at work and keeping her awake at night with headache from occiput to frontal area.

She has been to a chiropractor six times who keeps 'cracking' her neck, but it only gives her temporary relief. She is taking nurofen tablets as required, up to six times a day.

She wants to know what is wrong. Should she consider suing the fairground operators? And what can you do to relieve her pain?

Examination reveals a tired, tense-looking woman with a forward head posture, asymmetric restriction of active movement, and a tendency to breathe in deep, impatient sighs, without any abnormal upper-limb neurology. Palpation finds the posterior neck muscles to be taut and tender, especially at the skull base. She exhibits general hypermobility.

---

What is your advice and management?

## Answers to case study 1

The most likely diagnosis is a lumbar disc syndrome (gross restriction of SLR, lumbar deviation, worse after sitting, precipitated by a prolonged flexion strain). No further investigation is necessary at this stage. X-rays show only bony changes and MRI will not alter management.

Your knowledge of local referral mechanisms will allow you to refer him on to a physiotherapist.

The physiotherapist may suggest McKenzie exercises[19] to centralise pain and maintain spinal posture. These are repeated active movements of the spine into either extension, flexion or side gliding, which the patient is taught to do for himself after initial assessment has identified the preferred direction to centralise the pain. This would be useful, together with strict advice on back care for disc problems (minimise sitting, avoid slouching, bend at the knees not the back).

He should be advised to stay at work with the proviso that prolonged sitting and driving will delay recovery, so he should try to stand, walk and be as active as possible. If that is not possible due to work constraints then a phased return to work is an option. Prolonged absence and certification should be avoided since it may lead to chronicity.

As part of the holistic care you should be offering in the consultation, you should ask about the effect this illness is having on his wife and family. Is he worried about losing his job? Does he have any co-morbidities such as depression or anxiety?

There is no evidence that moderate running is a risk factor for the development of degenerative disc disease or back pain from any cause.

### Analysis of case study 1 with respect to the six domains of Being a GP

#### DOMAIN 1: PRIMARY CARE MANAGEMENT

▷ To be able to triage back pain into red flags.
▷ To manage severe nerve root pain requiring adequate analgesic control and/or fast-track pain relief.
▷ To know how to manage simple back and neck pain appropriately, or where to refer for management.

#### DOMAIN 2: PERSON-CENTRED CARE

▷ To recognise the three components – disease, distress, dysfunction – that may present in varying proportions in each and every case, making every presentation unique.
▷ To appreciate the effects that the pain may have on the person and his or her family.

#### DOMAIN 3: SPECIFIC PROBLEM-SOLVING SKILLS

▷ To be able to identify which patients need investigations and specific referrals, physical therapy or self-management.
▷ To be able to identify red flags.

#### DOMAIN 4: A COMPREHENSIVE APPROACH

▷ To understand the roles that physical therapy, exercise both generally and specifically, musculoskeletal services, complementary practitioners and the pain clinic play in the management of the chronic and more complex cases.

## DOMAIN 5: COMMUNITY ORIENTATION

▷ To understand the vital role that staying active and maintaining employment plays in the overall wellbeing of the patient.
▷ To make every effort to liaise with employers and work supervisors as necessary.
▷ To certify sick for only short periods and to review frequently.

## DOMAIN 6: A HOLISTIC APPROACH

▷ To recognise that the patient needs to be 'heard' (given time), 'felt' (through adequate examination) and given control (guided towards independence and self-management), and to find meaning in his or her suffering (even when the cause and diagnosis can often not be specified).

### Answers to case study 2

You diagnose a strain of one of the joints of the neck with associated muscle tension leading to headache. The loss of sleep and worry about the pain is fuelling the problem. Using your competences in consultation, you have explored the holistic nature of this problem. You appreciate the stresses of being a single parent and you have empathised with her over this. You will allow the patient to verbalise her concerns and worries, using active listening, and then you will together form a treatment plan using her priorities as a starting point. You also point out that she is loose jointed, which makes her more vulnerable to sudden strains and jerks, and the muscles have to work harder to maintain posture.

You explain that she is chest breathing as result of anxiety and the muscles at the root of the neck (scalene on the right) have tightened in response to referred pain and the abnormal breathing pattern. This indirectly leads to elevation of the first rib and irritation of the lower nerve trunk going to the arm.

You suggest low-dose amitriptyline at night for a few weeks to improve sleep and reduce muscle tension, and refer her to a physiotherapist for postural training.[14] You teach her how to relax her breathing pattern to increase diaphragmatic movement and reduce the chest inspiration, which helps inactivate the accessory muscles of respiration. You also discuss referral to the practice counsellor to help with her anxiety problems; you will use the primary care multidisciplinary team to help her overcome this problem.

You will review her in three weeks to ensure progress is being made. You also mention that she may need to enquire about having her workstation assessed by her employer, as occupational aspects may be making this problem worse.

### Analysis of case study 2 with respect to the six domains of *Being a GP*

#### DOMAIN 1: PRIMARY CARE MANAGEMENT

▷ To be able to triage back pain into red flags.

▷ To manage severe nerve root pain requiring adequate analgesic control and/or fast-track pain relief.

▷ To know how to manage simple back and neck pain appropriately, or where to refer for management.

#### DOMAIN 2: PERSON-CENTRED CARE

▷ To recognise the three components – disease, distress, dysfunction – that may present in varying proportions in each and every case, making every presentation unique.

▷ To understand in this case that the strains of being a single parent are exacerbating the problem.

#### DOMAIN 3: SPECIFIC PROBLEM-SOLVING SKILLS

▷ To be able to identify, by history taking and examination, which patients need investigations and specific referrals, physical therapy or self-management.

▷ To know how to get the investigations done and how to fast track referrals.

#### DOMAIN 4: A COMPREHENSIVE APPROACH

▷ To understand the roles that physical therapy, exercise both generally and specifically, musculoskeletal services, complementary practitioners and the pain clinic play in the management of the chronic and more complex cases.

#### DOMAIN 5: COMMUNITY ORIENTATION

▷ To understand the vital role that staying active and maintaining employment plays in the overall wellbeing of the patient.

▷ To make every effort to liaise with employers and work supervisors as necessary.

▷ To certify sick for only short periods and to review frequently.

▷ To appreciate the link with work and obtain a workplace assessment.

## DOMAIN 6: A HOLISTIC APPROACH

▷ To recognise that this patient has more than just a physical problem.
An assessment of the biopsychosocial issues of the case indicates that
a holistic management strategy is required. This patient has many
difficulties in her own personal life that must be addressed before her
pain will resolve.

### References

1 • Clinical Standards Advisory Group. *Back Pain: report of a CSAG Committee on Back Pain*
London: HMSO, 1994.

2 • Department of Health. *The Musculoskeletal Services Framework* London: DH, 2006.

3 • Bernstein I, Dunbar A, Ketkar V, *et al.* Looking at ourselves: what are musculoskeletal
doctors doing in the UK? [reports of six services] *International Musculoskeletal Medicine*
2009; **31(2)**: 80–94.

4 • Buchbinder R, Jolley D, Wyatt M. Population based intervention to change back
pain beliefs and disability: three part evaluation *British Medical Journal* 2001; **322(7301)**:
1516–20.

5 • Waddell G. *Working Backs Scotland* 2003, www.workingbacksscotland.scot.nhs.uk
[accessed October 2011].

6 • Williams N. Managing back pain in general practice: is osteopathy the new
paradigm? *British Journal of General Practice* 1997; **47(423)**: 653–5.

7 • Burton C. Beyond somatisation: a review of the understanding and treatment of
medically unexplained physical symptoms (MUPS) *British Journal of General Practice* 2003;
**53(488)**: 231–9.

8 • Haefeli M, Kalberer F, Saegesser D, *et al*. The course of macroscopic degeneration in
the human lumbar intervertebral disc *Spine* 2006; **31(14)**: 1522–31.

9 • Waddell G. *The Back Pain Revolution* Edinburgh: Churchill Livingstone, 1998.

10 • Linton S J. Occupational and risk factors for back pain: a systematic review *Journal
of Occupational Rehabilitation* 2001; **11(1)**: 53–66.

11 • Helman C G. Disease versus illness in general practice *Journal of the Royal College of
General Practitioners* 1981; **31(230)**: 548–52.

12 • MacDonald R. *The Ten Minute Back Examination* Bushey, Herts: BIMM, 2008,
www.bimm.org.uk [accessed October 2011].

13 • Guez M, Hildingsson C, Nilsson M, *et al*. The prevalence of neck pain *Acta
orthopaedica scandinavica* 2002; **73(4)**: 455–9.

14 • Hoffman J R, Mower W R, Wolfson A B, *et al*. Validity of a set of criteria to rule out
injury to the cervical spine in patients with blunt trauma *New England Journal of Medicine*
2000; **343(2)**: 94–9.

15 • Spitzer W O, Skovron M L, Salmi L R, *et al*. The Quebec Task Force on whiplash-
associated disorders *Spine* 1995; **20(Suppl. 8)**: 1S–73S.

16 • Lord S, Barnsley L, Wallis B J, *et al*. Chronic cervical zygapophysial joint pain after whiplash: a placebo controlled prevalence study *Spine* 1996; **21(15)**: 1737–44.

17 • Little P, Lewith G, Webley F, *et al*. Randomised controlled trial of Alexander technique lessons, exercise, and massage for chronic and recurrent back pain *British Medical Journal* 2008: **337**; 438–45.

18 • The Complete Guide to the Alexander Technique. Available at: www.alexander technique.com [accessed October 2011].

19 • McKenzie R. *The Lumbar Spine: mechanical diagnosis and therapy* Wellington: Spinal Publications, 1981.

# Chronic back and neck pain

**2**

*Steve Longworth*

## Introduction

There are many reasons for patients to consult their doctor with pain. They may be seeking cure or symptomatic relief, diagnostic clarification, reassurance, 'legitimisation' of symptoms, medical certification for work absence, or to express distress, frustration or anger. Doctors need to clarify which of these reasons apply to an individual and respond appropriately. GPs are potentially powerful therapeutic agents and can provide effective, immediate care, but they may also unintentionally promote progression to chronic pain.[1] For all these reasons patients with chronic back and neck pain are frequently seen as challenging, sometimes to the extent of being perceived as 'heartsink' patients. This need not be the case if the appropriate diagnostic and management strategies are applied.

Chronic pain in the back and neck is common but is not necessarily the same kind of problem as persistent acute pain. The key to understanding this issue is the meaning of the word 'chronic'.

Many of our patients use the word 'chronic' to mean 'severe' (and, confusingly, some patients use the word 'acute' to mean 'severe' as well). For most health professionals the word 'chronic' simply means 'longstanding'. In the context of longstanding back and neck pain, however, the word 'chronic', when used by health professionals, often carries extra meaning beyond simple longevity.

## When is chronic back pain chronic?

There are a number of definitions based on symptom duration (see Table 2.1 on p. 36).

In practice, however, it would appear that most clinicians define chronic low-back (and neck) pain not just in terms of duration, but also in terms of the presence or absence of *psychosocial factors* and *disability*. In other words, the label 'chronic low-back pain' often refers to a problem patient and a problem situation.[2] We need to distinguish these patients from the chronic group who are coping.

Table 2.1 ○ *Chronicity of low-back pain as defined by symptom duration*

| Duration | Authors |
|---|---|
| More than six weeks | NICE (2009)[3] |
| More than three months | Cohen *et al.* (2008)[4] |
| At least half the days in a 12-month period in a single or multiple episode(s) | Von Korff (1994)[5] |

Patients with longstanding back and neck pain may have continuous pain (often with acute exacerbations) or episodic pain of varying intensity. If these patients are *coping* with their pain and getting on with their lives then their treatment will be similar to patients with acute pain. Those patients who are *not* coping with their pain and who are *distressed* and *inappropriately disabled* by their symptoms require a different approach.

It is important at this point to emphasise that all chronic pain starts as an acute episode and that there is usually a physical initiator. It is extremely important not to mislabel the chronic-pain patient who is distressed by a potentially identifiable and treatable physical problem.

It is also very important to stress that there is no clinical dichotomy between organic disease and distress; it is not a question of a particular presentation being due to *either* a 'real' illness *or* to distress. Distress may exist in the presence or absence of clear-cut organic pathology.

The principles of diagnosis and management in patients with chronic back and neck pain are very similar, as are the risk factors for chronicity.

---

Box 2.1 ○ *Which anatomical areas are we talking about?*

▶ The neck is the region from the occiput to the top of the shoulder blades.
▶ The low back is the region from the 12th ribs to the gluteal folds.

NB: the thoracic spine is a 'red flag' area. While it is possible to have mechanical thoracic pain the GP needs to think hard about excluding serious organic pathology, not only spinal but also serious visceral pathology, e.g. lung and pancreas.

---

## The size of the problem

Most of us will experience at least one episode of low-back pain during our life. Reported lifetime prevalence varies from 49% to 70%, and point prevalence from 12% to 30% is reported in Western countries.[6]

Most people with acute back pain experience improvements in pain and disability, and return to work within one month. Further but smaller improvements occur up to three months, after which pain and disability levels remain almost constant. Low levels of pain and disability persist from three to at least 12 months. Most people will have at least one recurrence within 12 months.[7]

In the largest inception cohort study of patients with chronic low-back pain (where 'chronic' was defined as back pain present for three months) the cumulative probability of being pain free was 35% at nine months after the onset of chronicity (i.e. 12 months after the pain first started) and 41% at 12 months after the onset of chronicity. In this study only 11% of people had not returned to work in their previous capacity at the onset of chronicity. Of these, almost half had returned to work in their previous capacity within 12 months.[8]

Although many episodes of acute low-back pain will resolve rapidly, the proportion of people who develop chronic disabling back pain ranges from 1% to 30% in different studies.[9, 10]

Between 1987/8 and 1997/8 the one-year prevalence of back pain in adults in the UK aged between 20–59 years rose by 12.7%. A possible explanation is that cultural changes led to a greater awareness of more minor back symptoms and willingness to report them, and this cultural shift may also have rendered back pain more acceptable as a reason for work absence attributed to sickness.[11]

The 12-month prevalence of neck pain is between 30% and 50% but the 12-month prevalence of activity-limiting pain is 1.7% to 11.5%. Neck pain is more prevalent among women and prevalence peaks in middle age.[12]

Neck pain after a road traffic accident ('whiplash') is very common; 50% of those with whiplash-associated disorders (WAD) will report neck pain symptoms one year after their injuries.[13]

---

## Who develops chronic disabling back and neck pain?

The transition from acute to chronic disabling back or neck pain is a complex process and many individual, psychosocial and workplace factors may play a part.

Once back pain has been present for greater than one year few people with long-term pain and disability return to normal activities. It is this group who account for the majority of the health and social costs associated with low-back pain.[2]

Distress, depressive mood and somatisation (the tendency to experience and communicate bodily distress in response to psychosocial stress and to seek medical help for it) are associated with an increased risk of chronic low-back pain.[14] One study that collected prospective data on a general practice population before patients presented with back pain determined six key factors that had a high predictive value for back pain chronicity.[10] The likelihood of persistent disabling low-back pain increased with the number of factors reported. Only 6% of subjects who reported fewer than three factors had a poor outcome, compared with 70% of participants who reported more than four (Box 2.2).

---

**Box 2.2 ○ *Prospective predictors of low-back pain chronicity***

**1** ▶ Female sex (odds of a poor outcome – F:M = 2:1).

**2** ▶ Prior history of low-back pain.

**3** ▶ Dissatisfaction with current employment or work status.

**4** ▶ Widespread pain (axial skeletal pain in addition to pain above and below the waist and on the right and left side of the body).

**5** ▶ Radiating leg pain.

**6** ▶ Restriction of two or more spinal movements – standing extension, finger to floor distance, lateral flexion, knee extension and modified Shober's test.[15]

*Source*: Thomas E, Silman A J, Croft P R, *et al*. Predicting who develops chronic low back pain in primary care: a prospective study.[10]

---

In another primary care study, the perceived pain intensity at the initial presentation of a musculoskeletal pain problem, past experience of a chronic pain problem, and poor reliance on active coping strategies were predictive of pain maintenance and a poorer prognosis.[16]

The outcome of neck pain depends on the underlying cause, but acute neck pain usually resolves within days or weeks, although it can recur or become chronic. A UK survey of 7669 adults found that 18% had neck pain at the time of the survey, and half of those still had pain when asked one year later. Outcome is unpredictable once pain becomes chronic, and prognosis and the factors that influence it vary greatly. Reports on the importance of factors like age, sex, occupation, psychological factors and radiological findings are conflicting, but the quality of most studies is poor. The best predictors of an unfavourable outcome one year after presentation with neck pain are severity of the initial pain and concomitant back pain. At least 10% of affected people develop chronic neck pain with severe disability in 5% of affected people.[17]

After a whiplash injury following a road traffic accident (RTA) greater initial pain, more symptoms, and greater initial disability predict slower recovery. Few factors related to the collision itself (for example direction of the collision, headrest type) are prognostic; however, post-injury psychological factors such as passive coping style, depressed mood, and fear of movement are prognostic for slower or less complete recovery. There is also preliminary evidence that the prevailing compensation system is prognostic for recovery in WAD, i.e. consulting a lawyer after an RTA is associated with prolonged neck pain and associated disability.[13]

Ethnic and cultural factors greatly influence the presentation of chronic pain. Community and primary care-based studies have consistently demonstrated that South Asians and other immigrants from non-Western cultures tend to express psychological distress through somatisation or somatic metaphors more frequently than native Britons. It has also become apparent that this cultural variation in the expression of psychological distress does make it difficult for GPs to recognise the disorder in South Asian minorities, and that the standard screening instruments, such as the General Health Questionnaire,[18] may under-diagnose psychological distress in these ethnic minority groups.[19]

## Clinical assessment

The diagnosis should be kept under review at all times.[3] Once a patient has been diagnosed with chronic back or neck pain (with or without chronic disability and distress) it is important to be alert to changes in his or her clinical condition and to repeat the diagnostic triage (including investigations) if there is a 'signal change' such as worsening of current symptoms or signs or the development of new symptoms or signs.

Patients with chronic back and neck pain are often frequent consulters in primary care, and making a balanced and objective clinical assessment may be difficult and challenging even for experienced doctors. Patients with distress may transmit this feeling to their doctor, compounding the uncertainties that frequently surround diagnosis and clinical management. All doctors are wary of missing serious physical disease and we all have horror stories of 'mislabelling', where serious pathology was missed. Patients who have been medicalised by over-investigation and over-treatment may come less readily to mind.

One practical problem is that many patients with disabling chronic back and neck pain report that they are 'worse than ever' each time you see them, so self-reported increased pain intensity may be less helpful than asking about systemic upset, e.g. the 'Fever WARMS' questions (Box 2.3).

---

**Box 2.3  ○  *'Fever WARMS' questions for systemic illness***

**Ask about:**

▶ fever

▶ weight loss

▶ anorexia (loss of appetite)

▶ rigors

▶ malaise

▶ sweats.

---

### How not to miss serious disease

Make time. If *you* do not have the time, refer them to someone who does. This might be a GP colleague with a particular interest or expertise in musculo-skeletal problems in your own practice or a local General Practitioner with a Special Interest (GPwSI), but it might also be a non-medical colleague such as a community-based physiotherapist. If you do refer to a colleague then this may be a valuable learning opportunity, so do ask for feedback beyond the contents of a standard clinic letter.

Thoroughly review the patient's previous records.

Check his or her medication. Is the patient taking statins (potential myopathy) or systemic steroids (increased risk of osteoporotic wedge fracture and infection)? If the patient has sensory symptoms in a limb is he or she taking a drug that is known to cause neuropathy as a side effect (Box 2.4)?

---

**Box 2.4  ○  *Some drugs that may cause a neuropathy***

▶ Isoniazid.

▶ Nitrofurantoin.

▶ Statins.

▶ Pyridoxine.

▶ Phenytoin.

▶ Griseofulvin.

▶ Flecainide.

▶ Amiodarone.

▶ AIDS and cancer drugs.

▶ Allopurinol.

If you are not sure, check the small print in the *British National Formulary*.

---

Examine the patient thoroughly. Be alert for 'hard' signs and do not ignore them.

*In younger patients check for hypermobility. In patients over 65 do not forget poly-myalgia rheumatica. In patients of all ages be alert for features of a systemic inflamma-tory disorder (prolonged morning stiffness, objective joint swelling, etc.).*

Check the pulse, temperature and weight, and dip-test the urine.

Review previous investigations (Box 2.5). The choice of investigation depends upon the duration of symptoms and overall clinical picture. A patient with a four-month history of back pain might conceivably have a myeloma, but this would be highly unlikely in a patient with a ten-year his-tory. The shorter the history the harder you need to look for red flags.

A patient with neck pain and brachialgia (cervical nerve root pain felt in the upper limb) or low-back pain and sciatica (lumbar nerve root pain felt in the lower limb) lasting more than three months should be considered for a magnetic resonance imaging (MRI) scan.

---

Box 2.5 ○ *Investigations to consider*

**In patients with chronic back and neck pain**

▶ If not previously checked (and depending on symptom duration) consider full blood count (FBC), renal and liver function, prostate-specific antigen (PSA) (men), immunoglobulin electrophoresis and urine for Bence Jones protein.

▶ Vitamin D.

▶ Erythrocyte sedimentation rate (ESR)/PV/C-reactive protein.

▶ CPK.

▶ Plain X-ray to exclude osteoporotic fracture(s) in older patients or in younger patients with significant risk factors for osteoporosis.

**In patients with neuropathic or sensory limb symptoms**

▶ Blood sugar.

▶ Vitamin B12 + folate.

▶ Thyroid function tests.

▶ Coeliac screen.

▶ Gamma GT.

▶ Bone profile.

**In patients with red flags or brachalgia / sciatica >three months**

▶ MRI scan of the neck/lumbar spine.

**In patients with thoracic spine pain**

▶ Chest X-ray (?HRCT – high-resolution CT chest scan, especially in smokers).

## The identification of distress

There is a sliding scale of distress severity that for the vast majority of patients is not linked to secondary gain. Distress is related to severe pain in association with honest misunderstandings and misattributions that then lead to fear, catastrophising (focusing upon the worst possible outcomes or interpreting uncomfortable experiences as unbearable), and low mood. This highly dynamic process is influenced by an individual's beliefs, emotions and coping responses.

Someone who is distressed in the absence of clear-cut organic pathology, or whose distress appears disproportionate to the physical disorder, is having a very real and unpleasant experience, and the doctor's task is to find the best way to help. Problems may arise when patients come with expectations about interventions (e.g. scans, injections, surgery) that are unlikely to be helpful and when doctors fail to consider psychosocial factors.

It is also important to stress that if distress is present in association with clearly identifiable organic pathology, the distress must be addressed in its own right.

There are three possible scenarios to bear in mind when managing distress:

1 ▷ Effectively treating any associated organic disorder may diminish or abolish the distress; if the distress is primarily pain related there is a good chance it can be successfully addressed
2 ▷ The distress may persist despite apparently effective treatment of associated organic pathology. The distress will influence the persistence of the pain from the organic disorder unless treatment is effectively targeted at both aspects of the problem
3 ▷ The distress may exist in the absence of any identifiable organic disorder.

## Assessment of distress

Many of the following features will be present.[20] The more of these features that are present, the more you need to consider the possibility that the patient is distressed. However, there are some caveats (Box 2.6).

## History

The more of the following features that are present, the more you need to consider the possibility that the patient is distressed:

42

---

Box 2.6 ○ *Caveats when assessing distress*

---

▶ Do not make any assumptions and forget to perform a thorough clinical assessment or you may miss the patient who is distressed by serious pathology (a relatively short history and consistent organic physical signs may be present, as well as the 'distress signals').

▶ No one feature of distress *on its own* is necessarily diagnostic of anything.[21]

▶ Differing cultural responses to pain may make it difficult to interpret 'distressed' behaviour in some patient populations.

▶ *Vitamin D deficiency* frequently presents with widespread non-specific pain (including the spine) and no hard signs; do not diagnose a chronic pain syndrome without ruling this out.

▶ Primary vitamin D deficiency is common in adults of all ages in the UK and other developed countries. People particularly at risk include: certain ethnic minority groups (e.g. South Asian, African Caribbean, Middle Eastern); housebound people; those aged over 65 years; those in residential care; and those inadequately exposed to spring/summer sunshine. Secondary vitamin D insufficiency can occur with fat malabsorption (e.g. due to coeliac disease, pancreatic insufficiency); gastrointestinal bypass surgery; gastrectomy; parenteral nutrition; or medication (e.g. carbamazepine, phenytoin). Hepatic disorders impair vitamin D hydroxylation and renal failure impairs vitamin D activation.[22]

▷ often there is a long history with extensive medical records and the patient has 'done the rounds' of multiple specialists and specialties (the 'revolving door' phenomenon).
▷ past history of other chronic pains or functional problems, e.g. irritable bowel syndrome, chronic tension headaches, perhaps with a history of childhood headaches, chronic fatigue, fibromyalgia, premenstrual syndrome, dysfunctional uterine bleeding, etc.
▷ 'What's the pain like?' is a key question (Box 2.7).

---

Box 2.7 ○ *Is the patient describing the pain in a physical or affective manner?*

---

**Physical**

Mild/moderate/severe, burning/aching/throbbing, etc. (organic descriptors).

**Affective**

Purgatory/hell/torture/murder/makes me feel suicidal/I feel like I've been dipped in a vat of pain (emotional descriptors).

---

Pain may also be:

▷ Continuous pain ('never free of it') or located to the coccyx;
   nondermatomal numbness may also be described.

Other features in the history may be:

▷ emergency admissions with back pain and/or whole lower limb
▷ no treatment helps (and treatments have often made it worse) and every
   time you see the patient he or she is 'worse than ever'
▷ correspondence from the clinicians who have seen him or her before
   refers to behaviour that is 'inappropriate' or 'out of proportion'
▷ significant 'downtime' is reported, i.e. the average number of hours
   spent lying down between 7 a.m. and 11 p.m.
▷ late for his or her appointment (or has missed lots of appointments in
   primary and secondary care) and may be highly critical of previous
   doctors/therapists
▷ compensation claim outstanding.

## Examination

Features in the examination may be:

▷ patient accompanied by another person (e.g. spouse) who helps him or
   her into the room, does a lot of the talking ('Something must be done!')
   and helps the patient to undress and onto the examination couch (the
   'partner in pain')
▷ antalgic (painful) gait and slow, deliberate movements
▷ props – collar/stick/crutches/lumbar corset/TENS machine, which may
   be 'distress signals'
▷ inappropriate demeanour and appearance, e.g. smiling patient who is
   'in agony'
▷ discrepancies between the patient's behaviour before and during the
   formal examination, i.e. look for these by asking the patient to undress
   while you write in his or her notes, but observe how he or she does this
   when thinking your attention is elsewhere
▷ overt pain behaviour – guarding, bracing, rubbing, grimacing and
   sighing.[23] Also during the examination, the patient may call out,
   make jumpy, startled movements, keep his or her eyes closed, grab
   the clinician's hand to stop a test being performed, touch the clinician
   to indicate the site of the pain, laugh or cry inappropriately
▷ Waddell's signs – the pain is made worse by axial loading (vertical
   skull compression, or pressure over the shoulders if the patient has

neck pain), and also by pseudorotation of the spine (hold the patient's arms down by his or her sides at the hips, ask the patient to keep his or her feet still, and rotate them left and right – rotation occurs at the hips, not the spine). Pinching a fold of skin over the lumbar area in prone is painful (the 'ground-glass back'), and the flip test is positive (straight-leg raise (SLR) in lying is restricted and/or painful or impossible, but the patient can sit up and lean forwards). Sensory disturbances are regional (stocking), not dermatomal, and any motor disturbances are also regional, not myotomal (often global with jerky giving way – 'the judders')[24]

▷ tests that do not hurt are never reported as being painless, but 'not too bad'[25]

▷ Kummel's signs – in a hospital out-patient setting, if all of Waddell's signs are present the patient's chance of ever returning to work is 50%. This falls to 25% if two further signs are present, i.e. the back pain is made worse by neck rotation and shoulder abduction[26]

▷ afterwards, the patient feels exhausted and it has made the pain worse.

---

## Investigations

▷ Radiography of the lumbar spine in primary care patients with low-back pain of at least six weeks' duration is not associated with improvement in patient functioning, severity of pain or overall health status, but is associated with an increased workload for doctors. However, patients receiving radiography are more satisfied with the care they receive. The challenge for primary care is to increase satisfaction without recourse to radiography.[27]

▷ If the diagnosis is secure, GPs should avoid ordering more tests, as this may increase the patient's distress ('I need another scan – there must be something *really* wrong with me!'),[28] may generate disappointment when the test is normal ('So what is the matter with me then?') and delays the day when the GP has to 'bite the bullet' and deal with the underlying issues.

▷ Doctors often seize on minor abnormalities and normal variants in test results to explain the patient's symptoms. This may mean that obstacles to recovery are unaddressed and the patient may receive inappropriate treatment.[29] The longer this goes on, the worse the patient's distress and he or she may become more difficult to help.

▷ If the test results do not fit the clinical picture then 'treat the man, not the scan'.

## Clinical assessment of risk factors for chronicity

The risk factors for the development of chronicity are listed in Box 2.8.

---

Box 2.8 ○ *Factors associated with development and persistence of low-back pain*

**Physical**

▶ Older age.*†
▶ Prior episode of back pain.*†
▶ Higher-pain intensity or disability.†
▶ Obesity.*†
▶ Poor physical fitness.
▶ Low baseline activity levels.*†
▶ Reduced trunk muscle strength and endurance.
▶ Neurological symptoms.†
▶ Signs of nerve root involvement.
▶ Radiating leg pain.
▶ Reduced SLR.

**Psychosocial**

▶ Manual labour or physically stressful job.*†
▶ Poor job satisfaction or low pay.*†
▶ Total work loss due to low-back pain in past year.
▶ Low educational level.†
▶ Self-rated health poor.
▶ Smoking.*†
▶ Inadequate coping skills.†
▶ Fear-avoidance behaviour.*†‡
▶ Anxiety.*†
▶ Depressed mood.†
▶ Emotional/psychosocial distress.*†
▶ Somatisation.*†
▶ Disproportionate illness behaviour.
▶ Personal problems (alcohol, marital, financial).
▶ Ongoing adversarial medico-legal proceedings.†

---

*Source*: modified from Rubinstein S M, van Tulder M. A best-evidence review of diagnostic procedures for neck and low-back pain.[30]

*Notes*: * Associated with *development* of low-back pain in some studies.
† Associated with *persistence* of low-back pain in some studies.
‡ The avoidance of physical activities that stems from a patient's fears that his or her pain will worsen.
NB: association does *not* imply causality. Evidence is mixed for some factors, including smoking, obesity and low educational level.

To elicit the psychosocial, psychiatric and occupational obstacles to recovery it may be helpful to use CERTIFICATE (Box 2.9).

---

**Box 2.9** ○ *CERTIFICATE – interview prompts to elicit psychosocial, psychiatric and occupational obstacles to recovery*

C ▷ What do you understand is the **Cause** of your back pain?

E ▷ Have you **Ever** had any other chronic pain problem (chronic whiplash, irritable bowel syndrome, tension headaches, fibromyalgia, repetitive strain injury, premenstrual syndrome, etc.) and what happened?

R ▷ How are others **Responding** to your back pain (family, co-workers, boss)? What are they doing at work to help?

T ▷ Have you ever had **Time** off work in the past with back pain?

I ▷ **If** you are currently off work, when do you expect to return? Ever? What do you feel about your job?

F ▷ **Financial**. Is time off work causing financial hardship? Any there outstanding legal/insurance claims? Are you receiving benefits (including Disabled Parking Badge)?

I ▷ What **Investigations** have you had so far and what did they show?

C ▷ What are you doing to **Cope** with the back pain?

A ▷ **Affective**. Some people with long-term pain get low, down or depressed; how is your mood at the moment?

T ▷ What have you been **Told** about your back pain by your GP/physiotherapist/osteopath/*et al.*?

E ▷ **Expectations**. What do you expect is going to happen? What were you hoping we might be able to do?

*Source*: adapted from Main CJ, Williams AC. ABC of psychological medicine: musculoskeletal pain.[1]

---

## Assessment tools

The recently developed Keele STarT Back Screening Tool, from the Arthritis Research Campaign National Primary Care Centre at Keele University, looks promising. It may provide GPs with a simple and useful tool to identify, at their initial presentation, patients with potentially treatment-modifiable prognostic indicators. Using the tool may allow GPs to allocate patients with back pain to one of three categories:[31]

1 ▷ A low-risk subgroup (patients with few negative prognostic indicators, suitable for primary care management according to best-practice guidelines, e.g. analgesia, advice and education)

2 ▷ A medium-risk subgroup (patients with an unfavourable prognosis with high levels of physical prognostic indicators, appropriate for physiotherapy)

3 ▷ A high-risk subgroup (patients with a very unfavourable prognosis, with consistently high levels across psychosocial prognostic indicators, appropriate for management by a combination of physical and cognitive behavioural approaches).

---

### Does early psychosocial intervention prevent chronicity?

Although psychosocial factors certainly contribute to the development of chronic low-back pain and disability, less is known about the efficacy of interventions aimed at patients identified with increased risk due to these factors. A clinical trial of a specifically designed intervention, to be applied by GPs, for patients with acute or subacute low-back pain did not find positive effects.[32] The intervention focused on the identification of psychosocial prognostic factors, discussing these factors with the patient, setting specific goals for reactivation, and providing an educational booklet. Compared with usual care, however, no differences were found on any outcome measure during a year-long follow-up.

The NICE guideline[3] recommends that, if significant psychological distress and/or high disability persist after receiving at least one of three less intensive physical interventions (structured exercise programme, manipulation or acupuncture), the patient should be considered for referral to a combined physical and psychological treatment programme, comprising around 100 hours of therapy spread over a period of up to eight weeks. This should include a cognitive behavioural approach and exercise.

The development and evaluation of interventions aimed at the prevention of chronicity is of utmost importance in the coming years.[6]

---

### An approach to management

One of the main management issues with distressed patients is the time it takes to effectively address their concerns one by one. The more chronic the problem, often the more time it takes to address and modify the patient's misunderstandings. This requires effective listening, communication and reassurance coupled with appropriate pain medication and advice about reactivation. Effective management means booking the more complex patients into longer

Figure 2.1 ○ *The Keele STarT Back Screening Tool*

**Patient name:** ........................................................................ **Date:** ..............

Thinking about the **last two weeks** tick your response to the following questions:

|  | Disagree 0 | Agree 1 |
|---|---|---|
| **1** My back pain has **spread down my leg(s)** in the last two weeks | ☐ | ☐ |
| **2** I have had pain in the **shoulder** or **neck** at some time in the last two weeks | ☐ | ☐ |
| **3** I have only **walked short distances** because of my back pain | ☐ | ☐ |
| **4** In the last two weeks, I have **dressed more slowly** than usual because of back pain | ☐ | ☐ |
| **5** It's not really safe for a person with a condition like mine to be physically active | ☐ | ☐ |
| **6** **Worrying thoughts** have been going through my mind a lot of the time | ☐ | ☐ |
| **7** I feel that **my back pain is terrible** and **it's never going to get any better** | ☐ | ☐ |
| **8** In general I have **not enjoyed** all the things I used to enjoy | ☐ | ☐ |

**9** Overall, how **bothersome** has your back pain been in the **last two weeks**?

| Not at all | Slightly | Moderately | Very much | Extremely |
|---|---|---|---|---|
| ☐ | ☐ | ☐ | ☐ | ☐ |
| 0 | 0 | 0 | 1 | 1 |

**Total score (all 9):** ............................. **Psych Score (Q5, 6, 7, 8, 9):** ....................

**The Keele STarT Back Tool Scoring System**

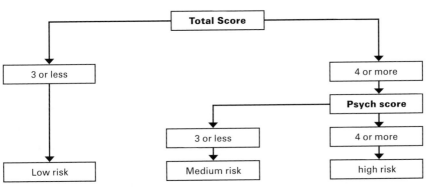

*Source*: Keele University,
www.keele.ac.uk/research/pchs/pcmrc/dissemination/tools/startback/.
This work was funded by Arthritis Research UK.

appointment slots to enable clinicians to effectively problem-solve the patient's individual issues. A rushed consultation may make the situation worse.

### Therapies for chronic back pain

#### PHARMACOTHERAPY

For oral non-steroidal anti-inflammatory drugs (NSAIDs) the evidence is greater for acute (where the treatment effect is small) than chronic back pain.[3] Paracetamol is slightly less effective than NSAIDs but has fewer or less severe side effects.[4] Minimal evidence exists that NSAIDs are effective for radiculopathy, or that one drug is better than any other.[4]

For chronic low-back pain the evidence supporting muscle relaxants (including benzodiazepines, which should only be prescribed with clearly defined goals and time frames) is less convincing than for acute pain.[4]

Most systematic reviews have found that tricyclic antidepressants, but not selective serotonin reuptake inhibitors, are more effective than placebo for chronic non-specific low-back pain. Antidepressants reduce pain severity but do not improve functional status in chronic back pain.[4]

Scant evidence exists to support any drug class for radiculopathy, but there is a small benefit for gabapentin.[4] Pregabalin may be a third-line choice for neuropathic symptoms if amitriptyline and gabapentin are not tolerated.

Opioids are generally regarded as a reasonable option for some episodes of acute back pain, but the evidence for use in chronic low-back pain is unclear. Although opioids can provide short-term relief in some patients with chronic low-back pain, their long-term benefits remain unproved. If strong opioids (e.g. morphine, fentanyl, oxycodone, buprenorphine, high-dose tramadol) are used for chronic low-back pain or other non-malignant conditions, many guidelines advocate their use only when more conservative treatments have failed, in conjunction with risk assessment tools and an opioids contract, and with clearly defined goals and exit strategies.[4] It may be sensible to have a written practice policy about this issue and to consider referral to a pain specialist before taking this step. Consider carefully whether prescribing strong opioids for chronic back pain is a rational pharmacological intervention or a hasty response to a patient's distress.

The 2009 NICE clinical guideline[3] advises starting with regular paracetamol as the first option. When this is insufficient, and taking into account individual risk of side effects and patient preference, offer NSAIDs and /or weak opioids (e.g. codeine, dihydrocodeine). Co-prescribe a proton pump inhibitor with the NSAID for patients aged over 45. Consider adding low-dose amitriptyline (initially 10 mg at night and gradually escalating the dosage until pain improves, the maximum antidepressant dosage is reached, or dosage is limited by unacceptable side effects).

Bearing in mind all of the above, my own approach is to try to involve the patient in making decisions about his or her drug therapy. At the outset I suggest that we try to erect an 'umbrella' of pain relief to reduce the frequency, duration and severity of any pain episodes, and allow the patient to start to mobilise, or maintain and improve upon their current level of mobility.

## INJECTION THERAPY FOR CHRONIC LOW-BACK PAIN

Facet joint, epidural, trigger point and sclerosant injections have not been shown to be effective for back pain and sciatica.[33] The NICE guideline recommends that therapeutic substances should not be injected for back pain.[3] This represents a major shift in the management of chronic back pain as many orthopaedic, rheumatology and chronic pain management services have been providing injection therapy for many years and may be reluctant to stop offering these interventions.

X-ray-guided nerve root block injections for brachialgia (cervical nerve root pain) and sciatica (lumbar nerve root pain) remain a reasonable option that may prevent some patients from progressing to surgery.[34]

## SURGERY FOR CHRONIC LOW-BACK PAIN

Surgical discectomy may be considered for selected patients with brachialgia or sciatica due to a disc prolapse that does not respond to initial conservative management, but this treatment is aimed at relieving limb pain, not spinal pain.[35]

Fusion surgery for chronic low-back pain may be no better than conservative treatment.[36] Recommendations that fusion surgery should be applied in carefully selected patients are difficult to follow because no clear and validated criteria exist to identify these patients in advance.[6] NICE has, however, recommended consideration of referral for an opinion on spinal fusion. This referral is for patients who have completed a comprehensive package of care, including a combined physical and psychological treatment programme, and who have persistent, severe, non-specific low-back pain for which the patient would consider surgery.[3]

## POPULATION-BASED MEASURES FOR BACK PAIN

A population-based strategy of provision of positive messages about back pain improves population and GP beliefs about back pain, and seems to influence medical management and reduce disability and workers' compensation costs related to back pain, at least in Australia. A public health campaign based on the messages in *The Back Book*[37] demonstrated that it is possible to intervene successfully at the population level.[38] The campaign included TV, radio, print and billboard advertisements, plus other interventions, including making multi-language versions of *The Back Book* widely available.

---

Box 2.10 ○ *Key priorities for implementation in the management of patients with persistent, non-specific, low-back pain lasting six weeks to 12 months*

---

▶ Consider offering a course of manual therapy including spinal manipulation of up to nine sessions over up to 12 weeks.

▶ Consider offering a course of acupuncture needling comprising up to ten sessions over a period of up to 12 weeks.

▶ Consider offering a structured exercise programme tailored to the individual.

▶ Offer supervised group exercise programmes in preference to one-to-one supervised exercise programmes.

▶ Consider referral for a combined physical and psychological treatment programme for patients who have high disability and/or significant psychological distress after having received less intensive treatments.

▶ Do not offer X-ray of the lumbar spine for the management of non-specific low-back pain.

▶ MRI for non-specific low-back pain should only be performed within the context of a referral for an opinion on spinal fusion.

▶ Consider referral for an opinion on spinal fusion for people who have completed a comprehensive package of care, including a combined physical and psychological treatment programme, and who have persistent, severe, non-specific low-back pain for which the patient would consider surgery.

▶ Do not offer injections of therapeutic substances into the back.

---

*Source*: National Institute for Health and Clinical Excellence. *Clinical Guideline 88, Low Back Pain: early management of persistent non-specific low back pain.*[3]

---

### Therapies for chronic neck pain

#### DRUG THERAPY FOR CHRONIC NECK PAIN

The major limitations of most studies are the lack of replication of the findings and sufficiently large trials. Muscle relaxants, analgesics and NSAIDs have limited evidence and unclear benefits. Lidocaine injection into myofascial trigger points appears effective in two trials. There is moderate evidence that botulinum toxin A is *not* superior to saline injection for chronic mechanical neck pain.[39]

## PHYSICAL TREATMENTS FOR CHRONIC NECK PAIN

Specific exercises may be effective for the treatment of acute and chronic mechanical neck pain, with or without headache. To be of benefit, a stretching and strengthening exercise programme should concentrate on the musculature of the cervical, shoulder–thoracic area, or both. A multimodal care approach to exercise, combined with mobilisation or manipulation for subacute and chronic neck pain (with or without headache), reduces pain, improves function, and improves global perceived effect in the short and long term. The relative benefit of other treatments (such as physical modalities) compared with exercise or between different exercise programmes is not known.[40]

Hard and soft collars have traditionally been used for whiplash-related neck pain and for neck pain in general, but neither hard nor soft collars immobilise the spine. Collars yield poorer outcomes than prescribed activity and mobilising exercises, and may promote inactivity with the adoption of the sick role and a prolongation of the recovery period.[41]

In patients with brachalgia (cervical nerve root pain) one study compared three management strategies comprising either three weeks of rest and immobilisation in a semi-hard cervical collar followed by three weeks of weaning off the collar; six weeks of physiotherapy, twice weekly, focused on graded activity exercises and education with a physiotherapist; or advice to continue normal activities. After six weeks patients in all groups had improved, but improvement was faster in the two intervention groups, which were equally effective. Patient satisfaction, use of medication and work absenteeism were similar for all three groups during the six-week follow-up period. By six months most patients in all groups had little or no pain or disability. Only 6% of patients were treated surgically, and these were equally distributed among the three groups.[42] A pragmatic approach might be to explain the findings of this study to the patient and allow him or her to choose which strategy to adopt, with the option to change the strategy if recovery is slow.[43]

Caution is needed when drawing a valid conclusion on the efficacy of conservative treatments in patients with whiplash injury. It appears that 'rest makes rusty', whereas active interventions have a tendency to be more effective in patients with whiplash injury.[44]

### Routine NHS physiotherapy referral

In a well-conducted study, referral for routine physiotherapy interventions for patients with back pain for more than six weeks seemed to be no more effective than one session of assessment and advice from a physiotherapist.[45]

Although in this study patients felt better after the interventions, objective outcomes did not improve, putting into doubt the utility of this approach.

Referral to physiotherapy is an easy option. It gives the doctor some time, and the patient is having treatment, but NHS physiotherapy adds little to giving the patient an advice sheet. In a resource-limited health service we might ask serious questions about the use of these resources, appropriate management of patients, and referral patterns.[46] NICE, however, in the guidance for chronic back pain includes management options that might be addressed by physiotherapy referral (Box 2.10).

### Pain management programmes

If one is available, then referral to a multidisciplinary chronic pain management programme may be a useful option. Exercise programmes and physical reconditioning can improve pain and functional levels in patients with chronic low-back pain.[3]

Cognitive behavioural therapy can be of value in improving the day-to-day functioning and quality of life of patients with chronic pain when other conventional treatments have apparently failed. However, such treatment is intensive, expensive and not widely available, and it is still unknown what type of patients benefit most from what type of behavioural treatment.

While intensive daily multidisciplinary biopsychosocial rehabilitation with functional restoration ($>100$ hours) reduces pain and improves function in chronic low-back pain patients, less intensive interventions do not show improvements in clinically relevant outcomes.[47]

---

### Occupational aspects

When people do not return to work with back and neck pain, psychosocial obstacles are often more important than biomedical factors. Yellow, blue and black flags are warning signals that psychosocial issues are acting as obstacles (Box 2.11).[48]

All parties need to identify the flags and develop a plan to overcome the obstacles.

GPs are in a pivotal position to emphasise these key messages:

▷ remind the patient that symptoms are common and usually short term
▷ while some people need treatment many settle with self-management
▷ activity is helpful and prolonged rest is not
▷ most people can stay at work, perhaps with adjustment to tasks

> Box 2.11 ○ *Psychosocial flags for the clinic and workplace*
>
> **Yellow flags (related to the person)**
>
> **1** ▸ Thoughts, e.g. catastrophising, dysfunctional beliefs and expectations about pain, work and health care, negative expectation of recovery, preoccupation with health.
>
> **2** ▸ Feelings, e.g. worry, distress, low mood, fear of movement, uncertainty about the future.
>
> **3** ▸ Behaviours, e.g. extreme symptom report, passive coping strategies, serial ineffective therapy.
>
> **Blue flags (related to the workplace)**
>
> **1** ▸ Employee, e.g. fear of re-injury, high physical job demand, low expectation of resuming work, low job satisfaction, low social support or social dysfunction in the workplace, perception of high job-related 'stress'.
>
> **2** ▸ Workplace, e.g. lack of job accommodation or modified work or employer communication with employee.
>
> **Black flags (related to the context)**
>
> Examples of these are misunderstandings and disagreements between key players (including health care), financial and compensation problems, process delays, over-reactions to sensationalist media reports, spouse or family member with negative expectations, fears or beliefs, social isolation or dysfunction, unhelpful policies or procedures used by the employer.

or schedules

▷ an early return to work/activity helps recovery and usually does no harm

▷ long-term inactivity and time of work is detrimental to health and wellbeing

▷ *do not* tell the patient that work was the cause – it probably was not.

Guidance from NICE recommends that doctors should not automatically write a sickness certificate and should instead discuss with their patients any obstacles to returning to work. The guidance includes a number of recommendations for employers and GPs and other NHS professionals. The aim is to reduce the number of employees moving to long-term absence because of sickness and to promote a return to work.[49]

It might be helpful to liaise with the company medical officer or occupational health department. Encourage employers to implement the Faculty of Occupational Medicine guidelines for the management of low-back pain at work (www.facoccmed.ac.uk).

A decision to stop work because of a chronic medical condition or disability is often made by the patient, with or without the advice or agreement of a health professional or employer. The key factors believed to influence this decision are the perceived symptoms (e.g. pain, disability, anxiety), the nature of the work demands and the sociodemographic context. There is now considerable evidence that the decision to retire early on health grounds due to chronic low-back pain is predominantly based on factors of which the medical condition is the least important.[50] Chronic low-back pain has become a diagnosis of convenience for many people who are actually disabled for socioeconomic, work-related or psychological reasons.[51]

Long periods of sick leave without a clearly defined diagnosis or a treatment or rehabilitation plan can lead to disability that is difficult to salvage.

---

**A strategy for dealing with chronic spinal pain[52]**

1 ▶ **Treat physical disease (if present) and dysfunction**
  ▷ 'Disease' means organic or structural pathology.
  ▷ 'Dysfunction' refers to the deconditioning and maladaptive changes in physical functioning that are maintaining the pain, i.e. the back hurts because it doesn't work properly. This concept requires a paradigm shift in our diagnostic thinking.[53]

2 ▶ **Manage the illness**
  ▷ Illness means symptoms and behaviours.
  ▷ Use the Keele STarT Back Tool to guide management.
  ▷ Follow the NICE management pathway.
  ▷ Every consultation is an opportunity for simple cognitive behavioural therapy.
  ▷ Give the patient positive messages (Box 2.12).
  ▷ Explain what has happened to the patient. Patients with somatisation disorders feel satisfied and empowered by medical explanations that are tangible (easily understood), exculpating (i.e. don't blame the patient for the problem) and involving.[54]
  ▷ Empathise – those patients who describe more pain or disability seek more types of diagnostic and therapeutic measures, while those who feel they have been understood seek less.[55]
  ▷ Medication is important but is only one aspect of patient management.
  ▷ Reflect upon your own attitude to pain; GPs who report high levels of pain-related fear are more likely to recommend rest and sick leave for their patients with back pain.[56]
  ▷ Don't give up on the possibility of helping patients with chronic pain.

3 ▶ **Negotiate the sick role**

▷ Use the yellow, blue and black flags to identify obstacles to a return to work and explore ways to remove them; CERTIFICATE may help to do this.

▷ Stress the positive aspects of remaining in employment.

▷ Challenge negative beliefs (especially about work) in a non-confrontational way.

▷ Don't let the patient become a chronic invalid by default.

---

Box 2.12  ○  *Positive messages*

---

▶ It's hurting but it's not harming.

▶ The pain does not mean serious damage.

▶ Use it or lose it.

▶ If you rest you rust.

▶ Maintain normal activities – do what you normally do.

## Conclusion

There is a continuum of chronic pain, rather than a distinct class of chronic pain patients. Because pain outcomes are highly variable between people and over time, chronic pain should be viewed as having an inherently uncertain prognosis, not as a static trait that identifies patients whose pain is intractable.

The term 'chronic pain' carries negative connotations for patients and clinicians alike. By shifting the focus from pain duration to prognosis, and by defining chronic pain in probabilistic terms, based on an assessment of the risk of an unfavourable outcome (e.g. by using the Keele STarT Back Tool), the assessment of chronic pain may be refocused from labelling patients as having intractable pain to focusing on steps that might be taken to reduce risks of an unfavourable outcome.[57]

Box 2.13 ○ *Case study*

Mr Hall is a 42-year-old man who came to see a GP registrar about his ongoing back pain. He has had pain now for nine months and seen a variety of other GPs in the practice. He was still working, but had had three episodes of sick leave when his back had 'seized' and he could not stand up straight. He believed that the cause of his pain was having to move a heavy refrigerator at work ten months previously. He explained that he worked on a production line with mostly female operatives and had moved the heavy fridge because no one else was strong enough. Now his female colleagues help him out when his back hurts and sometimes do part of his job for him. He was extremely worried about the next episode of back pain and the damage that this may do to him. Although he had been referred to a physiotherapist, he felt that this had made things much worse and had stopped going. He was married with two sons and his wife did not work, so there were issues over money at home and marital relations were strained.

The GP registrar attempted to examine Mr Hall, but he demanded another sick note and the registrar felt forced to give him a certificate for two weeks. The next day, the registrar discussed the case with his trainer and they decided to refer Mr Hall on to the local Musculoskeletal Service, which was lead by a GPwSI and physiotherapist. They had correctly identified that Mr Hall had a lot of 'yellow flags' that were interfering with his recovery. He had concerns over the cause of his pain being related to his job; he had some fear-avoidance behaviour that was preventing him from working; he had financial worries and marital problems.

## *Analysis of case study with respect to the six domains of Being a GP*

### DOMAIN 1: PRIMARY CARE MANAGEMENT

The registrar was aware that Mr Hall had a chronic back problem and was aware of some of the implications of this. He struggled with the management of this complex case, though, and was able to ask his trainer for help. He had reviewed Mr Hall's notes and seen that he had consulted frequently for the back problem and had failed to gain benefit from physiotherapy.

### DOMAIN 2: PERSON-CENTRED CARE

Despite seeing many of the doctors in the practice, no one had really been able to get to the bottom of Mr Hall's problem. The registrar had noted the 'yellow flags' in the presentation and appreciated that more expert help was required. The registrar had also noted the distress in the patient's presentation.

### DOMAIN 3: SPECIFIC PROBLEM-SOLVING SKILLS

Using the previous records and the registrar's consultation, the GP trainer was able to assess the case so far and see that onward referral was necessary to address the psychological issues.

## DOMAIN 4: A COMPREHENSIVE APPROACH

This is a complex case and needs to be managed well at this point or Mr Hall will have lifelong ill health and sickness absence. The GP trainer is aware of the prognosis of someone like Mr Hall, who has a chronic back problem and many yellow flags.

## DOMAIN 5: COMMUNITY ORIENTATION

The GP trainer considered other patients he knew who worked at the same factory as Mr Hall and whether there were workplace issues that could affect the whole community. He wondered whether to involve the occupational health services.

## DOMAIN 6: A HOLISTIC APPROACH

Using the methods described in this chapter, the approach to Mr Hall's back pain has been holistic, considering the biopsychosocial aspects of the case.

---

## Summary

▷ Persistent back and neck pain is common.
▷ Patients with chronic back and neck pain consult for many reasons.
▷ The diagnosis should be kept under review at all times.
▷ Management is frequently challenging.
▷ The transition from acute to chronic disabling back or neck pain is a complex process and many individual, psychosocial and workplace factors may play a part.
▷ The term 'chronic pain' often implies the presence of significant psychosocial factors and disproportionate disability.
▷ Patients with chronic back and neck pain may be distressed and coping poorly with their situation.
▷ There is no clinical dichotomy between organic disease and distress, and both must be addressed if present.
▷ Someone who is distressed in the absence of clear-cut organic pathology, or whose distress appears disproportionate to the physical disorder, is having a very real and unpleasant experience, and the GP's job is to find the best way to help.
▷ Distress is related to severe pain in association with honest misunderstandings and misattributions that then lead to fear,

catastrophising and low mood; this highly dynamic process is influenced by an individual's beliefs, emotions and coping responses.

▷ When assessing distress no one feature of the history or examination by itself is necessarily diagnostic of anything.

▷ To elicit the psychosocial, psychiatric and occupational obstacles to recovery it may be helpful to use CERTIFICATE.

▷ Use the Keele STarT Back Tool to help with prognosis and management.

▷ The choice of investigation depends upon the duration of symptoms and overall clinical picture; beware medicalisation by ordering inappropriate tests.

▷ Follow the NICE guidelines on the early management of persistent non-specific low-back pain.

▷ When people do not return to work with back and neck pain psychosocial obstacles are often more important than biomedical factors.

▷ Yellow, blue and black flags are warning signals that psychosocial issues are acting as obstacles.

▷ GPs are in a pivotal position to facilitate a timely return to work.

▷ Pain outcomes are highly variable between people and over time.

▷ Focus on steps to reduce the risks of an unfavourable outcome, e.g. give positive messages about work and activity.

## Acknowledgements

Louise Warburton, Jonathan Hill and Kate Dunn for their feedback and helpful suggestions.

### References

1 • Main C J, Williams A C. ABC of psychological medicine: musculoskeletal pain *British Medical Journal* 2002; **325(7363)**: 534–7.

2 • Cedraschi C, Robert J, Goerg D, *et al.* Is chronic non-specific low back pain chronic? Definitions of a problem, and problems of a definition *British Journal of General Practice* 1999; **49(442)**: 358–36.

3 • National Institute for Health and Clinical Excellence. *Clinical Guideline 88, Low Back Pain: early management of persistent non-specific low back pain* London: NICE, 2009, http://guidance.nice.org.uk/CG88 [accessed October 2011].

4 • Cohen S P, Argoff C E, Carragee E J. Management of low back pain *British Medical Journal* 2008; **337**: a2718.

5 • Von Korff M. Studying the natural history of back pain *Spine* 1994; **19(suppl. 18)**: S2041–6.

6 • Koes B W, van Tulder M W, Thomas S. Diagnosis and treatment of low back pain *British Medical Journal* 2006; **332(7555)**: 1430–4.

7 • Pengel L H, Herbert R D, Maher C G, *et al.* Acute low back pain: systematic review of its prognosis *British Medical Journal* 2003; **327(7410)**: 323.

8 • Costa L, Maher C G, McAuley J H, *et al.* Prognosis for patients with chronic low back pain: inception cohort study *British Medical Journal* 2009; **339**: b3829.

9 • van den Hoogen H J, Koes B W, van Eijk J T, *et al.* On the course of low back pain in general practice: a one year follow up study *Annals of the Rheumatic Diseases* 1998; **57(1)**: 13–19.

10 • Thomas E, Silman A J, Croft P R, *et al.* Predicting who develops chronic low back pain in primary care: a prospective study *British Medical Journal* 1999; **318(7199)**: 1662–7.

11 • Palmer K T, Walsh K, Bendall H, *et al.* Back pain in Britain: comparison of two prevalence surveys at an interval of 10 years *British Medical Journal* 2000; **320(7249)**: 1577–8.

12 • Hogg-Johnson S, van der Velde G, Carroll L J, *et al.* The burden and determinants of neck pain in the general population: results of the Bone and Joint Decade 2000–2010 Task Force on Neck Pain and Its Associated Disorders *Spine* 2008; **33(suppl. 4)**: S39–51.

13 • Carroll L J, Holm L W, Hogg-Johnson S. Course and prognostic factors for neck pain in whiplash-associated disorders (WAD): results of the Bone and Joint Decade 2000–2010 Task Force on Neck Pain and Its Associated Disorders *Spine* 2008; **33(suppl. 4)**: S83–92.

14 • Pincus T, Burton A K, Vogel S, *et al.* A systematic review of psychological factors as predictors of chronicity/disability in prospective cohorts of low back pain *Spine* 2002; **27(5)**: E109–20.

15 • Waddell G. Diagnostic triage. In: *The Back Pain Revolution* (2nd edn) London: Churchill Livingstone, 2004.

16 • Potter R G, Jones J M, Boardman A P. A prospective study of primary care patients with musculoskeletal pain: the identification of predictive factors for chronicity *British Journal of General Practice* 2000; **50(452)**: 225–7.

17 • Binder A I. Cervical spondylosis and neck pain *British Medical Journal* 2007; **334(7592)**: 527–31.

18 • Jackson C. The General Health Questionnaire *Occupational Medicine* 2007; **57(1)**: 79.

19 • Njobvu P, Hunt I, Pope D, *et al.* Pain amongst ethnic minority groups of South Asian origin in the United Kingdom: a review *Rheumatology* 1999; **38(12)**: 1184–7.

20 • Longworth S. Chronic back pain disability: a review article: 1. Mechanisms and diagnosis *Journal of Orthopaedic Medicine* 2004; **26(1)**: 2–6.

21 • Main C J, Waddell G. Behavioral responses to examination: a reappraisal of the interpretation of 'nonorganic' signs *Spine* 1998; **23(21)**: 2367–71.

22 • Anon. Primary vitamin D deficiency in adults *Drug and Therapeutics Bulletin* 2006; **44(4)**: 25–9.

23 • Keefe F J, Block A R. Development of an observation method for assessing pain behaviour in chronic low back pain patients *Behavioural Therapy* 1982; **13**: 363–75.

24 • Waddell G. Illness behaviour. In: *The Back Pain Revolution* (2nd edn) London: Churchill Livingstone, 2004.

25 • Cyriax J H. Psychogenic pain. In: *Textbook of Orthopaedic Medicine* (8th edn) London: Baillière-Tindall, 1982.

26 • Kummel B. Nonorganic signs of significance in low back pain *Spine* 1996; **21(9)**: 1077–81.

27 • Kendrick D, Fielding K, Bentley E, *et al.* Radiography of the lumbar spine in primary care patients with low back pain: randomised controlled trial *British Medical Journal* 2001; **322(7283)**: 400–5.

28 • Turner J. Medically unexplained symptoms in secondary care *British Medical Journal* 2001; **322(7289)**: 745–6.

29 • Deyo R A. Magnetic resonance imaging of the lumbar spine: terrific test or tar baby? *New England Journal of Medicine* 1994; **331(2)**: 115–16.

30 • Rubinstein S M, van Tulder M. A best-evidence review of diagnostic procedures for neck and low-back pain *Best Practice & Research Clinical Rheumatology* 2008; **22(3)**: 471–82.

31 • Hill JC, Dunn K M, Lewis M, *et al.* A primary care back pain screening tool: identifying patient subgroups for initial treatment *Arthritis & Rheumatism* 2008; **59(5)**: 632–41.

32 • Jellema P, van der Windt D A W M, van der Horst H E, *et al.* Should treatment of (sub) acute low back pain be aimed at psychosocial prognostic factors? Cluster randomised clinical trial in general practice *British Medical Journal* 2005; **331(7508)**: 84–90.

33 • van Tulder M W, Koes B, Seitsalo S, *et al.* Outcome of invasive treatment modalities on back pain and sciatica: an evidence-based review *European Spine Journal* 2006; **15(suppl. 1)**: S82–92.

34 • Riew K D, Park J B, Cho Y S, *et al.* Nerve root blocks in the treatment of lumbar radicular pain: a minimum five-year follow-up *Journal of Bone and Joint Surgery (American)* 2006; **88(8)**: 1722–5.

35 • Fairbank J. Prolapsed intervertebral disc *British Medical Journal* 2008; **336(7657)**: 1317–18.

36 • Koes B W. Surgery versus intensive rehabilitation programmes for chronic low back pain: spinal fusion surgery has only modest if any effects *British Medical Journal* 2005; **330(7502)**:1220–1.

37 • Burton K, Cantrell T, Klaber Moffett J, *et al. The Back Book* (2nd edn) London: The Stationery Office, 2002.

38 • Buchbinder R, Jolley D, Wyatt M. Population based intervention to change back pain beliefs and disability: three part evaluation *British Medical Journal* 2001; **322(7301)**: 1516–20.

39 • Peloso P, Gross A, Haines T. Medicinal and injection therapies for mechanical neck disorders *Cochrane Database of Systematic Reviews* 2007; **3**: CD000319.

40 • Kay T M, Gross A, Goldsmith C. Exercises for mechanical neck disorders *Cochrane Database of Systematic Reviews* 2005; **3**: CD004250.

41 • Muzin S, Isaac Z, Walker J, *et al.* When should a cervical collar be used to treat neck pain? *Current Reviews in Musculoskeletal Medicine* 2008; **1(2)**: 114–19.

42 • Kuijper B, Tans J T, Beelen A, *et al.* Cervical collar or physiotherapy versus wait and see policy for recent onset cervical radiculopathy: randomized trial *British Medical Journal* 2009; **339**: b3883.

43 • Cassidy D J. Mobilisation or immobilisation for cervical radiculopathy? *British Medical Journal* 2009; **339**; b3952.

44 • Peeters G G, Verhagen A P, de Bie R A, *et al.* The efficacy of conservative treatment in patients with whiplash injury: a systematic review of clinical trials *Spine* 2001; **26(4)**: E64–73.

45 • Frost H, Lamb S E, Doll H A, *et al.* Randomised controlled trial of physiotherapy compared with advice for low back pain *British Medical Journal* 2004; **329(7468)**: 708–11.

46 • MacAuley D. Back pain and physiotherapy *British Medical Journal* 2004; **329(7468)**: 694–5.

47 • Guzman J, Esmail R, Karjalainen K, *et al.* Multidisciplinary rehabilitation for chronic low back pain: systematic review *British Medical Journal* 2001; **322(7301)**: 1511–16.

48 • Kendall N A S, Burton A K, Main C J, *et al.* on behalf of the Flags Think-Tank. *Tackling Musculoskeletal Problems: a guide for the clinic and workplace* London: The Stationery Office, 2009.

49 • National Institute for Health and Clinical Excellence. *Management of Long-Term Sickness and Incapacity for Work* London: NICE, 2008.

50 • Sawney P. Current issues in fitness for work certification *British Journal of General Practice* 2002; **52(476)**: 217–22.

51 • Andersson G B J. Epidemiological features of chronic low back pain *Lancet* 1999; **354(9178)**: 581–5.

52 • Longworth S. Chronic back pain disability: a review article: 2 *Management Journal of Orthopaedic Medicine* 2004; **26(2)**: 42–50.

53 • Williams N. Managing back pain in general practice: is osteopathy the new paradigm? *British Journal of General Practice* 1997; **47(423)**: 653–5.

54 • Salmon P, Peters S, Stanley I. Patients' perceptions of medical explanations for somatisation disorders: qualitative analysis *British Medical Journal* 1999; **318(7180)**: 372–6.

55 • Hermoni D, Borkan J M, Lahad A, *et al.* Doctor–patient concordance and patient initiative during episodes of low back pain *British Journal of General Practice* 2000; **50(459)**: 809–10.

56 • Coudeyre E, Rannou F, Tubach F, *et al.* General practitioners' fear avoidance beliefs influence their management of patients with low back pain *Pain* 2006; **124**: 330–7.

57 • Von Korff M, Dunn K M. Chronic pain reconsidered *Pain* 2008; **138(2)**: 267–76.

# The principles of physiotherapy

**3**

*Krysia Dziedzic and Lindsay M. Bearne*

## Aims of this chapter

▶ To give an understanding of how physiotherapy is an essential component in the management of musculoskeletal conditions in primary care.

▶ To outline the principles of physiotherapy for commonly used core interventions in primary care, e.g. education and advice, exercise, manual therapy.

▶ To summarise the current evidence base for the treatment options to relieve pain and stiffness, improve movement and function, and increase participation and quality of life.

## Introduction

Physiotherapy is an essential component in the management of musculoskeletal conditions in primary care. The commonest musculoskeletal conditions seen in physiotherapy departments are low-back pain and osteoarthritis (OA), and recent NICE recommendations have highlighted the benefits of non-pharmacological treatments as front-line approaches.[1,2] This chapter reviews the role of exercise and physical therapies (electrotherapy, thermotherapy, cryotherapy, manual therapy and acupuncture) in common musculoskeletal conditions and considers the current evidence for these treatment options.

### The aims of physiotherapy

The aims of physiotherapy can be considered in relation to the International Classification of Functioning (ICF),[3] which describes a model based on disease, impairment, activities and participation. Treatment options aim to relieve pain and stiffness, improve movement and function, and allow people to participate in aspects of their life as and when they want to.

The clinical assessment is an important starting point of the physiotherapy management plan and embraces a holistic biopsychosocial approach. A detailed subjective and objective assessment includes psychosocial and health-related quality of life evaluation. Assessments are individualised to take account of presenting features and individual needs. The physiotherapy assessment may be informed by a detailed referral from a GP, which could include an account of the current complaint and a print-out of the patient's medical and medication history. Physiotherapists work with the patient and his or her GP to identify the key problems and develop realistic, achievable and measurable patient-oriented goals.

When considered in a biopsychosocial context, physiotherapy treatments predominantly address the 'bio' elements with the least adverse treatment effects. However, if applied appropriately, physiotherapy treatments can help maximise function and health-related quality of life, and contribute to a holistic approach to patient management.

The modern approach to physiotherapy delivery includes triage clinics, group work, telephone advice lines, accident and emergency services, and evening and weekend sessions within the public and private sector, including sports and occupational settings. Alterative triage systems for musculoskeletal conditions have been developed to allow direct access by telephone to physiotherapy, e.g. Physio Direct (www.csp.org.uk). There is a multicentre randomised controlled trial of Physio Direct in musculoskeletal pain conditions presenting in primary care, which should be reporting in 2011. Findings from this study will inform future services of this kind.

Such approaches potentially balance the needs of the individual, community and a health system with finite resources. However, there is limited evidence that any one approach is beneficial over another. The evidence-based practice groups at the Arthritis Research UK Primary Care Centre (www.keele.ac.uk/research/pchs/pcmrc/EBP/index.htm) recently addressed the question of models of referral to other healthcare professionals from GPs. A critically appraised topic has been developed and there is limited evidence to support one model over another (www.keele.ac.uk/research/pchs/pcmrc/EBP/MRF/bank/Models_Access_CD.pdf).

Physiotherapists have recognised the importance of evaluating such diverse approaches in terms of patient and service outcomes, including in-house physiotherapy services, and in the future evidence will be available to support (or refute) such approaches. Any service that is proven to be cost-effective and rated highly by users should be retained. In general, feedback about in-house services is very positive. Patients value an on-site, accessible physiotherapy service.

The principles of physiotherapy are outlined for the following interventions: education and advice; exercise; electrotherapy; acupuncture; thermotherapy and cryotherapy; splints, strapping, bracing and orthoses; manual therapy; massage.

---

## Education and advice

Patient education and advice forms part of the fundamental armoury of many physiotherapy treatments. It can include one-to-one instruction, group sessions or self-management plans. Any or all of oral, written, audio or visual material can be used. Convincing evidence to support the use of education and advice alone in reducing pain and functional limitation in regional musculoskeletal pain has yet to be established. However, education and advice does improve anxiety and depression, self-efficacy, vitality and knowledge, e.g. Buszewicz *et al.*[4] OA guidelines recommend that accurate written and verbal information should be offered to all people with OA to enhance their understanding and counter misconceptions, and this should be an integral part of the management plan rather than a single event at one point in time.[1]

---

## Theme – giving advice and information

Which is the **single most** appropriate management option when considering giving advice and information to a 57-year old woman with peripheral joint pain in both knees and hands, with no red flags (e.g. signs of rheumatoid arthritis (RA))?

1 ▷ Give a brief verbal description of the likely course and prognosis.
2 ▷ Give a brief verbal description of the likely course and prognosis and back this up with written information (e.g. Arthritis Care leaflet on OA and Arthritis Research UK leaflets).
3 ▷ Give a brief verbal description of the likely course and prognosis, and suggest the physiotherapist might be a possible source of further information.
4 ▷ Give nothing and explain it is all part of getting older and that nothing can be done.

*Correct answer* ▷ **2** ▶ This is the best-practice approach. However, in usual practice there is evidence to suggest that answer 4 is most likely to be done.

## Exercise

Exercise therapy is a management strategy that is widely used by physio-therapists for common musculoskeletal conditions and encompasses a broad spectrum of specific interventions and approaches. It can range from specific strengthening exercises, balance and flexibility exercises on land and in water, as well as more general physical activity.[5] Exercise can be prescribed and delivered by physiotherapists or it can be conducted by individuals within their own home or community, e.g. yoga, Pilates, postural training such as the Alexander Technique (see below). Exercise is a safe treatment, relieving pain and improving function.[1] Certain health beliefs can prevent the uptake of exercise, e.g. exercise is wearing out the joint, causes pain, has risks. The long-term effectiveness of exercise interventions is largely determined by patient adherence and concordance with the exercise programme. However, there is scarce evidence for either long-term effectiveness or strategies that may enhance long-term adherence to exercise.

There have been three previous summaries of systematic reviews of physiotherapy evidence for exercise therapies in musculoskeletal conditions demonstrating the benefits on pain relief and functional limitation.[5-7] For example, the recent NICE low-back pain guidelines recommend exercise classes for persistent or recurrent back pain as a cost-effective approach for such patients,[2] with individually tailored exercises for those who prefer a one-to-one approach. The benefit of general exercise in *sub-acute* low-back pain (6 to 12 weeks) has yet to be confirmed. In *acute* low-back pain (<6 weeks) general back exercises appear to be unhelpful, but the 'McKenzie' approach, which is prescribed by physiotherapists with specialist training, is beneficial compared with passive approaches.[8] The McKenzie Method is a system of evaluating and treating spinal disorders developed by Robin McKenzie, a physiotherapist from New Zealand. It is practised extensively throughout the world (www.mckenzieinstitute. ca/details.htm). It is an active treatment philosophy that emphasises teaching the patients how to manage and treat pain themselves, how to prevent the pain from occurring again and how to maintain an active lifestyle. Patients are encouraged to take an active role in their own recovery, with an emphasis on self-treatment (www.mckenziemdt.org).

The McKenzie Method is based on assessment and simple classification of mechanical syndromes: Postural, Dysfunction and Derangement. Each one is uniquely approached using mechanical procedures, movement and positions. A certified McKenzie physiotherapist will know when the patient can successfully manage these approaches on his or her own.

For neck pain, the benefit of exercise can be combined with manual therapy.

## Theme – referring for exercises for low back pain

Which is the **single most** inappropriate scenario to suggest general physiotherapy exercises classes for?

1 ▷ Episode of non-specific low-back pain lasting fewer than six weeks.
2 ▷ Episode of non-specific low-back pain lasting more than six weeks but fewer than 12 weeks.
3 ▷ Episode of non-specific low-back pain lasting more than 12 weeks but fewer than 12 months.
4 ▷ Episodes of intermittent non-specific low-back pain lasting more than 12 months.

*Correct answer* ▷ **1** ▶ There is evidence to suggest that general back exercises are unhelpful in acute back pain. A more tailored approach would be required and would be at the discretion of the physiotherapist.

69

In OA, systematic reviews confirm that strengthening, stretching and functional exercises are beneficial compared with no exercise and that aerobic exercise is beneficial for knee OA.[5-7] Superiority of one approach over another is unknown. Systematic reviews of patellofemoral pain syndrome conclude that there are benefits for quadriceps exercises.[5-7]

## Theme – referring for exercises for osteoarthritis

A 57-year-old woman with knee pain and clinical signs of OA mentions to you that her pain is limiting her everyday activities and she wishes to have a safe and effective pain-relieving treatment. She has never received a referral for treatment before. Which is the **single most** appropriate scenario to suggest?

1 ▷ A prescription of oral non-steroidal anti-inflammatory drugs (NSAIDs).
2 ▷ Referral to physiotherapy for exercises.
3 ▷ A trial of Transcutaneous Electrical Nerve Stimulation (TENS).
4 ▷ Referral for arthroscopic lavage.

*Correct answer* ▷ **2** ▶ NICE recommends exercise as a core treatment for OA. Refer to Chapter 8 for further detail on the NICE OA guidelines.[1]

While there is a lack of systematic reviews in upper-limb conditions, there is evidence that exercise is beneficial in specific conditions,[5] for example subacromial impingement syndrome where pain is thought to come from degeneration of the rotator cuff and overuse or encroachment of the subacromial soft tissue.

There are limited reviews of hydrotherapy in the field of non-inflammatory musculoskeletal pain. However, the beneficial effects for some individuals warrant its consideration. Community pools may be able to offer continued programmes[1] and with the government's pledge for free swimming for the over-sixties this may be a form of exercise to promote in primary care and the community.

Lessons in the Alexander Technique, which teaches individuals to identify and correct poor postural habits, may offer a self-management approach that improves functional limitation and reduces pain in patients with chronic or recurrent low-back pain.[9] The Alexander Technique is distinct from manual therapy, back schools and conventional physiotherapy (www.viddler.com/explore/atbmj/videos/1/)[9] although physiotherapists may be trained in this technique. The technique uses continuous individualised assessment of a patient's habitual musculoskeletal movement and posture, and guides new movements and postures in order to reduce muscle spasm and improve co-ordination, flexibility and postural strength.[9] Six sessions followed by exercise prescription from registered teachers are beneficial for patients with chronic back pain.[9]

*The long-term effectiveness of exercises is based on patients' adherence to the programme.*

Many randomised controlled trials of exercise, e.g. Hurley *et al.*,[10] demonstrate a dose effect of exercise adherence. However, long-term studies are lacking. Strategies for maintaining exercise in the longer term for people with musculoskeletal conditions may require multimodal interventions, possibly including cognitive behavioural approaches, and may need to be considered alongside management of other long-term conditions in primary care, e.g. heart disease, diabetes.

Expert patient programmes or lay-led self-management programmes specifically for people living with long-term conditions, where there is active engagement of physiotherapists, or other community initiatives (e.g. exercise on prescription) may be ways of supporting maintenance of exercise programmes.

*In summary, exercise is a core treatment for musculoskeletal conditions irrespective of age, co-morbidity, pain severity or disability and it is up to the physiotherapist and GP to make a judgement on how best to ensure participation.*

## Electrotherapy

Electrotherapy includes ultrasound, short-wave diathermy (SWD), interferential therapy and low-level laser therapy. Electrotherapy is considered a passive treatment approach and although widely used with a sound biological rationale there is limited evidence to support many of the electrotherapy modalities in the treatment of musculoskeletal pain.

### Transcutaneous electrical nerve stimulation

TENS is a small battery-operated machine, which produces selected pulsed currents delivered via electrode placement on the skin. The currents can activate specific nerve fibres producing analgesic responses.[11,12] The intensity and frequency of the currents can be varied to maximise treatment response.

In people with inflammatory disease, acupuncture-like TENS reduces pain and increases muscle power, whilst conventional TENS improves self-reported disease activity but not pain.[13] It also relieves pain and stiffness in knee OA, especially in the short term.[1] Longer courses of treatment (>4 weeks) and greater-intensity protocols (high burst or low frequency) may produce greatest pain relief,[14] and proper training in the placing of pads and selection of stimulation intensity can also enhance the response of patients with knee OA.[1]

Clinical guidelines recommend acupuncture-like TENS for improving pain, oedema and muscle power in patients with RA.[15] For short-term symptomatic relief TENS is a relatively safe adjunct therapy for the relief of pain in patients with OA [1,16] and for patients with osteoporosis with intractable pain, chronic low-back pain and recent vertebral factures.[17]

Good-practice guidance recommends an assessment by a physiotherapist with proper training in the selection of stimulation intensity, with reinforcement with an instruction booklet. Patients should be encouraged to experiment with dosages if the desired relief of symptoms is not initially achieved. This enables patients to control their symptoms as part of a self-management approach. A further follow-up visit is essential, allowing the health professional to check patients' usage of TENS, resolve any problems [1] and provide guidance on purchase of TENS machines, if appropriate.

One of the main indications for using TENS for pain control is when other management techniques are contraindicated or not desirable, e.g. manual therapy (in osteoporotic patients) or medication (in those people with allergies or previous addictions to analgesics).

Contraindications include active implants (pacemakers, devices with batteries giving active medication). Whilst adverse events from the small battery-operated TENS machines are known, such as local skin reactions and allergies to the adhesive pads, they are rare and TENS is recognised as a useful and safe treatment modality.[18] It has been widely cited that TENS is contraindicated during pregnancy. However, a recent review suggests that, although not an ideal (first-line) treatment option, the application of TENS around the trunk during pregnancy is safe.[19]

---

**Theme – referring for a trial of TENS**

Which is the **single most** appropriate scenario for referral to physiotherapy for a trial of TENS for pain management?

1 ▷ 20-year-old male with a chronic lateral ligament sprain of the ankle.
2 ▷ A woman with pelvic girdle pain during the second trimester of pregnancy.
3 ▷ A 55-year-old man with well-controlled RA but persistent knee pain.
4 ▷ A 30-year-old with chronic tennis elbow (lateral epicondylitis of the elbow).

*Answer* ▷ **3** ▶ Clinical guidelines recommend acupuncture-like TENS for improving pain in patients with RA.[2,15]

### Interferential therapy

Interferential therapy (IFT) can be described as the transcutaneous application of alternating medium-frequency electrical currents and may be considered as a form of TENS. Its potential for pain relief may relate to an ability to promote healing and produce muscular contraction.

Evidence for the effectiveness of IFT in musculoskeletal conditions is limited. Due to the size of the apparatus, application of IFT is restricted to use within the physiotherapy department and therefore encourages reliance on physiotherapists rather than promoting self-management.

### Low-level laser therapy

Laser (light amplification by the stimulated emission of radiation), at low-intensity or low-level doses considered too low to affect any detectable heating of the tissue, is used to treat disease and injury.

Low-level laser therapy (LLLT) utilises a pencil-like beam of light energy to promote tissue healing and pain relief in a broad spectrum of soft-tissue injuries and diseases. The effects of LLLT are not thermal but termed 'photobioactivation', which are thought to control the inflammatory response, promoting healing and pain relief.[20,21]

In patients with OA, LLLT is ineffective for pain relief.[1,22] However, LLLT improves pain and morning stiffness in people with RA, but not function or range of movement.[15]

## Ultrasound therapy

In the management of musculoskeletal conditions, ultrasound therapy is commonly used as an adjunctive therapy for its proposed effects on inflammation and tissue repair as well as for pain relief.[23] Ultrasound produces thermal and non-thermal effects. When passed through tissue, a percentage of the ultrasound energy is absorbed, generating heat; this is potentially useful in pain relief since it reduces joint stiffness and increases blood flow. Other, non-thermal, mechanisms (bio-effects) might theoretically aid pain relief. If applied in high doses, the absorption of ultrasound results in heating that increases metabolic rate and blood flow (thermal effects).[24]

While there is evidence to support the physiological effects of ultrasound in experimental studies,[25] evidence for its clinical effectiveness in people with musculoskeletal conditions is limited.[15,26–28] Despite being a frequently used electrophysical modality in musculoskeletal conditions[23,29] ultrasound may only be effective for people with carpal tunnel syndrome and those with calcific tendonitis of the shoulder.[30]

## Short-wave diathermy diatherapy

Short-wave diathermy (SWD) produces its physiological and therapeutic effects by rapidly alternating electrical and magnetic currents at short-wave frequencies. SWD energy can be delivered in either a pulsed or a continuous mode, setting up both electric and magnetic fields in human tissues. The level of heat generated depends upon the conductivity of the tissues. Continuous SWD is applied to tissues usually for 20–30 minutes. Pulsed SWD (PSWD or pulsed electromagnetic energy (PEME)) is the application of a series of short bursts of energy, the patient receiving a lower dose of energy for the equivalent time.

The evidence for the clinical effectiveness of short-wave therapy is mixed. Some studies report no benefit of PSWD for people with lower-limb OA,[31–34] while others conclude that pulsed SWD may be beneficial.[35,36] SWD is not normally included in physiotherapy guidelines for the management of musculoskeletal conditions.

## Acupuncture

Acupuncture is used by many physiotherapists with specialist training and the Acupuncture Association of Chartered Physiotherapists (AACP) (www.aacp.uk.com) is a recognised special-interest group within the profession.

There is growing evidence that acupuncture is beneficial for pain management in musculoskeletal conditions and a course of acupuncture needling should be considered for people with low-back pain.[2] However, the addition of acupuncture to a course of physiotherapy advice and exercise for OA of the knee gives no further improvement in function and pain.[37] While NICE recommends acupuncture for low-back pain, it does not for OA.[1,2] While adverse reactions to acupuncture have been reported, when applied by trained practitioners acupuncture is very safe.[38]

## Theme – referring for pain relief in low-back pain

A 40-year-old patient with back pain of less than 12 months' duration would like another referral to physiotherapy. He has attended an exercise class but this was not beneficial for pain relief. Which is the **single most** appropriate management to suggest to the patient?

1 ▷ A course of ultrasound.
2 ▷ A course of interferential therapy.
3 ▷ A course of acupuncture.
4 ▷ A course of pulsed SWD.

*Correct answer* ▷ **3** ▶ Another course of physiotherapy would be indicated and acupuncture is recommended by NICE, along with exercise and manipulation.[2]

## Thermotherapy and cryotherapy

Thermotherapy (the therapeutic application of a heating agent) and cryotherapy (the therapeutic application of a cooling agent) are widely used physiotherapy treatments to reduce pain, oedema and muscle spasm, improve tissue healing and facilitate range of motion and function.

Clinically, superficial heating can be achieved by heat pads or paraffin wax baths, by radiation such as infrared light therapy and by convection, such as sauna or steam room.[39] Cryotherapy includes the use of ice packs and ice baths, commercially available gel packs or sprays, and massage with ice over acupuncture points or painful areas.

Prior to application of either therapy, skin testing is recommended as patients with abnormal sensation (e.g. diabetic neuropathy) are at risk of damage.[40]

Thermotherapy increases tissue temperature and blood flow, while cryotherapy decreases tissue blood flow by initially causing vasoconstriction followed by vasodilatation. While there are differences in physiological responses, both therapies can be used in patients with musculoskeletal conditions, and patient preference as well as physiological response should be considered when selecting which therapy to use.

Despite being used for years as a safe and effective symptomatic treatment of acute and chronic musculoskeletal conditions, systematic reviews of thermotherapy and cryotherapy highlight a lack of good-quality research.[41,42] Based on anecdotal reports and some evidence of effectiveness, thermotherapy and cryotherapy are useful palliative self-management therapies for patients' musculoskeletal conditions and should be included in the management of patients with RA,[15] OA[1,15,28] and osteoporosis.[17]

---

**Theme – giving advice for an acute sport injury (soft-tissue injury)**

A footballer complains of pain and stiffness of the knee after sustaining a 'dead leg' in a Sunday league football match. Following a thorough examination, which excludes serious injuries (including fracture and knee ligament damage), what is the **single most** appropriate advice to provide?

1 ▷ Just ignore it and keep it moving – it will get better in its own time.
2 ▷ PRICE – protection, rest, ice therapy, compression and elevation of affected area – and begin early range of motion exercises as soon as possible.
3 ▷ Apply topical skin creams to reduce the pain and inflammation.
4 ▷ Buy a knee support.

*Correct answer* ▷ **1** ▶ Early reassessment is recommended. If considerable recovery has not occurred in a few days referral to a physiotherapist should be recommended.

## Splints, strapping, bracing and orthoses

There are few rigorous studies of the efficacy of splints, strapping, bracing and orthoses in musculoskeletal pain.[5,43] However, while these techniques and devices are widely used and expensive, they should be considered in people with biomechanical joint pain or instability.[1] Physiotherapists frequently refer patients to occupational therapy, orthotic and podiatry colleagues for specialist assessment and advice.

## Theme – referral for an acute soft-tissue injury

A 36-year-old woman with a sprained first carpometacarpal joint following a basketball injury has been to casualty where they have strapped her hand. She wants to know what she can do to get her hand moving as soon as possible.

Which is the **single most** inappropriate management to suggest to the patient?

1  ▷ A course of ice packs to reduce the swelling and improve the pain.
2  ▷ Elevation of the hand when resting, and keeping the fingers
       and thumb moving as much as possible within the limits of pain.
3  ▷ Topical NSAIDs to relieve pain and inflammation.
4  ▷ Referral to physiotherapy.

*Correct answer* ▷ **4** ▶ At this early stage, with correct advice on management of an acute soft-tissue injury, the patient should make a good recovery. A review could be suggested if full range of movement does not return within a couple of weeks.

## Manual therapy

Manual therapy is the application of passive movement to a joint either within ('mobilisation') or beyond its active range of movement ('manipulation'). This includes oscillatory techniques, high-velocity low-amplitude thrust techniques, sustained stretching and muscle energy techniques.[44] Manual therapy can be applied to joints, muscles or nerves and the aims of treatment include pain reduction, increasing range and quality of joint movement, improving nerve mobility, increasing muscle length and restoring normal function.

A systematic review of manipulation and mobilisation of the cervical spine assessed the evidence for their efficacy and safety in neck pain.[45] The review suggested that mobilisation might be beneficial in acute neck pain compared with neck collars and TENS. In subacute and chronic pain, manual therapy in general is probably superior in producing a short-term relief of pain compared with other studied interventions (muscle relaxants, usual general practice care, massage, traction, electrical stimulation, heat, cold packs and acupuncture).

Manual traction and stretching was shown to be superior to exercise in hip OA[46] and the NICE OA guidelines recommend that this should be considered as an adjunct to other core treatments in the hip.[1]

In chronic low-back pain a course of manual therapy including spinal manipulation should be considered.[2]

While mobilisations (application of movement to a joint within its physiological range of movement) are not associated with serious complications, manipulations (high-velocity low-amplitude thrust techniques applied beyond active joint range of movement) can have severe adverse reactions. Spinal manipulation, particularly when performed on the cervical spine, is associated with mild to moderate adverse effects (30–61% of all patients) and can result in serious complications such as vertebrobasilar artery dissection followed by stroke.[47,48] Consequently premanipulative testing protocols attempt to identify patients at risk of vertebrobasilar artery insufficiency,[49] although the effectiveness of this screening has yet to be established. All guidelines contraindicate the use of manipulation in patients with RA due to the risk of joint instability, particularly in the upper cervical spine,[50] and caution should be exercised when considering the use of manipulation in other inflammatory rheumatic conditions.

In addition to the biomechanical and *physiological* effects of manual therapy, the psychological effect of any therapy that has direct physical contact, for example massage, produces a response to the 'laying on of hands'. This placebo response – a response produced by a mechanism with incidental ingredients or components that have no remedial effect for the disorder but result in a positive effect of treatment – is enhanced by 'learned expectancy' (previous experience of a stimulus establishes a habitual direction of response) and the therapeutic benefits of the patient–therapist interaction and relationship.[51]

---

## Theme – referring for hip osteoarthritis

A 60-year-old woman with a clinical diagnosis of hip OA is limping because of her hip pain. She has tried all the core treatments recommended in the NICE guideline and you feel that a referral for further treatment is warranted. You arrange for provision of a walking stick.

Which is the **single most** appropriate management to suggest to the patient?

1 ▷ A course of physiotherapy – manipulation and stretching to the hip.
2 ▷ A hip joint replacement.
3 ▷ A course of hydrotherapy.
4 ▷ Advice to lose weight.

*Correct answer* ▷ **1** ▶ The NICE OA guideline recommends manipulation and stretching for the hip as an adjunct to core treatment for pain relief for hip OA.[2]

---

## Massage

Massage has been used for years to reduce pain and oedema, increase circulation, improve muscle tone and enhance joint flexibility. Its effect may be explained by the pain gate theory[52] but it is also likely to have a placebo response similar to other manual therapies.

Sport massage is a popular and widely used modality for recovery after intense exercise, and there are some data supporting its use to facilitate recovery from repetitive muscular contractions.[53] However, evidence of its efficacy in patients with chronic musculoskeletal conditions is limited; a course of massage improves function and pain in patients with OA knee[54] and pain and quality of life in patients with fibromyalgia,[55] although it is ineffective in patients with neck pain.[56] A systematic review of nine studies suggests massage is beneficial in patients with *subacute* and *chronic* low-back pain especially when combined with exercise and education but it was no better than manipulation and inferior to TENS for back pain relief.[57] Furthermore, massage produces only short-term improvement in disability in patients with recurrent or chronic low-back pain.[9]

While massage is not often recommended in clinical guidelines, as it has high patient satisfaction and low adverse effects, it is a viable adjunct to therapy for patients with musculoskeletal conditions.

---

## Models of multidisciplinary working in primary care

People with musculoskeletal conditions need a wide range of high-quality support and treatment from simple advice to highly specialised treatments. Physiotherapists often work in partnership with General Practitioners with a Special Interest (GPwSIs) – a GP who has additional expertise and advanced practice in the management of, for example, musculoskeletal conditions.

The Musculoskeletal Services Framework (MSF) [58] describes best practice, built around evidence and experience. It has prompted the organisation of the 'Multidisciplinary Interface Clinic'. Physiotherapists are already working in 'interface'-style clinics assessing a range of musculoskeletal conditions, mostly within primary care.[59]

---

## Conclusions

Physiotherapy is an essential component in the management of musculoskeletal conditions in primary care. It is estimated that up to 30% of all general practice consultations are for musculoskeletal problems.[58] The ageing population will further increase the demand for treatment of age-related disorders such as OA.[58]

In recent years there has been an explosion of high-quality evidence to support the core approaches of physiotherapy, including education and advice, exercise and manual therapy.[5-7] Multidisciplinary services are central to the provision of high-quality care for people with musculoskeletal conditions, with physiotherapists working in partnership with GPs and their patients to deliver high-quality care.

### Key learning points

▶ Physiotherapy is an essential component in the management of musculoskeletal conditions in primary care.
▶ Physical therapies aim to control pain, minimise joint stiffness and limit joint damage, improve function and enhance participation with the least adverse treatment effects.
▶ There is good evidence for the effectiveness of core treatment approaches such as exercise and manual therapy.
▶ Physical therapies offer popular and beneficial approaches to the multidisciplinary, patient-centred management of musculoskeletal conditions.

### Further reading

▷ Bearne L, Hurley M. Physical therapies: treatment options in rheumatology. In: K Dziedzic, A Hammond (eds). *Rheumatology: evidence-based practice for physiotherapists and occupational therapists* Edinburgh: Elsevier, 2010, pp. 111–22.

▷ Dziedzic K, Jordan J, Foster N. Land and water based exercise therapies for musculoskeletal conditions. In: P Brooks, P Conaghan (eds). *Principles of Non-Pharmacological Management of Musculoskeletal Conditions* [Baillière's Best Practice and Research in Clinical Rheumatology] Edinburgh: Elsevier, 2008, pp. 407–18.

▷ Hurley M, Bearne L. The principles of therapeutic exercise and activity. In: K Dziedzic, A Hammond (eds). *Rheumatology: evidence-based practice for physiotherapists and occupational therapists* Edinburgh: Elsevier, 2010, pp. 99–110.

▷ National Institute for Health and Clinical Excellence. *Rheumatoid Arthritis: the management of rheumatoid arthritis in adults* London: Royal College of Physicians, 2009, www.nice.org.uk/CG79 [accessed October 2011].

## Useful websites

▷ Chartered Society of Physiotherapists, **www.csp.org.uk**.

▷ National Institute for Health and Clinical Excellence, **www.nice.org.uk**.

▷ Electrotherapy on the Web, **www.electrotherapy.org**.

▷ British Acupuncture Council, **www.acupuncture.org.uk**.

**References**

1 • National Institute for Health and Clinical Excellence. *Osteoarthritis: national clinical guideline for care and management in adults* London: Royal College of Physicians, 2008, www.nice.org.uk/CG059 [accessed October 2011].

2 • National Institute for Health and Clinical Excellence. *Low Back Pain: early management of persistent non-specific low back pain* London: NICE, 2009, www.nice.org.uk/ CG88 [accessed October 2011].

3 • World Health Organization. *International Classification of Functioning, Disability and Health* Geneva: WHO, 2001.

4 • Buszewicz M, Rait G, Griffin M, *et al.* Self management of arthritis in primary care: randomised controlled trial *British Medical Journal* 2006; **333(7574)**: 879.

5 • Dziedzic K, Jordan J, Foster N. Land and water based exercise therapies for musculoskeletal conditions. In: P Brooks, P Conaghan (eds). *Principles of Non-Pharmacological Management of Musculoskeletal Conditions* [Baillière's Best Practice and Research in Clinical Rheumatology] Edinburgh: Elsevier, 2008, pp. 407–18.

6 • Smidt N, de Vet H C W, Bouter L M, *et al*. Effectiveness of exercise therapy: a best evidence summary of systematic reviews *Australian Journal of Physiotherapy* 2005; **51(2)**: 71–85.

7 • Taylor N F, Dodd K J, Shields N, *et al*. Therapeutic exercise in physiotherapy practice is beneficial: a summary of systematic reviews 2002–2005 *Australian Journal of Physiotherapy* 2007; **53(1)**: 7–16.

8 • Long A, Donelson R, Fung T. Does it matter which exercise? A randomized control trial of exercise for low back pain *Spine* 2004; **29(23)**: 2593–602.

9 • Little P, Lewith G, Webley F, *et al*. Randomised controlled trial of Alexander technique lessons, exercise, and massage (ATEAM) for chronic and recurrent back pain *British Medical Journal* 2008; **337**; a884.

10 • Hurley M V, Walsh N E, Mitchell H L, *et al*. Clinical effectiveness of a rehabilitation program integrating exercise, self-management, and active coping strategies for chronic knee pain: a cluster randomized trial *Arthritis and Rheumatism* 2007; **57(7)**: 1211–19.

11 • Cheing G, Hui-Chan C. Analgesic effects of transcutaneous electrical nerve stimulation and interferential currents on heat pain in healthy subjects *Journal of Rehabilitation Medicine* 2003; **35(1)**: 15–19.

12 • Cheing G L, Tsui A Y, Lo S K, *et al*. Optimal stimulation duration of TENS in the management of osteoarthritic knee pain *Journal of Rehabilitation Medicine* 2003; **35(2)**: 62–8.

13 • Brosseau L, Judd M G, Marchand S, *et al*. Transcutaneous electrical nerve stimulation (TENS) for the treatment of rheumatoid arthritis in the hand *Cochrane Database of Systematic Reviews* 2003; **3**: CD004377.

14 • Osiri M, Welch V, Brosseau L, *et al*. Transcutaneous electrical nerve stimulation for knee osteoarthritis *Cochrane Database of Systematic Reviews* 2000; **4**: CD002823.

15 • Brosseau L, Wells G A, Tugwell P, *et al*. Ottawa panel evidence based clinical practice guidelines for electrotherapy and thermotherapy interventions in the management of rheumatoid arthritis *Physical Therapy* 2004; **8(11)**: 1016–143.

16 • Philadelphia Panel. Philadelphia Panel evidence-based clinical practice guidelines on selected rehabilitation interventions for knee pain *Physical Therapy* 2001; **81(10)**: 1675–1700.

17 • Chartered Society of Physiotherapy. *Physiotherapy Guidelines for the Management of Osteoporosis* London: CSP, 1999.

18 • Walsh D M. *TENS: clinical applications and related theory* New York: Churchill Livingstone, 1997.

19 • Coldron Y, Crothers E, Haslam J, *et al*. *ACPWH Guidance on the Safe Use of Transcutaneous Electrical Nerve Stimulation (TENS) for Musculosketal Pain during Pregnancy*, 2007, www.electrotherapy.org/downloads/Modalities/TENS%20in%20pregnancy%20 guidelines.pdf [accessed October 2011].

20 • Robertson V, Ward A, Low J, *et al*. *Electrotherapy Explained: principles and practice* (4th edn) Philadelphia, PA: Butterworth-Heinemann Elsevier, 2006.

21 • Watson T. The role of electrotherapy in contemporary physiotherapy practice *Manual Therapy* 2000; **5(3)**: 132–41.

22 • Brosseau L, Wells G A, Tugwell P, *et al*. Ottawa panel evidence-based clinical practice guidelines for therapeutic exercises and manual therapy in the management of osteoarthritis *Physical Therapy* 2005; **85(9)**: 907–71.

23 • Watson T. *Electrotherapy on the Web: an educational resource*, 2008, www.electrotherapy.org/modalities/ultrasound.htm [accessed October 2011].

24 • Nussbaum EL. Ultrasound: to heat or not to heat – that is the question *Physical Therapy Reviews* 1997; **2**: 59–72.

25 • Mortimer AJ, Dyson M. The effect of therapeutic ultrasound on calcium uptake in fibroblasts *Ultrasound in Medicine and Biology* 1998; **14(6)**: 499–506.

26 • Ainsworth R, Dziedzic K, Hiller L, *et al.* A prospective double blind placebo-controlled randomized trial of ultrasound in the physiotherapy treatment of shoulder pain *Rheumatology* 2007; **46(5)**: 815–20.

27 • Van Der Windt DA, Van Der Heijden GJ, Van Den Berg SG, *et al.* Ultrasound therapy for acute ankle sprains *Cochrane Database of Systematic Reviews* 2002; **2**: CD001250.

28 • Zhang W, Doherty M, Leeb BF, *et al.* EULAR evidence based recommendations for the management of hand osteoarthritis: report of a Task Force of the EULAR Standing Committee for International Clinical Studies Including Therapeutics (ESCISIT) *Annals of Rheumatic Diseases* 2007; **66(3)**: 377–88.

29 • Kitchen S, Partridge C. A survey to examine clinical use of ultrasound, shortwave diathermy and laser in England *British Journal of Therapy and Rehabilitation* 1996; **3(12)**: 644–50.

30 • Robertson VJ, Baker KG. A review of therapeutic ultrasound: effectiveness studies *Physical Therapy* 2001; **81(7)**: 1339–50.

31 • Callaghan MJ, Whittaker PA, Grimes S. An evaluation of pulsed shortwave on knee osteoarthritis using radioleucoscintigraphy: a randomised, double blind, controlled trial *Joint Bone Spine* 2000; **72(2)**: 150–5.

32 • Klaber Moffett J, Richardson P, Frost H, *et al.* A placebo controlled double blind trial to evaluate the effectiveness of pulsed short wave therapy for osteoarthritic hip and knee pain *Pain* 1996; **167(1)**: 121–7.

33 • Laufer Y, Zilberman R, Porat R, *et al.* Effect of pulsed shortwave diathermy on pain and function of subjects with osteoarthritis of the knee: a placebo-controlled, double-blind clinical trial *Clinical Rehabilitation* 2005; **19(3)**: 255–63.

34 • Thamsborg G, Florescu A, Oturai P, *et al.* Treatment of knee osteoarthritis with pulsed electromagnetic fields: a randomized, double-blind, placebo-controlled study *Osteoarthritis and Cartilage* 2005; **13(7)**: 575–81.

35 • Jan MH, Chai HM, Wang CL, *et al.* Effects of repetitive shortwave diathermy for reducing synovitis in patients with knee osteoarthritis: an ultrasonographic study *Physical Therapy* 2006; **86(2)**: 236–44.

36 • Van Nguyen J, Marks R. Pulsed magnetic fields for treating osteoarthritis *Physiotherapy* 2002; **88**: 458–70.

37 • Foster NE, Thomas E, Barlas P, *et al.* Acupuncture as an adjunct to exercise based physiotherapy for osteoarthritis of the knee: randomised controlled trial *British Medical Journal* 2007; **335(7617)**: 436.

38 • White A, Hayhoe S, Hart A, *et al.* Adverse events following acupuncture: prospective survey of 32 000 consultations with doctors and physiotherapists *British Medical Journal* 2001; **323(7311)**: 485–6.

39 • Hicks JE, Gerber LH. Rehabilitation of patients with osteoarthritis. In: RW Moskowitz, DS Howell, VM Goldberg, *et al.* (eds). *Osteoarthritis: diagnosis, medical and surgical management* Philadelphia, PA: WB Saunders Co., 1992, pp. 427–64.

40 • Fox J, Sharp T. *Practical Electrotherapy: a guide to safe application* London: Churchill Livingstone Elsevier, 2007.

41 • Brosseau L, Yonge K A, Robinson V, *et al.* Thermotherapy for treatment of osteoarthritis *Cochrane Database of Systematic Reviews* 2003; **4**: 1–8.

42 • Collins N C. Is ice right? Does cryotherapy improve outcome for acute soft tissue injury? *Emergency Medicine Journal* 2008; **25(2)**: 65–8.

43 • Brouwer R W, Jakma T S, Verhagen A P, *et al.* Braces and orthoses for treating osteoarthritis of the knee *Cochrane Database of Systematic Reviews* 2005; **1**: CD004020.

44 • Bearne L, Hurley M. Physical therapies: treatment options in rheumatology. In: K Dziedzic, A Hammond (eds). *Rheumatology: evidence-based practice for physiotherapists and occupational therapists* Edinburgh: Elsevier, 2010, pp. 111–22.

45 • Gross A, Hoving, J L, Haines T A, *et al.* A Cochrane Review of manipulation and mobilization for mechanical neck disorders *Spine* 2004; **29(14)**: 1541–8.

46 • Hoeksma H L, Dekker J, Ronday H K, *et al.* Comparison of manual therapy and exercise therapy in osteoarthritis of the hip: a randomised clinical trial *Arthritis and Rheumatism* 2004; **51(5)**: 722–9.

47 • Ernst E. Adverse effects of spinal manipulation: a systematic review *Journal of the Royal Society of Medicine* 2007; **100(7)**: 330–8.

48 • Taylor A J, Kerry R. Neck pain and headache as a result of internal carotid artery dissection: implications for manual therapists *Manual Therapy* 2005; **10(1)**: 73–7.

49 • Magarey M E, Rebbeck T, Coughlan B, *et al.* Pre-manipulative testing of the cervical spine review, revision and new clinical guidelines *Manual Therapy* 2004; **9(2)**: 95–108.

50 • Neva M H, Hakkinen A, Makinen H, *et al.* High prevalence of asymptomatic cervical spine subluxation in patients with rheumatoid arthritis waiting for orthopaedic surgery *Annals of Rheumatic Diseases* 2006; **65(7)**: 884–8.

51 • Roche P. Placebo and patient care. In: L Gifford (ed). *Topical Issues in Pain: placebo and nocebo, pain management, muscles and pain* (vol. 4) Falmouth: CNS Press, 2002, pp. 19–41.

52 • Melzack R, Wall P D. Pain mechanisms: a new theory *Science* 1965; **150(699)**: 971–9.

53 • Best T M, Hunter R, Wilcox A, *et al.* Effectiveness of sports massage for recovery of skeletal muscle from strenuous exercise *Clinical Journal of Sports Medicine* 2008; **18(5)**: 446–60.

54 • Perlman A L, Sabina A, Williams A L, *et al.* Massage therapy for osteoarthritis of the knee: a randomised controlled trial *Archives of Internal Medicine* 2006; **166(22)**: 2533–8.

55 • Brattberg G. Connective tissue massage in the treatment of fibromyalgia *European Journal of Pain* 1999; **3(3)**: 235–44.

56 • Ezzo J, Haraldsson B G, Gross A R, *et al.*; Cervical Overview Group. Massage for mechanical neck disorders: a systematic review *Spine* 2007; **32(3)**: 353–62.

57 • Furlan A D, Brosseau L, Imamura M, *et al.* Massage for low back pain (Cochrane Review) *Cochrane Database of Systematic Reviews* 2003; **2**: CD001929.

58 • Department of Health. *The Musculoskeletal Services Framework: a joint responsibility: doing it differently* London: DH, 2006, www.dh.gov.uk/en/Publicationsandstatistics/Publications/PublicationsPolicyAndGuidance/DH_4138413 [accessed October 2011].

59 • Stevenson K, Hay E. Do physiotherapists' attitudes towards evidence-based practice change as a result of an evidence-based educational programme? *Journal of the Evaluation of Clinical Practice* 2004; **10(2)**: 207–17.

# Primary care diagnosis and management of shoulder disorders

# 4

*Caroline Anne Mitchell and Ade Adebajo*

## Aims of this chapter

▶ Describe the epidemiology of shoulder disorders.

▶ Show the common risk factors for shoulder disorders.

▶ Demonstrate how to take a clinical history that includes a holistic assessment of the impact of the shoulder problem on the individual, including psychosocial issues and individual prognostic risk factors.

▶ Enable a practitioner to perform a brief but relevant physical examination in order to identify joint or soft-tissue shoulder disorders and differentiate from other causes of shoulder pain.

▶ Enable a practitioner to identify 'red flag' symptoms and signs of potentially serious causes of shoulder disorders that require primary care investigation and/or urgent specialist assessment.

▶ Enable a practitioner to plan and discuss with the patient an evidence-based management plan for the treatment of common shoulder problems in primary care.

▶ Describe a typical care pathway for more complex shoulder problems that require the input of musculoskeletal specialists, including referral pointers for imaging, review by an allied health professional, and routine review by a secondary care specialist.

## Introduction

Shoulder pain is a common presenting complaint in primary care, with an annual consultation rate of 1–2% in adults over the age of 45 years. There is a self-reported prevalence of shoulder pain of between 14% and 26% in the general population, so this rate might be lower than expected.[1,2] The prevalence and functional impact of shoulder problems increase with age.

Shoulder disorders typically cause pain, sleep disturbance and significant functional impairment. A wide range of activities may be impaired, including self-care, driving and work.

---

## Outcomes of presentation with a shoulder disorder in primary care

A large prospective multicentre primary care study investigated treatment and referral outcomes following initial presentation with a shoulder disorder. Approximately half of the people with a new episode of shoulder disorder consulted the GP only once, but a substantial number (14%) were still consulting with a shoulder problem during the third year of follow-up. Older age had the strongest association with likelihood to be still consulting. Most treatment and follow-up occurred in primary care, for example non-steroidal anti-inflammatory drugs (NSAIDs) (30%) or a 'shoulder injection' by the GP (10%). A minority of patients (22%) were referred to physiotherapy, orthopaedic specialists, rheumatologists or other secondary care services such as a pain clinic, or for imaging.[3] The largest proportion of referrals made by the GP was to a physiotherapist (63.9%), followed by referral to an orthopaedic or rheumatology clinic (26.9%).

Other studies report complete resolution of shoulder disorders in about 50% of patients within three months of onset, but likewise acknowledge that chronicity and recurrence are a significant problem. It has been reported that up to a quarter of people presenting in primary care with a new episode of shoulder pain had experienced shoulder pain in the past. In this group of patients with a recurrent shoulder problem, only a fifth had recovered at six months and up to a half still had symptoms at 18 months after presenting with the new episode.[4,5] Psychosocial and occupational factors may also influence prognosis.[6,7]

---

## The shoulder joint: structure and function

There are four articulations of the shoulder joint:

▷ glenohumeral
▷ acromioclavicular
▷ sternoclavicular
▷ scapulothoracic.

86

Figure 4.1 ○ *The anatomy of the shoulder*

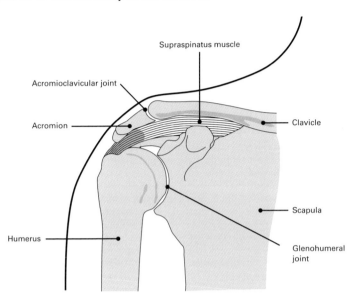

Supraspinatus muscle

Acromioclavicular joint

Acromion

Clavicle

Humerus

Scapula

Glenohumeral joint

*Source*: Hazleman B. Shoulder problems in general practice.[8] Illustration reproduced by kind permission of Arthritis Research UK.

The glenohumeral joint allows the greatest freedom of movement of any joint of the body (flexion, extension, abduction, adduction, circumduction and rotation). The hemispherical head of the humerus sits in the relatively shallow glenoid cavity of the scapula, protected above by an arch formed by the coracoid process, the acromion and the coracoacromial ligament. Additional strength and stability of the joint is provided by the surrounding ligaments, tendons (of the supraspinatus, infraspinatus, subscapularis and teres minor muscles) and other soft tissues that blend into the shoulder capsule and comprise the rotator cuff.

**Risk and prognostic factors for shoulder pain**

The movement of the shoulder joint through several planes enables a wide range of complex upper-limb activities but at risk of injury to the rotator cuff and to the stability of the shallow glenohumeral joint.

Physical factors such as injury (acute or minor repetitive trauma), heavy manual work, prolonged overhead activities, and working in other awkward positions are all implicated in the development of shoulder disorders. However, individuals may develop shoulder pain and dysfunction without an obvious precipitant. Changes occur with ageing and include greater laxity of soft tissues and changes in the healing processes. Familial predisposition to rotator cuff tendinopathy has also been described.

Risk factors that predispose the individual to onset, recurrence and chronicity of shoulder pain are summarised in Table 4.1.[9, 10]

Table 4.1  ○  ***Risk factors***

| | |
|---|---|
| Occupational factors | Working overhead, heavy manual work, repetitive upper-arm movements, for example as carried out by builders, plumbers, engineers, hairdressers, factory assembly workers |
| Sporting activities | Involving upper-arm use or risk of injury, for example in golf, tennis, squash, climbing, team sports |
| Diabetes | Increased risk of adhesive capsulitis ('frozen shoulder') |
| Prolonged immobility of the joint | For example stroke, fracture, soft-tissue trauma, breast cancer surgery |
| Genetic predisposition (rare) | |

*Source*: reproduced from e-GP: e-Learning for General Practice/Rheumatology and Musculoskeletal Problems/Shoulder Pain (www.e-GP.org).[11]

---

Box 4.1  ○  ***Adverse prognostic factors***

▶ Older age.

▶ Severe or recurrent symptoms at presentation.

▶ Late presentation.

▶ Associated neck pain.

▶ Female gender.

▶ Diabetes.

---

## The comprehensive primary care assessment

Most shoulder problems are effectively managed in primary care, as functional recovery is usual. Diagnosis is pragmatic and based on clinical assessment, rather than blood tests and radiography, once red-flag causes and pain derived from systemic or distant disease are excluded. Red-flag referral and investigation triggers are summarised in Table 4.2. New onset of bilateral shoulder pain and stiffness should prompt consideration of polymyalgia

Table 4.2 ○ *Red-flag triggers for referral and/or investigation*

| | |
|---|---|
| Tumour | Unexplained deformity, mass or swelling |
| | Lymphadenopathy |
| | History of cancer |
| | Symptoms and signs of cancer and/or paraneoplastic syndrome |
| | Blood or imaging investigations suggestive of malignancy |
| Acute rotator cuff tear | Recent trauma |
| | Acute disabling pain and significant weakness |
| | Positive 'drop arm' test |
| Polymyalgia rheumatica | Bilateral shoulder pain with or without pelvic girdle symptoms or temporal headache |
| | Visual symptoms |
| | Older adult |
| | Raised erythrocyte sedimentation rate (ESR) or C-reactive protein (CRP) |
| Systemic illness, autoimmune disorder, inflammatory arthritis | Systemically unwell |
| | Other or generalised arthropathy |
| | Proximal pain and weakness |
| | Weight loss |
| | Rash |
| | Significantly elevated ESR and/or CRP |
| Infection | Red skin |
| | Fever |
| | Systemically unwell |
| Unreduced dislocation | Loss of external rotation |
| | Abnormal shape following recent trauma |
| | Epileptic fit |
| | Electric shock |
| Neurological lesion | Unexplained wasting |
| | Significant sensory or motor deficit |
| Age | Under 16 years |

rheumatica in those over 50 years of age, with or without proximal lower-limb symptoms.

---

### Defining shoulder pain

The causes of shoulder pain may usefully be divided into two categories.

#### Shoulder problems that arise from the shoulder joint

▷ Rotator cuff disorders – rotator cuff tendinopathy, impingement, subacromial bursitis, rotator cuff tears.
▷ Glenohumeral disorders – adhesive capsulitis ('frozen shoulder', arthritis – degenerative or inflammatory).
▷ Acromioclavicular disease.
▷ Trauma, dislocation, fracture, tendon rupture.
▷ Infection.

#### Shoulder problems that arise from elsewhere

▷ Referred pain – neck pain, acute myocardial ischaemia, referred diaphragmatic pain.
▷ Systemic disorders – polymyalgia rheumatica.
▷ Malignancy – apical lung cancer, metastases.

#### History

All GP consultation models emphasise the importance of facilitating the patient's account of events through an open and empathic communication style, rather than imposing the doctor's agenda too early in the process. The overall aim in addition to a clinical diagnosis is to explore the patient's concerns and expectations, the characteristics of the pain, functional and psychosocial impairment, impact on work and social activities, and individual risk and prognostic factors (see Table 4.1).

Subsequently a focused exploration of the character of the shoulder pain should be undertaken, looking at the mode of onset (acute or subacute), duration, nature, site, radiation and exacerbating and relieving factors, sleep disturbance and associated symptoms.

Specific questions should be incorporated into the consultation to exclude 'red flag' referral pointers. Significant trauma, past history of cancer, intractable pain increasing in severity, systemic symptoms of fever, sweats, weight loss, rash, swollen lymph glands, unusual or recent-onset respiratory symptoms, localised swelling or deformity of the joint should be excluded (see Table 4.2).

Previous musculoskeletal problems, in particular a previous episode of shoulder pain, minor trauma, hand dominance, sporting and occupational activities (repetitive arm movements, heavy lifting, regular stretching or the use of arms overhead) should also be asked about directly if not already covered. Review the notes summary and ask about the presence of significant past and current medical conditions such as diabetes, stroke, ischaemic heart disease, respiratory disease, cancer, inflammatory arthritis, gastrointestinal or renal disease, and psoriasis. Also, check prescribed and 'over the counter' drugs and adverse reactions.

## Examination

Observe the general appearance of the patient, for example pallor. Examine the neck (including range of movement of cervical spine), upper limbs, axillae and chest wall for local sources of referred pain. Examine other joints, the skin for rash, the chest, the abdomen and for generalised lymphadenopathy, if the history suggests constitutional symptoms.

### *Examination of the shoulder joint*

#### INSPECTION

▷ From the front, side and behind for deformity, muscle wasting, swelling or signs of trauma.
▷ Palpation of the shoulder bones and joints. Compare both shoulders for any swelling, deformity, or warmth and crepitus. Palpate for local lymphadenopathy.

#### MOVEMENT

▷ Compare the full range of passive, active and resisted movements, and stability of both shoulder joints: flexion, extension, abduction, adduction, internal rotation and external rotation.
▷ Observe movement of the scapula.

#### RECORD

▷ Limitation of range.

▷ Reported discomfort.

▷ Whether active movements are affected more than passive movements.

It is usual to assess whether the patient has a 'painful arc' (70 to 120° of active abduction); this clinical sign, while strongly suggestive of a rotator cuff disorder, is neither sensitive nor specific.[12] If a large rotator cuff tear is suggested by the history and examination (trauma in a young person, significant weakness associated with pain at onset and on examination), the 'drop arm' test may be performed. The drop arm test is a feature of a complete rotator cuff tear; if present, the patient will be unable to support the affected arm, abducted to 90°. On releasing the arm, the patient's arm drops suddenly without any control by the patient. In the normal situation, the arm drops gradually.[12] Otherwise specific tests of the function of joints and tendons are not currently recommended for a GP consultation as there is no evidence that these tests are discriminating enough to be of diagnostic or prognostic value in primary care.[13, 14]

## Diagnosis

There is a range of diagnostic labels derived from clinical observations, for example painful arc syndrome. Some examples from pathophysiology are rotator cuff tears, subacromial bursitis, impingement syndrome caused by pressure upon the cuff tendons by the acromion and head of the humerus (in association with subacromial osteophytes, muscle weakness and soft-tissue laxity). An example from radiographic evidence is glenohumeral arthritis.

The commonest causes of shoulder pain and dysfunction are: rotator cuff disorders, glenohumeral disorders (including 'frozen shoulder'), acromioclavicular disorders and referred neck pain. It is useful to discriminate between these four broad categories of shoulder disorder. However, over-differentiation of diagnostic categories does not influence early, largely conservative, management. Furthermore, research has demonstrated that mixed shoulder disorders are common[15] and that there may be a lack of concordance between clinicians using 'diagnostic' tests.[15]

A clinical algorithm based on history, examination (with an emphasis on comparison of active and passive movements and functional limitation) and specific enquiry about 'red flags' is a pragmatic and rigorous approach to primary care assessment and formulation of a management plan (see Figure 4.2).

Figure 4.2 ○ *Clinical assessment algorithm*

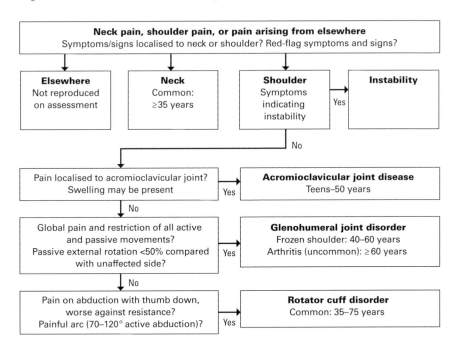

*Source*: reproduced from e-GP: e-Learning for General Practice/Rheumatology and Musculoskeletal Problems/Shoulder Pain (www.e-GP.org).[11]

## Rotator cuff disorders

Rotator cuff disease is diagnosed in up to 70% of people with shoulder pain.[16] Rotator cuff tendinopathy is the commonest disorder and is often associated with a relevant history of repetitive or awkward overhead movements and lifting. The patient typically complains of pain felt in the shoulder and lateral aspect of the upper arm that is worse with overhead activities and at night, particularly when lying on the affected side. Active movements are typically more painful and restricted than passive movements, which are usually full, if painful. Muscle wasting may occur with longstanding symptoms due to relative disuse of the affected upper limb.

A rotator cuff tear may be suggested by:

▷ the age of the patient; it may be a consequence of a 'normal' ageing process as up to half the population aged 70 to 80 years have tears
▷ the mode of onset and character of the pain (acute onset, history of trauma) – the patient may describe a severe 'searing' pain at the onset of the shoulder problem

▷ functional impairment (exacerbation with overhead activities and significantly disabling *painful weakness* of shoulder movements).

Partial tears are commoner than full-thickness tears. Rotator cuff tears in the elderly are attributed to repetitive minor trauma from bony spurs on the under-surface of the acromion, intrinsic degeneration of the cuff, or secondary to inflammatory arthritis. Research has shown that these tears, as detected by MRI scan, are commonly asymptomatic and usually compatible with normal painless function.[17] Occasionally, longstanding tears can be associated with glenohumeral arthritis.

In younger adults rotator cuff tears are usually related to acute trauma. Earlier referral for intensive rehabilitation would usually be indicated and in some cases consideration of surgery.

## Glenohumeral disorders

Glenohumeral disorders cause deep joint pain and sleep and significant functional impairment, for example difficulties with dressing due to restricted external rotation. There is global pain and significant (>50%) restriction of active and passive movements in the affected shoulder.

The aetiology of the 'frozen shoulder' (adhesive capsulitis) is unknown, but risk factors have been identified, such as prolonged immobilisation (for example following a stroke, breast surgery or forearm fracture) and diabetes. True glenohumeral arthritis is rare and incidence increases with age. Isolated osteoarthritis of the shoulder may occur following fractures of the humeral head or neck, large rotator cuff tears, or due to rheumatoid arthritis. It may be suspected if there is a limited range of painful movement sometimes accompanied by crepitus. Plain radiographs are useful in this instance.

Adhesive capsulitis is generally reported to run a self-limiting course over two to three years, but some studies have found that up to 40% of patients have persistent symptoms and restricted movement lasting beyond three years.

Three classical phases of the 'frozen shoulder' have been described:

▷ initial gradual development of generalised and severe shoulder pain, worse at night with inability to lie on the affected side, lasting between two and nine months
▷ a stiff phase with less severe pain, characterised by global stiffness and severe loss of shoulder movement, lasting between four and 12 months
▷ finally a recovery phase characterised by a gradual improvement of range of movement and function over five to 24 months.

There is significant impairment of activities of daily living and work during the early phases.

---

## Acromioclavicular disorders

Acromioclavicular disease is usually secondary to trauma (joint dislocation may occur) or secondary to osteoarthritis. There is localisation of pain, tenderness and, occasionally, swelling of the acromioclavicular joint and restriction of passive, horizontal adduction (flexion) of the shoulder, with the elbow extended, across the body (the scarf test). Acromioclavicular osteoarthritis may also be associated with rotator cuff tendinopathy and subacromial impingement.

---

## Referred mechanical neck pain

The patient will typically describe symptoms arising from the neck as well as the shoulder and upper-limb area. The pain and tenderness is localised to the lower neck and suprascapular area, and may be referred to the shoulder and upper limb. Upper-limb paraesthesia may occur and it is important to enquire about motor symptoms.

Movement of the cervical spine and shoulder will usually produce more generalised upper-back, neck and shoulder pain, and consequently shoulder movements may be restricted. If there are symptoms of paraesthesiae and/or motor symptoms, perform an appropriate neurological assessment.

### Investigations

The diagnosis of shoulder pain is usually by clinical assessment alone. Blood tests and plain radiographs are not necessary in the absence of 'red flags' unless there is a failure to respond to treatment. Plain radiographs may exclude causes of shoulder pain, such as significant glenohumeral osteoarthritis, so some clinicians would advocate a plain X-ray for just suspected glenohumeral problems in primary care.

Due to the high prevalence of asymptomatic abnormalities in the rotator cuff, shoulder ultrasound and MRI have little to add to the largely conservative management of rotator cuff disease in primary care. Ultrasound and MRI can detect full-thickness rotator cuff tears but have less accuracy for detecting partial-thickness tears. In Australia where direct access to radiological investigations is more common (over 40% in the study sample), a research study reported that increased use of radiological intervention (plain films and ultrasound) did not improve patient-reported outcomes and the authors reinforced guidance that imaging does not alter management in acute mechanical shoulder problems and should be reserved for 'red flag' conditions.[18]

## Treatment

The aims of treatment are to understand the personal and social context of the patient's symptoms, control pain and restore movement and function of the shoulder. The GP should provide clear information about diagnosis, the natural course of symptoms and prognosis. Primary care guidelines emphasise 'watchful waiting' in the first instance with the promotion of informed self-care (through verbal, written and electronic patient information), analgesics if needed and open access for review if symptoms persist or change.[19] The local physiotherapy team will usually be able to provide copies of condition-specific exercise sheets as an early intervention for shoulder problems. If there is a failure to respond to the above measures after four to six weeks or the interim development of concerning 'red flag' symptoms and signs, the GP should reassess the patient.

## Analgesia

Paracetamol is suitable as a first-line treatment and may be supplemented by mild opiates such as codeine phosphate (prescribed or over the counter). Opiate prescribing should be at the lowest effective dose and patients need to be counselled about side effects such as constipation and the potential for tolerance and dependence.

If no contraindications exist, NSAIDs may be used short term. The GP should explore the potential for interaction with other prescribed drugs and in the elderly, specifically counselling about the increased risk of upper gastrointestinal side effects, cardiovascular events and the impact on renal function associated with NSAIDs. The MHRA advises that diclofenac (150 mg daily) has an increased risk of cardiovascular disease compared with low-dose ibuprofen (1200 mg daily or less) and naproxen (1000 mg daily).[20]

## Occupational and lifestyle issues

Initially patients may need to modify exacerbating activities and address occupational or sporting factors ('relative rest'), but the focus should be on encouraging the patient to maintain movement of the joint as much as possible. There is a risk of loss of employment and income, which may cause significant anxiety. It may also interfere with patient adherence to the advice of relative rest and the avoidance of exacerbating factors. GP advice and active rehabilitation should focus on a return to work as early as possible when medical certification is provided. As the shoulder problem improves, options may be discussed with the patient such as a return to work with temporary respite from work involving repetitive shoulder movements or heavy lifting, or alternatively a phased return to work.[21] Formal occupational health advice and assessment may be appropriate within the workplace.

Treatment is largely determined by diagnostic triage into the four common presentations, but there is a role for physiotherapy in the two commonest conditions: rotator cuff disorders and adhesive capsulitis (in certain phases). A randomised, controlled trial recruiting participants with undifferentiated shoulder problems from primary care showed that those who were allocated to a physiotherapy treatment group were less likely to re-consult with a GP than those receiving steroid injections alone.[22] Physiotherapists diagnose, treat and advise patients on self-management of shoulder problems, including exercise programmes and strategies to manage pain and impaired function. In many Primary Care Trusts 'extended-scope physiotherapists', usually working within musculoskeletal triage/referral management services, diagnose the full range of shoulder problems. This includes recognition of red-flag symptoms and signs, ordering investigations as appropriate and formulating a management plan with the patient that may include injection of the joint, other conservative physiotherapy treatments and, if necessary, referral on to a rheumatologist or orthopaedic surgeon.

Rotator cuff disorders can be treated by: physiotherapy, steroid injection, other non-operative treatments (including complementary therapy) or surgery. Systematic reviews suggest equivalent short-term benefit for physiotherapy (incorporating supervised exercise) and steroid injections in the management of shoulder disorders.[23,24] Physiotherapy treatment would usually comprise a combination of mobilisations and directed exercises designed to strengthen and stabilise the cuff and scapular muscles, and may be used alone or combined with other measures such as steroid injection. The GP should discuss the relative advantages/disadvantages and potential risks associated with steroid injections and physiotherapy in order to facilitate informed patient choice.

The advantage of a physiotherapy referral is that the patient will be given information and an active management plan for the current shoulder problem and advice on how to prevent and treat recurrences. Working patients, patients and those with cognitive impairment may however find it difficult to complete a supervised rehabilitation and treatment programme. The GP should ensure that the patient wishes and is able to do this before making the referral.

The GP should have a clear diagnosis and management plan before considering a subacromial or intra-articular steroid injection, based on differentiation between rotator cuff disorders and glenohumeral disorders, and exclusion of red-flag features. While there is no reported harm in steroid injections where there is a coexisting minor rotator cuff tear, this intervention should be avoided if the history and examination (positive drop arm test) suggests an acute/large rotator cuff tear.

For rotator cuff disorders, subacromial injection of depot corticosteroid and local anaesthetic up to 10 ml in volume (BNF) may provide relief of pain and enable active rehabilitation, but the effect may be small and last just a few weeks. Injections may be repeated up to two or three times at six-weekly intervals, if initial response is good. In patients with a recurrent shoulder problem that has responded well to local steroid injections in the past, it is appropriate to repeat effective treatment. Many specialists would recommend avoiding more than three injections in a single episode of a shoulder problem without onward referral for specialist musculoskeletal assessment.

A steroid injection should not be repeated if the initial response is poor or very short-lived. In this case, the patient should be reassessed, red-flag symptoms excluded and a consideration of alternative approaches, including referral to a musculoskeletal interface service, made.

There is limited evidence for several alternative non-operative treatments for shoulder pain.[25,26] Overall the evidence base is dominated by small, underpowered studies with different end points, which often exclude important, patient-reported functional outcomes. Systematic reviews report short-term pain relief following acupuncture, and suprascapular nerve block. Randomised clinical trials have failed to establish the efficacy of heat or ice packs, low-power laser, ultrasound and pulsed electromagnetic field therapy, and extracorporeal shockwave therapy.

Referral to a musculoskeletal interface clinic or orthopaedic surgeon may be required when symptoms associated with rotator cuff disorder fail to respond to conservative treatment in primary care. Operative treatment involves decompression of the subacromial space, with or without rotator cuff repair. Some procedures can be performed arthroscopically, which can mean a shorter recovery time. Research of limited quality (observational, small numbers, short-term follow-up, differing end points) has suggested that surgical interventions for significant persistent pain and disability associated with impingement and rotator cuff tear may be effective in reducing pain and improving function. However, three randomised, controlled trials found that surgery was not superior to treatment with supervised exercises.[27]

## Glenohumeral disorders

Treatment may be tailored to the presenting phase of glenohumeral disorders. The aim of treatment is to control severe pain, improve range of movement and promote function. Patients should be informed of the usual time course and generally favourable prognosis of adhesive capsulitis. The clinical evidence base is limited in terms of guidance about frequency, dose and type of corticosteroid for adhesive capsulitis. Intra-articular injection of corticosteroid combined with local anaesthetic, using either an anterior or posterior approach into the glenohumeral joint, may provide short-term pain relief (six to eight weeks) during the early stages of adhesive capsulitis and facilitate some maintenance of mobility and function.

There is some evidence that physiotherapy mobilisation and strengthening exercises following steroid injection in the early stages may provide additional benefits over these treatments alone.[28] Otherwise, physiotherapy in the early, painful phase of the condition may aggravate the pain. However, in the later phases, gentle mobilisation and strengthening exercises can improve mobility and reduce the duration of disability. An intra-articular steroid injection may provide short-term pain relief in glenohumeral arthritis and likewise facilitate exercise and improvement of mobility and function of the joint.

There is a lack of evidence from good-quality clinical trials of long-term symptomatic and functional improvement following surgical intervention for adhesive capsulitis, for example manipulation under anaesthesia or arthroscopic capsular release. Manipulation under anaesthesia (MUA), possibly combined with intra-articular steroid injection and/or arthroscopic debridement of adhesions, and subsequent mobilisation through physiotherapy, may be helpful if conservative options have failed. MUA can be complicated by fractures, haemarthroses and tears of the labrum, tendons or ligaments.

## Acromioclavicular disorders

Symptoms usually respond to rest and simple analgesia. Otherwise, a local steroid injection may be considered. Often this is easier to perform under ultrasound control in the musculoskeletal interface clinic. An arthroscopic excision of the distal clavicle is rarely performed for resistant acromioclavicular joint pain.

## Shoulder instability

Recurrent shoulder instability is usually secondary to trauma and is treated by surgery or alternatively specialist physiotherapy.

## Referral pointers for shoulder pain

Musculoskeletal referral assessment service or sports and exercise medicine.

▷ Any active or exercising individual of any age whose symptoms affect exercise performance or occupation, or daily function if not employed, providing there is no direct indication for direct surgical referral.
▷ They have had two months of structured rehabilitation and are not improving, or two to four months of structured rehabilitation and suboptimal improvement.

## Rheumatology

▷ Any patient with existing inflammatory diagnosis under specialist review.
▷ Shoulder symptoms associated with systemic symptoms suggestive of connective tissue disorder, symptoms and signs of inflammatory arthritis, significantly elevated ESR and/or CRP.
▷ Bilateral shoulder symptoms associated with pelvic symptoms (polymyalgia rheumatica possible). The GP should exclude malignancy red flags and discuss rather than refer. This is because a trial of steroids is diagnostic and follow-up in primary care is appropriate.

## Orthopaedics

▷ Recurrent dislocation of shoulder.
▷ Trauma with no significant improvement after four to six weeks; consider rotator cuff tear.
▷ Previous malignancy.
▷ Acute onset/exacerbation/severe pain and limitation/pain associated with weakness.
▷ Osteoarthritis of the shoulder with pain and functional limitations.

## Case studies

The first curriculum statement, *Being a GP*, lists six domains of competence for the primary care consultation.[29] These are:

1 ▷ Primary care management
2 ▷ Person-centred care
3 ▷ Specific problem-solving skills
4 ▷ A comprehensive approach
5 ▷ Community orientation
6 ▷ A holistic approach.

Standard considerations are listed below and the cases are summarised in relation to the domains.

---

Box 4.2 ○ **Case study 1**

A 35-year-old builder presents with a two-week history of right-sided shoulder pain that is causing him difficulties at work. He had been helping to erect scaffolding prior to the subacute onset of pain on certain right-shoulder movements.

On examination he has a full range of pain-free movement of the cervical spine and >50% range of all shoulder movements (there is more passive movement than active), with greatest restriction on abduction and external rotation. His drop arm test is negative. (In a positive test, on releasing the arm, the patient's arm drops suddenly without any control.)

What key factors are likely to influence your diagnosis in this case? Try to list all the relevant considerations from this patient's history together with any red-flag referral pointers. Will you request investigations?

The key issues in this case are the patient's age and occupation. As a builder there is the likelihood of causation through trauma. Also, because his job involves heavy lifting, it is likely that not only will his ability to do this be impaired, but that it will also aggravate his shoulder problem.

What occupational and prognostic advice will you give him? What sources are helpful for written patient information? Consider your follow-up plans: Would they include physiotherapy and/or specialist referral?

---

### Analysis of case study 1 with respect to the six domains of Being a GP

#### DOMAIN 1: PRIMARY CARE MANAGEMENT

This builder presents with shoulder pain. The GP is able to take a history and perform an examination, which rules out a likely rotator cuff tear but points at rotator cuff tendinopathy as a possible cause of the pain. He has a high-risk occupation for rotator cuff problems (erecting scaffolding). The GP is not confident of his diagnostic skills, so asks a colleague who is a GP with a Special Interest (GPwSI) in musculoskeletal disorders to see the patient. The GPwSI confirms a rotator cuff problem and refers the patient to the hospital physiotherapy department. He also discusses the advantages and disadvantages of a steroid injection, which could be performed at reassessment in the practice in the future. In his referral letter he is able to postulate a diagnosis and suggest a treatment plan.

### DOMAIN 2: PERSON-CENTRED CARE

The builder is concerned about taking time off work as he does not receive sick pay from the building company. He opts to stay at work and try to modify his working patterns. His GP is aware that this may exacerbate the shoulder problem.

### DOMAIN 3: SPECIFIC PROBLEM-SOLVING SKILLS

The first GP whom the builder sees is aware of his lack of knowledge in musculoskeletal problems and enlists the help of a GPwSI colleague from the practice. The GPwSI is able to formulate a treatment plan. The GPwSI suggests a clinical practice meeting for the team to discuss primary care diagnosis and management of shoulder problems, including 'hands on' examination practice and referral pointers, using her as an 'expert' resource.

### DOMAIN 4: A COMPREHENSIVE APPROACH

The GP has considered all the relevant features of the case, including the lack of sick pay and the patient's future in the building industry.

### DOMAIN 5: COMMUNITY ORIENTATION

The GP is aware that his patient's employers are a large local building firm whose treatment of sick employees is usually not good. He makes a mental note of this for future reference. He may be required to act as the patient's advocate in any future disputes over work.

### DOMAIN 6: A HOLISTIC APPROACH

All the possible factors that may impinge on the builder's treatment and future have been taken into consideration.

---

Box 4.3 ○ **Case study 2**

---

A 52-year-old diabetic woman presents with a six-month history of left-sided shoulder pain and stiffness, but no history of trauma. She has seen a couple of other GPs several times at the surgery. She had a steroid injection three months ago with limited benefit and was referred to physiotherapy, but again feels that she has really made no progress with this. Her pain is interfering with sleep and she has been signed off work – she is a social care worker – for five months. There is no past history of cancer, nor any other red-flag features. She asks if you would recommend that she goes to see a private acupuncturist. She has no systemic symptoms of illness.

On examination there was global pain and restriction of all left-shoulder movements (>50%), both active and passive. There was some discomfort on movement of her cervical spine, but no restriction in range of movement.

What key factors are likely to influence your diagnosis in this case? Try to list all the relevant considerations from this patient's history together with any red-flag referral pointers.

▶ You should consider the patient's age. This woman is 52 years' old.
▶ She is diabetic.
▶ She has had pain for six months but no history of trauma.

What occupational and prognostic advice will you give her? What sources are helpful for written patient information? Consider your follow-up plans: Would they include physiotherapy and/or specialist referral?

**103**

## Analysis of case study 2 with respect to the six domains of Being a GP

### DOMAIN 1: PRIMARY CARE MANAGEMENT

This diabetic patient presents with shoulder pain that has been present for six months and has responded poorly to primary care interventions to date. The history and examination suggest adhesive capsulitis as a cause of the pain. Diabetes is both a risk factor for adhesive capsulitis and also an adverse prognostic factor in terms of time to functional improvement of symptoms. While glenohumeral osteoarthritis is highly unlikely in this age group, many specialists would advocate a plain X-ray of the shoulder for glenohumeral problems.

### DOMAIN 2: PERSON-CENTRED CARE

There is a significant impact on activities of daily living and work absence of six months with potential financial problems. She wishes to explore the option of complementary therapy: acupuncture.

**DOMAIN 3: SPECIFIC PROBLEM-SOLVING SKILLS**

The first GP is aware of his lack of knowledge about acupuncture for shoulder problems – he uses clinical knowledge summaries, 'best evidence' and the *Cochrane Library* to research this. The *Cochrane Review* includes lay summaries of the evidence for acupuncture (and surgical interventions) for adhesive capsulitis, which he can share with the patient. The GP records the work he has undertaken as part of a structured case review for his annual appraisal, with evidence of applying the reading/internet research to patient care. He could also undertake an online learning module.

The GP reflects on the management of shoulder problems in the practice and discusses with his partners initiating a practice-based audit of shoulder injections, to review indications for and outcomes of shoulder injections over the next 12 months.

**DOMAIN 4: A COMPREHENSIVE APPROACH**

The GP has considered all the relevant features of the case, including the impact of the pain and function on activities of daily living and prolonged sick leave.

A referral to a musculoskeletal interface service is appropriate at this stage, particularly if the GP is not confident in intra-articular injections. An extended-scope physiotherapist could offer both injection therapy and specialist physiotherapy rehabilitation follow-up. Musculoskeletal interface services typically comprise extended-scope practitioners in podiatry and physiotherapy, a GPwSI and close links to orthopaedic and rheumatology departments. There would usually be a standard referral *pro forma* for this service.

**DOMAIN 5: COMMUNITY ORIENTATION**

At this stage it would be helpful for the patient to consider approaching her employers to discuss adaptations to her working environment to enable a phased return to work that did not involve significant upper-limb activity and strain. The natural course of the shoulder problem is long, but she should soon be entering a less painful, albeit stiff phase of her 'frozen' shoulder. In large organisations, there may be an occupational health service to facilitate this.

**DOMAIN 6: A HOLISTIC APPROACH**

Most of the possible factors that may impinge on treatment and the person's future employment have been taken into consideration. Chronic daily pain, disability and work absence may have a significant psychological impact; consider using the two standard depression screening questions to identify associated low mood and treat any associated depression according to the recently updated NICE guideline.[30]

---

## Summary

Shoulder pain is a common presenting complaint in primary care that causes pain and in some cases severe functional impairment. This chapter describes four common causes of shoulder pain and the characteristics in the history and examination that help to differentiate between these conditions. However, mixed shoulder disorders are common and over-differentiation between categories does not change largely conservative primary care management. Red-flag symptoms and signs that warrant urgent follow-up and referral to specialist services are summarised.

### *Acknowledgements*

Thanks to Prof. E Hay and Prof. A Carr for their input to a clinical review undertaken for the BMJ in 2005.

### *Useful websites and professional resources*

▷ RCGP interactive e-Learning module, *Primary Care Management of Shoulder Pain* [includes video clips of examination techniques and case scenarios].
▷ Arthritis Care, **www.arthritiscare.org.uk** [accessed October 2011].
▷ Arthritis Research UK, **www.arthritisresearchuk.org/** [accessed October 2011].
▷ Carr A J, Hamilton W H. *Orthopaedics in Primary Ca*re (2nd edn) Oxford: Butterworth-Heinemann, 2004.
▷ Hazleman B. *Shoulder Problems in General Practice* (Collected Reports on the Rheumatic Diseases, Series 4) Chesterfield: ARC, 2005, **www.arthritisresearchuk.org/arthritis_information/information_ for_medical_profes/hands_on,_syn_and_topical_revi.aspx** [accessed October 2011].
▷ National Institute for Health and Clinical Excellence, **www.nice.org.uk** [accessed October 2011].

▷ New Zealand Guidelines Group. *The Diagnosis and Management of Soft Tissue Shoulder Injuries and Related Disorders* Wellington: NZGG, 2004, **www.nzgg.org.nz/guidelines/0083/040715_FINAL_Full_ Shoulder_GL.pdf_1.pdf** [accessed October 2011].

▷ *BMJ learning:* useful online module 'The Frozen shoulder', with certificate, on completion, for a personal development plan; **www.bmjlearning.com** [accessed October 2011].

## Patient references

▷ Arthritis Research Campaign. *The Painful Shoulder,* 2004 [leaflet, also available by post], **www.arthritisresearchuk.org/arthritis_ information/arthritis_types_symptoms/shoulder_pain. aspx** [accessed October 2011].

▷ NHS Direct, **www.nhsdirect.nhs.uk** [accessed October 2011].

### References

1 • Urwin M, Symmons D, Allison T, *et al.* Estimating the burden of musculoskeletal disorders in the community: the comparative prevalence of symptoms at different anatomical sites, and the relation to social deprivation *Annals of the Rheumatic Diseases* 1998; **57(11)**: 649–55.

2 • Badcock LJ, Lewis M, Hay EM, *et al.* Consultation and the outcome of shoulder-neck pain: a cohort study in the population *Journal of Rheumatology* 2003; **30(12)**: 2694–9.

3 • Linsell L, Dawson J, Zondervan K, *et al.* Prevalence and incidence of adults consulting for shoulder conditions in UK primary care: patterns of diagnosis and referral *Rheumatology* (Oxford) 2006; **45(2)**: 215–21.

4 • Croft P, Pope D, Silman A. The clinical course of shoulder pain: prospective cohort study in primary care *British Medical Journal* 1996; **313(7057)**: 601–2.

5 • Kuijpers T, van der Windt DA, van der Heijden GJ, *et al.* Systematic review of prognostic cohort studies on shoulder disorders *Pain* 2004; **109(3)**: 420–31.

6 • Bongers PM. The cost of shoulder pain at work *British Medical Journal* 2001; **322(7278)**: 64–5.

7 • Masters S, O'Doherty L, Mitchell G, *et al.* Acute shoulder pain in primary care *Australian Family Physician* 2007; **36(6)**: 473–6.

8 • Hazleman B. *Shoulder Problems in General Practice* (Collected Reports on the Rheumatic Diseases, Series 4) Chesterfield: ARC, 2005, www.arc.org.uk/arthinfo/ documents/6502.pdf [accessed October 2011].

9 • Reilingh ML, Kuijpers T, Tanja-Harfterkamp AM, *et al.* Course and prognosis of shoulder symptoms in general practice *Rheumatology* (Oxford) 2008; **47(5)**: 724–30.

10 • Thomas E, van der Windt D A, Hay E M, *et al*. Two pragmatic trials of treatment for shoulder disorders in primary care: generalisability, course, and prognostic indicators *Annals of the Rheumatic Diseases* 2005; **64(7)**:1056–61.

11 • Mitchell C, Adebajo A O. Shoulder pain, www.e-GP.org.

12 • Calis M, Akgun K, Birtane M, *et al*. Diagnostic values of clinical diagnostic tests in subacromial impingement syndrome *Annals of the Rheumatic Disease* 2000; **59(1)**: 44–7.

13 • Bamji A N, Erhardt C C, Price T R, *et al*. The painful shoulder: can consultants agree? *British Journal of Rheumatology* 1996; **35(11)**: 1172–4.

14 • New Zealand Guidelines Group. *The Diagnosis and Management of Soft Tissue Shoulder Injuries and Related Disorders* Wellington: NZGG, 2004, www.nzgg.org.nz/guidelines/0083/040715_FINAL_Full_Shoulder_GL.pdf_1.pdf [accessed April 2011].

15 • Ostor A J, Richards C A, Prevost A T, *et al*. Diagnosis and relation to general health of shoulder disorders presenting to primary care *Rheumatology* (Oxford) 2005; **44(6)**: 800–5.

16 • Speed C. Shoulder pain *Clinical Evidence* 2006; 14: 1543–60, http://clinicalevidence.bmj.com/ceweb/conditions/msd/1107/1107.jsp [accessed April 2011].

17 • Sher J S, Uribe J W, Posada A, *et al*. Abnormal findings on magnetic resonance images of asymptomatic shoulders *Journal of Bone and Joint Surgery* 1995; **77(1)**: 10–15.

18 • Masters S, O'Doherty L, Mitchell G, *et al*. Acute shoulder pain in primary care *Australian Family Physician* 2007; **36(6)**.

19 • Winters J C, Van der Windt D A W M, Spinnewijn W E M, *et al*. NHG standaard Schouderklachten [clinical guideline shoulder pain of the Dutch College of General Practice] *Huisarts wet* 2008; **51(11)**: 555–65.

20 • Medicines and Healthcare Products Regulatory Agency. *Cardiovascular Safety of COX – 2 Inhibitors and Non-selective NSAIDs*, www.mhra.gov.uk/Safetyinformation/Generalsafetyinformationandadvice/Product-specificinformationandadvice/Product-specificinformationandadvice-A-F/CardiovascularsafetyofCOX-2inhibitorsandnon-selectiveNSAIDs/index.htm [accessed April 2011].

21 • Karjalainen K, Malmivaara A, van Tulder M, *et al*. Multidisciplinary biopsychosocial rehabilitation for neck and shoulder pain amongst working age adults *Cochrane Database of Systematic Reviews* 2003; **2**: CD002194.

22 • Hay E M, Thomas E, Paterson S M, *et al*. A pragmatic randomised controlled trial of local corticosteroid injection and physiotherapy for the treatment of new episodes of unilateral shoulder pain in primary care *Annals of the Rheumatic Diseases* 2003; **62(5)**: 394–9.

23 • Green S, Buchbinder R, Hetrick S. Physiotherapy interventions for shoulder pain. *Cochrane Database of Systematic Reviews* 2003; **2**: CD004258.

24 • Buchbinder R, Green S, Youd J M. Corticosteroid injections for shoulder pain *Cochrane Database of Systematic Reviews* 2003; **1**: CD004016.

25 • Green S, Buchbinder R, Glazier R, *et al*. Interventions for shoulder pain *Cochrane Database of Systematic Reviews* 2000; **2**: CD001156.

26 • Green S, Buchbinder R, Hetrick S. Acupuncture for shoulder pain *Cochrane Database of Systematic Reviews* 2005; **2**: CD005319.

27 • Coghlan J A, Buchbinder R, Green S, *et al*. Surgery for rotator cuff disease *Cochrane Database of Systematic Reviews* 2008; **1**: CD005619.

28 • Carette S, Moffet H, Tardif J, *et al*. Intraarticular corticosteroids, supervised physiotherapy, or a combination of the two in the treatment of adhesive capsulitis of the shoulder: a placebo-controlled trial *Arthritis and Rheumatism* 2003; **48(3)**: 829–38.

29 • Royal College of General Practitioners. *Being a General Practitioner* (curriculum statement 1) London: RCGP, 2007.

30 • National Institute for Health and Clinical Excellence. *Clinical Guideline 91, Depression in Adults with a Chronic Physical Health Problem: treatment and management*, London: National Collaborating Centre for Mental Health, 2009, http://guidance.nice.org.uk/ CG91 [accessed October 2011].

# Hip and knee problems

**5**

*Martyn B. Speight and Jon Greenwell*

## Aims of this chapter

This chapter is intended to give an overview of the hip and knee conditions that commonly present in primary care. It lists the key questions to ask when taking a history, enabling differentiation between the conditions affecting the hip or knee. It will allow the clinician to perform a proficient and focused examination of both joints. The management of common conditions affecting the hip and knee is also discussed.

The chapter does not focus on traumatic injuries, as these usually present to A&E departments. This chapter should be read alongside the chapters on osteoarthritis (OA), tendonopathy and inflammatory joint disease, as a number of complaints appear in both chapters.

### Key learning points

▶ The ability to take an accurate and focused history from a patient presenting with knee or hip pain.
▶ The ability to perform a proficient examination of a patient presenting with knee or hip pain.
▶ To enable an understanding of the different knee conditions that may present in primary care, and the ability to create a differential diagnosis.
▶ To enable an understanding of the different hip conditions that may present in primary care, and the ability to create a differential diagnosis.
▶ To facilitate an appreciation of the imaging modalities available to investigate patients presenting with knee and hip pain, and the limitations of those investigations.
▶ To understand the role that other healthcare professionals play in the management of patients with either knee or hip pain.

## Introduction to the knee joint

The presentation of pain around the knee joint is one of the most common musculoskeletal complaints presenting to general practice, and may arise due to a wide range of pathologies. In the younger patient pain most commonly arises from sporting or overuse injuries, which may affect the intra-articular or extra-articular structures of the knee.

The knee is also a common site for inflammatory and infective pathologies. The commonest cause of knee pain arising in older patients is from OA and degenerative disease. This is a major cause of disability and morbidity in the older patient, the prevalence and healthcare costs of which continue to rise as the population ages.

### *Basic functional anatomy*

The knee is a synovial, modified hinge joint. It is the most commonly injured joint in the body, formed at the end of the two largest mechanical levers. It is tri-compartmental, made up of two tibiofemoral and one patellofemoral joints.

The overall function of the knee is a combination of movement and stability. The most stable position is full extension with external tibial rotation and internal femoral rotation. At the opposite extreme is the vulnerable or loose-packed position, usually at about 25° flexion, when ligaments are relaxed. Stability of the knee is mainly derived through the quadriceps muscles, supported by the anterior and posterior cruciate ligaments and the medial and lateral collateral ligaments. The anterior cruciate ligament (ACL) is essential for control in pivoting movements. When injured it may lead to rotation of the tibia in an anterolateral direction, as occurs in landing from a jump, pivoting or a sudden deceleration. The posterior cruciate ligament (PCL) serves to stabilise the femur above the tibia. The medial collateral ligament provides medial stability against valgus loads, and passes from the medial femoral condyle downwards as a thickened band to attach to the anteromedial tibia. The deep fibres are contiguous with the medial meniscus. The lateral collateral ligament is a thin cord-like structure, passing from the lateral border of femur to the head of the fibula, resisting varus loads. Joint congruence, stability and load absorption are aided by the lateral and medial menisci, the medial being more firmly attached and less mobile, contributing to a far greater incidence of injury.

There are five commonly symptomatic bursae around the knee; pre-patellar, supra-patellar, infra-patellar, pes anserine and the semimembranosus or gastrocnemius bursa, often known as a Baker's cyst.

The patella is a bony ossicle, having facets to its posterior aspects as it glides twice its length through full flexion/extension. The main function of the patella is to improve the efficiency of the last 30° of extension, as it holds the quadriceps tendon away from the axis of movement, increasing the lever arm and aiding extension.

## History taking

History taking in knee conditions follows the same principles as other regions of the body: keeping the history focused, allowing (if not a diagnosis) a differential diagnosis to be constructed, before considering a focused examination. Before the specifics of the symptoms, a GP should always remember the age, sex, occupation and context of the patient's pain, and assess the impact on the patient's quality of life.

The location, character, severity and behaviour of the pain are important.

▷ Is the pain local or referred from the hip or lumbar spine?
▷ Is the pain of sudden or gradual onset?
▷ Is there any night pain?
▷ Enquire about any trauma or swelling; immediate swelling suggests cruciate ligament injury whereas next-day swelling suggests a meniscal injury.
▷ Often, the mechanism of the injury can immediately raise the index of suspicion of a specific diagnosis.
▷ Always enquire about any mechanical symptoms such as locking, suggesting meniscal damage, or giving way, suggesting ligament instability.

Enquire about any specific sports or leisure activities, and the ability to pursue such activities. The knee is a common initial presentation for inflammatory arthritis. Ask about prolonged early-morning stiffness, and warmth or redness in the joint, which suggest inflammatory or infective aetiologies. Check whether the patient is well and if there are systemic symptoms including eyes, skin, genitourinary or gastroinitestinal, which could suggest rheumatoid or reactive arthritis. The knee can also be an initial presentation of gout and a sudden onset of a severely painful swollen knee that resolves spontaneously over a few days does need screening for gout.

### Knee pain

#### Anterior knee pain

Anterior knee pain is most commonly due to patellofemoral joint maltracking and is more common in females. It can also be caused by OA of the patellofemoral joint. Enquire about pain around the patella with descents or ascents, with the knee feeling weak or unstable, and ask if the knee has given way whilst descending hills or stairs. The patient may also report pain on prolonged sitting (movie-goer's knee) or kneeling.

If the pain is localised to the infra-patellar region in an active patient, and there is a complaint of stiffness in the morning, or on commencing activity, think of a patellar tendinopathy. Anterior knee pain in children aged 9–16 years, during a growth spurt, with exercise-induced pain, localised around the patellar tendon at its tibial insertion, is due to Osgood–Schlatter's disease. This is a form of traction apophysitis at the insertion of the patellar tendon. Finally, patients presenting with a warm red lump to the front of their knee invariably have a pre-patellar or supra-patellar bursitis, and the GP should enquire about occupational risk factors (housemaid's knee).

#### Medial knee pain

Medial knee pain of gradual onset in an older patient, which is worse in the morning, eases with time and returns at the end of the day, is the commonest presentation of early OA. Associated effusions can occur with sudden increases in activity. Night pain and a diffuse stiffness are common features in OA, as is popliteal fossal pain from a Baker's cyst.

In the younger patient with gradual-onset medial knee pain, with no history of recent trauma, the GP should always ask about previous meniscal surgery. OA can occur early in patients who have had a meniscectomy. Reactive effusions are very common in this subpopulation of early OA patients., Following meniscectomy, coronary ligament sprain can quite commonly persist, despite numerous treatments, and can be a cause of pain.

Slightly inferior and anterior to the medial joint is the pes anserinus, and bursitis at this point can be difficult to differentiate in the history. The GP should enquire about sudden knee flexion movements in exercise (i.e. walking or running uphill on slippery/muddy ground), as this can cause bursitis. It can present right across the age range.

### Lateral knee pain

Lateral knee pain has a limited differential diagnosis. The two commonest causes are OA and iliotibial band friction syndrome in runners. GPs should ask about a running-induced, often downhill, sharp pain around the lateral knee. Pain ceases immediately upon stopping running. Recurrent, localised swelling over the lateral knee with mechanical symptoms is usually a meniscal cyst.

### Red flags

Red flags in knee pain include the child with a limp and referred knee pain from the hip region. This usually indicates serious hip pathology.

Night pain in a child with a limp and bony swelling is strongly suspicious of malignancy.

An isolated swollen knee in an adult, some two weeks after foreign travel and gastrointestinal upset, is usually a reactive arthritis and needs rheumatological input. A patient presenting with delayed onset of pain and loss of function in sport/exercise, following an awkward twist or impact/compression (jump from a height) type injury, could have an osteochondral injury and needs an orthopaedic opinion.

## Examination

### Inspection

Initial examination of the knee involves observation; both knees should be exposed, ideally from mid-thigh downwards and the feet should also be visible. The knees should be observed in both the standing and supine positions. The examiner should be looking for any effusion or swelling around the knee and any erythema or bruising. The feet should also be examined, with the GP looking for excessive pronation or supination.

### Range of movement

The range of movement should then be assessed. A good screening test is to ask the patient to squat fully, and then to take a few steps; this is often known as 'duck walking'. This test excludes significant meniscal injury. The range of movement is then checked with the patient supine. The normal range of movement is from 10° of hyperextension through to 140° of flexion.

### Palpation

Palpation of the knee should be used to look for warmth around the knee, indicating inflammation or infection, and also to assess for an effusion. There are two techniques to assess for an effusion, the patellar tap or by 'milking' the knee. The milking technique is more sensitive and enables the examiner to detect a much more subtle effusion. To perform the test, manually drain the medial patellar pouch by stroking the fluid in a superior direction. Then milk the fluid back into the knee from above on the lateral side while observing the medial pouch, looking for the re-accumulation of any fluid. To complete palpation the medial and lateral joint lines should be assessed with the knee flexed to 30°.

The soft tissue around the knee should also be palpated for the presence of any bursae. Finally, the patellofemoral joint and surrounding structures should be examined. The patella, medial and lateral facets should be palpated for tenderness, and the inferior pole of the patella, the patella tendon and the tibial tubercle should also be assessed for swelling or tenderness.

### Special tests

Special tests of the knee assess the stability of the ligaments, and examine the medial and lateral menisci and the patellofemoral joint.

The medial and collateral ligaments should be assessed with the knee flexed to 30° and a valgus and then a varus force applied respectively to the knee.

The PCL is assessed using the sag sign. Both knees are flexed to 90° and the position of the tibia in relation to the femur is assessed. The tibia is more posterior in a PCL-deficient knee.

The anterior drawer test is used to examine the ACL. Again the knee is flexed to 90°, and the patient's foot is stabilised. The examiner's hands are then placed around the femoral condyles, ensuring the hamstrings are relaxed. The tibia is then drawn anteriorly using a gentle but firm pressure. Then the limit of forward excursion compared with the femur is assessed and compared with the opposite leg.

Finally, the medial and lateral menisci are assessed. Two techniques are utilised; Thessaly's test is a recent innovation and is thought to be more sensitive and specific than McMurray's test. To perform McMurray's test the knee is flexed, and then at varying degrees of flexion an internal and external rotational force is applied to the knee. A positive test is seen if a clunk is detected or the patient's symptoms are re-created.

Thessaly's test is performed with the patient standing, with the knee at approximately 5 and 20° of flexion. The examiner helps the patient to balance by supporting him or her and then asks the patient to rotate internally and externally the knee and trunk, three times in both directions. The patient may experience joint line pain or clicking or catching.

If examination of the knee does not reveal any obvious abnormality then it is important to perform an examination of the hip joint to exclude OA of the hip as a cause of referred pain to the knee.

To assess for patellofemoral pain Clarke's test is performed. This involves the examiner placing his or her hand superior to the patella, over the distal quadriceps muscle, and pressing down with a moderate pressure. The patient is then asked to contract his or her quadriceps muscle, causing the patella to move superiorly towards the examiner's hand, and consequently being forced down to the femoral condyles. If the back of the patella is inflamed or irritable this causes pain and reproduces the patient symptoms.

## Investigations of knee disorders

As with any other investigations in medicine, a clinical diagnosis should first be reached using the history and examination. Then, relevant investigations can be requested and unnecessary investigations avoided.

### X-rays

X-rays have a role to play in confirming or excluding disease in conditions such as OA, looking for loose bodies, or excluding other bone pathology. Calcium deposits can clearly be seen in conditions such as calcium pyrophosphate disease. Radiographic OA affects about 25% of adults aged 50 and over.[1] There is a consistent association between pain severity, duration, stiffness, physical function and radiographic OA.[2] Concordance between symptoms and radiographic OA seems to be greater with more advanced structural damage.[1] A more recent study (Neogi T *et al.*)[3] demonstrated a strong dose–response relationship between severity of radiographic knee OA and knee pain, even in the mild stages of knee OA.

### Ultrasound scanning

Ultrasound scanning of the knee is the investigation of choice in suspected soft-tissue pathology around the knee, mainly because of its superior spatial resolution and because it is real-time imaging. As a rule of thumb, radiologists use ultrasound scanning for relatively superficial structures, when a small and discrete area is affected. In deciding if ultrasound scanning is appropriate, remember that, in addition to diagnosis, one of its main applications is to guide interventions. Around the knee, probably its greatest application is assessing tendon disease or looking for bursitis.

### Magnetic resonance imaging of the knee

Magnetic resonance imaging (MRI) of the knee is accurate and helps in making therapeutic decisions. The applications are numerous, but it is particularly good for assessing the nature of suspected internal derangement of the knee such as meniscal tears, cruciate ligament injuries and bone and cartilage pathology such as osteochondral lesions or osteochondritis dissecans.

The diagnostic accuracy of MRI scanning has been shown to be of the order of 94% for medial meniscus and ACL pathology, and slightly less for the lateral meniscus. This level of accuracy has been shown to have a major impact on decision-making processes. One study looked at orthopaedic diagnoses before and after MRI in 332 patients.[4] Clinicians indicated their clinical diagnosis, level of confidence and proposed management before imaging. In meniscal tears, 57 of 113 pre-imaging diagnoses were no longer considered after imaging, resulting in a change in management for 62% of patients. For confirmed diagnoses, confidence in the diagnosis improved significantly. The proportion of patients for whom arthroscopy was being considered changed considerably, with only 38% proceeding to arthroscopy after imaging. Similar studies have repeated such findings.[5]

More recently, the accessibility of MRI scans for GPs has been studied.[6-10] Studying direct access to MRI for GPs has revealed the following: it did not significantly alter GPs' diagnoses or treatment compared with direct referral to orthopaedics, but it significantly increased their confidence in their decisions. It yielded small but statistically significant benefits in patients' knee-related quality of life but non-significant improvements in physical functioning (DAMASK trial).[11] The results of a similar study, retrospectively analysing 12 years of GP open access to MRI scans, revealed a large variation in requesting patterns between GPs, suggesting the need for increased communication between GPs and imaging departments to optimise the use of the service.[12]

### Joint aspiration and blood tests

Joint aspiration for an effused joint can be both therapeutic as well as diagnostic. A tense effusion suggests haemarthrosis, which following aspiration should receive X-ray and prompt orthopaedic referral. Cruciate ligament injury or osteochondral injury need to be excluded. Joint aspiration from a non-inflammatory and non-infected joint is clear and viscous with a white cell count of less than 2000/mm.[3] Opaque aspirate suggests septic arthritis, and samples should be sent for laboratory microscopy, culture and sensitivities. If gout is suspected then microscopy for birefringent crystals should be requested.

If a patient has a suspected inflammatory component to his or her knee pain, then blood tests for inflammatory markers, urate and auto-immune status should be performed.

## Management of knee conditions

### Osteoarthritis

For the management of OA of the knee, please refer to the specific chapter covering this condition and to recent NICE guidance (NICE 2008).[13] NICE has discouraged arthroscopy for the very common scenario of the patient with OA with no mechanical signs or effusions.

A common association with an OA knee is a Baker's cyst, although these can occur in isolation. Management would discourage referral for aspiration as they tend to recur.

### Tendinopathies of the knee

For the detailed management of tendinopathies of the knee, please refer to the specific chapter covering tendinopathies.

### Bursitis

The most common bursitis around the knee is from the pre- and supra-patellar bursae. As an initial management, a trial of non-steroidal anti-inflammatory drugs (NSAIDs), ice and rest from provoking activity would be appropriate. Should this fail, the GP could consider local injection of corticosteroid. Aspiration is not recommended. For pes anserine bursitis, similar measures to the above should be advised. If not responding, a trial of a corticosteroid injection is advised. The GP should look for any predisposing factors in exercisers by ensuring adequate stretching of the appropriate muscles, pre- and post-exercise.

### Iliotibial band friction syndrome

This very painful condition is commonly found in runners, but also in patients taking part in other activities. First-line treatment should involve simple self-help measures of ice, NSAIDs, stretching and rest from pain-provoking activity. The GP should also look for precipitating factors, i.e. volume and intensity of running, and terrain. If symptoms fail to progress, patients should be referred for physiotherapy assessment. Assessment for bio-mechanical risk factors in the foot should be sought, with a view to referral to podiatry.

### Non-traumatic ligamentous pain

The soft tissues around the knee, such as ligaments and joint capsules, are a common source of pain, particularly in an unstable knee, or with minor sprains. The main ligaments are the medial collateral and the coronary (contiguous with joint capsule). Look for point tenderness over the joint line, or above the joint line on the medial femoral condyle and the absence of any other features of meniscal pathology or OA. If patients have already tried ice and/or NSAIDs, these conditions are usually successfully treated with corticosteroid injection, and some quadriceps-strengthening exercises.

### Non-traumatic meniscus

A non-traumatic meniscal problem usually presents with medial knee pain, reduced movements or a clicking/catching sensation; these are all usually against a background of some early OA. A persistently locked knee due to a meniscal injury requires urgent referral. If the patient is able to fully weight-bear, has a good range of movement and no recurrent effusions, a trial of conservative management involving analgesia, NSAIDs and physiotherapy referral is advised.

### Acute effusions

As referred to previously, GPs should consider aspirating an acutely effused knee. If a reactive effusion is suspected (i.e. to increased exercise), aspirate and consider a corticosteroid injection to promote healing. Advise relative rest and instruct on quadriceps exercises immediately. If infection, inflammation (e.g. a reactive arthritis) or gout is suspected, aspirate and arrange microbiology to tailor treatment specifically.

## Case histories

### *Anterior knee pain*

A 32-year-old woman presents to your surgery with a three-month history of left-knee pain. The pain came on gradually and she does not recall any traumatic events. She does not describe any locking or giving way. Neither does she report any swelling of the knee. She has noticed the knee has started clicking if she bends down. She finds kneeling on the floor painful, and has also noticed she has pain on walking down stairs or hills, but is pain free when walking on the flat. If she sits down for a prolonged period of time, for example at the cinema, the knee starts to feel uncomfortable.

She is normally very active and tries to go to the gym three times a week as she is trying to lose weight, but has had to stop this currently. She works as a primary school teacher.

On examination she does not have an effusion present, and she is able to perform a full squat; however, she is a little uncomfortable on full flexion. It is possible to hyper-extend her knees to 15°. You do notice that her patellae are small on both sides. There is no joint line tenderness but she is diffusely tender below the medial joint line anteriorly.

Testing the ligaments reveals no abnormality, and all meniscal tests are normal. There is some wasting of the quadriceps muscles when compared with the opposite side and Clarke's test is positive. A general hypermobility screen gives her a Beighton score of 6/9, with an increased range of movement in the thumbs and little fingers as well as the knees.

119

#### MANAGEMENT

As referred to in previous sections, this is a very common presentation in primary care, and is most commonly a biomechanical problem of maltracking/malalignment of the patellae in the intercondylar groove, leading to the patellofemoral pain syndrome. Occasionally, the diagnosis is OA of the patellofemoral joint, with no tibiofemoral joint involvement. Management is very much holistic; GPs should refer to physiotherapy for advice on a stretching and strengthening programme for the vastus medialis obliquus muscle, and possibly a McConnell taping regime (pain relief and improved neuromotor control). Refer for foot orthosis as an adjunct or alternative to physiotherapy. Foot orthoses produce earlier and larger improvements than flat inserts. However, adding foot orthoses to physiotherapy does not improve physiotherapy outcomes. Weight loss measures can be considered in the obese patient, but this is shown to have more impact on depression than on pain and function directly. Obesity is an established risk factor for the development and progression of both structural OA and knee pain.

### Osteoarthritis

A 78-year-old man has been to the surgery on a number of occasions over the past year complaining of bilateral knee pain. He says the pain is worse after resting and the knees are particularly stiff first thing in the morning, which takes around 30 minutes to improve. He reports some swelling to the knees, particularly the right one. He does not recall any locking or giving way of either knee. In the past he has had a lateral meniscectomy on the right side following an old football injury.

He lives alone and is having difficulty walking to the shops and carrying his shopping. He is not sleeping well and appears depressed.

He has tried simple analgesia but this does not help with his pain. He also complains of pain at the base of both thumbs.

On examination you notice he has a moderate effusion to the right knee, but no effusion to the left. The range of movement in the left knee is normal, but on the right side he is lacking any hyperextension beyond 0°, and flexion is only possible to 120°. You also notice he has a swelling in the popliteal fossa on the right side, consistent with a Baker's cyst.

He is tender over the right lateral joint line, and it feels narrowed compared with the left side. All meniscal tests are normal and Clarke's test is negative. He has marked wasting of the quadriceps muscles bilaterally, and these are weak on testing resisted knee extension.

You also notice he has squaring of the carpo-metacarpal joint of the left thumb and Heberden's nodes affecting some of the distal interphalangeal joints.

### MANAGEMENT

Using person-centred care, the GP should take a thorough history and screen for depression using a questionnaire tool such as the Patient Health Questionnaire 9 (PHQ9). If the patient scores highly, the GP may consider a referral to the psychiatrist with an interest in elderly care ('Working with colleagues and in teams'), but in this case the patient does not score too highly on the test. Instead, the GP refers to another member of his team, the health visitor with an interest in the elderly, who performs a home visit and arranges an assessment by social services. They can provide help with shopping and self-care.

The clinical assessment of his knee problem is strongly suggestive of OA ('Clinical management'). The GP explains his findings to the patient ('Communication and consultation skills') and the importance of the patient keeping active and losing some weight. He refers the patient to the physiotherapy department at the local community hospital ('Working with colleagues and in teams') and also arranges transport to enable the patient to attend ('Practising holistically').

The GP notes the patient has poor sleep, but feels that this is secondary to depression, rather than knee pain. However, he does arrange a follow-up consultation in six weeks, to assess if there has been any improvement in the symptoms ('A comprehensive approach', 'Managing medical complexity and promoting health'). The GP is also aware that, if symptoms do not eventually improve, then he may need to arrange further investigations such as X-ray and referral for a joint replacement ('Data gathering and interpretation'). He could use tools such as the Oxford Knee Score to assess the severity of the patient's symptoms and guide him on referral for further care (see appendix to this chapter).

### Meniscal tear

A 42-year-old woman returned from a skiing holiday six weeks ago. Whilst she was skiing she had to turn suddenly to avoid another skier and she fell, with her left leg getting stuck underneath her. She felt some pain initially but was able to carry on skiing after a short rest. Her knee did not swell immediately, but when she awoke the next morning she noticed it was swollen but thought nothing more of it.

Since her return the swelling has persisted despite taking ibuprofen. The knee has been painful, particularly when twisting or turning to the left-hand side. She does not report any locking of the knee but it has given way suddenly on one occasion when she turned to the left. She is also struggling to squat fully to get food out of the freezer, and is having to favour the opposite leg.

On examination there is still a moderate effusion to the left knee, with an inability to fully squat or duck walk. Flexion is also slightly limited. The medial joint line is significantly tender on palpation, and McMurray's test is positive when a valgus force is applied. Ligament testing and tests for the patellofemoral joint were normal.

Management of a meniscal tear involves early assessment of the patient's pain, any effusion present and whether or not the patient has loss of joint movement and loss of function. If the patient fails to progress over the first few days, referral for a surgical opinion should be made. Most surgeons now advise referral within two weeks. If the patient has a feature suggestive of a meniscal tear, but no loss of movement and can fully weight-bear, a trial of conservative treatment is advised over a four to six week period. A locked knee requires urgent orthopaedic opinion.

### Osgood–Schlatter's disease

A 14-year-old boy is brought to the surgery by his father. The father is concerned about the pain his son has had in his left knee for the past six months, which he describes as growing pains. The pain seems to be centred below the knee cap and he has noticed a swelling below the patella, which is tender to touch.

He is very keen on sport and plays football for his school and a local club, plays cricket in the summer, enjoys athletics and has tennis lessons. He reports the pain is worse both after exercise and the following morning, and he occasionally gets pain during the night. He finds it particularly uncomfortable to kneel on the floor. His father reports that he is in the middle of a growth spurt and has gained about 3 inches in height over the past six months.

On examination there is no effusion and a full range of movement. You do notice a prominent swelling below the patella on the left knee that is not present on the right knee. Joint line palpation reveals no abnormality and the knee is not hot or red. Ligament and meniscal tests are normal. When checking the length of the hamstring and quadriceps muscles these are found to be slightly short with a straight leg raise only possible to 30° bilaterally. You make a diagnosis of Osgood–Schlatter's disease.

#### MANAGEMENT

This is an osteochondritis of the growth plate of the tibial tuberosity where the patellar tendon attaches. It occurs during the adolescent growth spurt. It is a self-limiting condition, which settles with bony fusion of the tibial tuberosity. Management involves activity modification, usually advising relative rest from one or two types of activity involving running or jumping. There is no evidence that complete rest promotes healing. Advise ice after sport, refer to physiotherapy for muscle stretching and strengthening regimes. Inform the patient and his or her parents that symptoms can persist for up to two years.

---

### The hip joint

#### Introduction

The hip joint has fewer possible diagnoses than the knee, and is arguably more straightforward to examine. Most patients tend to present at an older age, with degenerative conditions. However, recently a new diagnosis of femoro-acetabular impingement (FAI) has been recognised, which can cause symptoms in younger, more active patients. In children and teenagers presenting

Table 5.1 ○ *Differential diagnosis of knee pain depending on location*

| Anterior knee pain | Medial knee pain | Lateral knee pain |
|---|---|---|
| Patellofemoral maltracking | OA | OA |
| Patellofemoral OA | Pes anserine bursitis | Iliotibial band friction syndrome |
| Patellar tendinopathy | Medial meniscal injury | Lateral meniscal injury |
| Osgood–Schlatter's disease | Medial collateral ligament strain | |
| Pre-patellar bursitis | Coronary ligament sprain | |
| OA | | |

Table 5.2 ○ *Knee pain associated with an effusion*

| Traumatic | Non-traumatic | Infective or inflammatory causes |
|---|---|---|
| Cruciate ligament rupture | OA | Rheumatoid arthritis |
| Meniscal tear | Degenerative meniscal tear | Seronegative arthritis |
| Patellar dislocation | | Gout |
| | | Reactive arthritis (Reiter's syndrome) |
| | | Infection |

with hip pain a referral to a paediatric orthopaedic surgeon should always be considered to exclude Perthes' disease and a slipped capital femoral epiphysis.

There is a similar situation with an increase in degenerative conditions presenting to primary care as the general population ages, as there is with the knee joint.

## Anatomy

The hip joint is a simple ball and socket joint, made up of the femoral head and the acetabulum of the pelvis. Both joint surfaces have a covering of articular cartilage. There is also an extension of the acetabular cartilage, making up the labrum, which increases the stability and congruence of the joint. There is a strong capsule that surrounds the joint. The alignment of the femoral head related to the neck of femur can be congenitally displaced, leading to possible FAI. The other cause of FAI is an extension of the bone around the acetabulum, which leads to over-coverage of the femoral head.

The main movements of the hip are flexion and extension, but the joint also allows for internal and external rotation, and abduction and adduction.

Over the lateral surface of the hip lies the trochanteric bursa. This is a fluid-filled sac that separates the gluteus maximus muscle from the posterior and lateral side of the greater trochanter of the femur. The iliotibial band also lies close to the greater trochanter of the femur.

### *History*

When taking a history in a patient with hip pain the routine is similar to that mentioned above of taking a knee history, in particular with regards to the pattern of pain, any night pain, symptoms in other joints and any trauma. The age of the patient and his or her occupation and hobbies should also be noted.

A patient with OA will often describe pain on standing and walking, with less pain at rest. In advanced arthritis, climbing the stairs becomes difficult, as does bending down to put on shoes and socks. The presence of night-time pain should be assessed. Pain on lying in the lateral position that is relieved by turning over suggests trochanteric bursitis, whereas generalised pain is more suggestive of arthritis.

FAI is more common in younger patients, and may follow a specific twisting injury, or can develop due to repetitive movement in a susceptible individual. The patients will describe clicking or snapping around the hip, with a dull ache that intensifies with certain activities and positions. The hip can be involved in an inflammatory polyarthropathy or septic arthritis, so these should be excluded in the history.

Another important cause of hip pain is pain referred from the lumbar spine. The patient should therefore be asked about any low-back pain, either current or in the past, and any other symptoms such as sciatica, suggestive of lumbar spine pathology.

In a patient with acute onset of hip pain following a fall, it is imperative that the symptomatic leg is assessed for a fracture of the neck of femur, looking for shortening and external rotation of the leg. If this is suspected he or she should be referred urgently for an orthopaedic opinion. The differential diagnosis of traumatic hip pain is a fracture to the inferior pubic ramus or dislocation of the hip.

### Examination

Examination of the hip starts as the patient walks into your consulting room. He or she may have a limp, or use a stick. The patient needs to be adequately exposed to allow for palpation and inspection of the joint, looking for redness, swelling or muscle wasting. The patient's leg length should also be formally assessed. The lateral thigh should be palpated behind and below the greater trochanter, to look for a possible bursitis. It is difficult to feel the joint line of the hip as it is deep, and covered by muscle and soft tissue.

The passive movement should be assessed in flexion, extension, rotation and abduction. Flexion is assessed by flexing the knee also and bringing the knee up towards the ipsilateral shoulder. Extension is assessed with the patient prone, and raising the knee from the couch.

Rotation in flexion is measured with the hip and knee flexed to 90°. Lateral movement of the foot pivoting at the knee should produce internal rotation of the hip. Medial movement of the foot produces external rotation at the hip.

Assessment of abduction requires that the pelvis first be immobilised. This is achieved either by placing one forearm between the iliac spines, or by placing the leg not being assessed over the side of the bed. With the pelvis fixed, the other leg is then abducted from the perpendicular to the pelvis as far as possible. The normal range is 40°. The other leg is then tested.

Normal ranges for passive movement (in degrees) in the hip are: flexion (130), extension (10), abduction (45), external rotation (40) and internal rotation (50). In OA flexion and internal rotation tend to be lost first (the capsular pattern for the hip).

The **FABER** test (**F**lexion **AB**duction and **E**xternal **R**otation) is a test looking for evidence of hip arthritis. In this manoeuvre the patient's pelvis is stabilised by placing a hand on the iliac crest (the side furthest from the examiner) and the patient flexes the hip joint nearer to the examiner; the flexed hip is then slowly abducted. If there is early hip OA then the abduction of the flexed hip will be restricted and painful. The FABER test may also be positive in a patient with FAI.

Trendelenburg's sign is a gait adopted by someone with an absent or weakened hip abductor mechanism. During the step, instead of the pelvis being raised on the side of the lifted foot, it drops. Thus it is seen as the patient's pelvis tilting towards the lifted foot, with much flexion needed at the knee on the affected side in order for the foot to clear the ground. The lesion is on the contralateral side to the sagging hip. A positive Trendelenburg sign is found in:

▷ subluxation or dislocation of the hip

▷ abductor weakness

▷ shortening of the femoral neck

▷ any painful hip disorder.

Trendelenburg's test can also be performed to formally assess the stability around the pelvis. The patient is asked to stand unassisted on each leg in turn, whilst the examiner's fingers are placed on the anterior superior iliac spines. The foot on the contralateral side is elevated from the floor by bending at the knee. An alternative approach is to have the patient undertake this manoeuvre facing the examiner and supported only by the index fingers of the outstretched hands; this accentuates any instability of balance shown during a positive test.

### Diagnosis and management of osteoarthritis

Management is along the lines of the recent NICE guidelines as outlined elsewhere in this chapter under knee and OA (see pp. 117–18). Physiotherapy can help to stretch and strengthen important muscle groups. If medication fails to control pain, and patients are unsuitable for surgery or it is contraindicated, then trial of an image-guided intra-articular injection can be effective. As with any joint injections, these are seen as 'circuit breakers' and not standalone therapy. 'Blind' joint injections in primary care are not recommended. With disease progression, the option of joint replacement surgery should be discussed, with onward referral to an orthopaedic hip surgeon for further assessment on suitability and to discuss pros and cons.

---

### Lateral hip pain/trochanteric bursitis

Historically, the vast majority of patients with lateral hip pain would have been diagnosed with trochanteric bursitis, a fairly non-specific term that is often misleading. More recently, various other diagnoses have been included, ranging from a specific gluteal tendinopathy, for which there is some MRI evidence to support clinical findings, to a much broader/all-encompassing 'greater trochanteric pain syndrome'. The latter presentation is very common in clinical practice, often chronic, and commonly with some low-back pain. One study revealed that one in five patients referred to a tertiary care orthopaedic spine centre for low-back pain were diagnosed with 'greater trochanteric pain syndrome'.[14] Another study estimated the incidence at 1.8 per 1000 patients per year, with 80% being female.[15] The pain often radiates posteriorly/postero-laterally to the point of attachment of the hip lateral rotators, into the hamstring/iliotibial band region; the patient sometimes experiences paraesthesiae. Symptoms are worse for standing, walking (particularly descents), laying on affected side and sitting cross-legged. The author finds these patients very different from those with a definite and discrete area of pain and tenderness laterally over the greater trochanter. Myofascial trigger points in the glutei/piriformis region are very common, in addition to tenderness over the greater trochanter. Spinal segmental dysfunctions are very common associations. There is no gold standard in investigations, with MRIs often only revealing an area of tendinopathy in the gluteal tendons in symptomatic patients; however, a very high percentage of asymptomatics have positive MRIs for tendinopathy.

A *British Medical Journal* editorial[16] reviewed the management of lateral hip pain and included reference to a randomised controlled trial,[17] which compared blind with X-ray-guided injections. They advised the following steps. First, take a detailed examination, where palpation and forced hip abduction should reproduce the patient's pain. Exclude an L3/4 intervertebral disc or facet joint as a source of referred pain. Since relevance of MRI findings is unknown, a blind injection is as effective as an X-ray guided one, and shows a 50:50 chance of positive outcome at three months. It seems reasonable to view some patients as having a gluteal tendinopathy, and therefore, by extrapolation of general principles of ameliorating tendon pain at various anatomical sites,[18] an eccentric exercise programme could be tried. The final resort is surgery to treat tendinopathy.

## Femoroacetabular impingement

Femoroacetabular impingement, as a concept and diagnostic entity, was first introduced in the late 1990s by Reinhold Ganz. It is regarded by many as a morphological condition that predisposes the hip to intra-articular pathology, which then becomes painful and is a precursor to OA.

There are two types of impingement: Cam deformity, in which there is an osseous ridge/bump at the femoral head/neck junction, and Pincer deformity, in which there is either a generalised or focal acetabular over-coverage. Cam is more common in young males, whilst Pincer is more common in middle-aged females. The clinical presentation can include: groin pain 48%, buttock/groin 7%, 'catching' sensation 56%, 'clicking' 23% and 'giving way' 7%.[19] Functionally, patients experience problems with dressing (socks/shoes), sitting for long periods and squatting. Examination is by passive flexion combined with adduction and internal rotation (positive in 95%) and/

or a positive (90%) FABER test. Investigations include plain X-rays reported by an experienced musculoskeletal radiologist. Second-line investigation is an MRI arthrogram. Management should include referral to an experienced hip surgeon practising hip arthroscopy, for full diagnostic work-up, which in some cases includes not just radiology but also intra-articular injection of local anaesthetic. There are still no long-term data on surgical outcomes of impingement surgery.

### References

1 • Peat G, McCarney R, Croft P. Knee pain and osteoarthritis in older adults: a review of community burden and current use of health care *Annals of the Rheumatic Diseases* 2001; **60(2)**: 91–7.

2 • Duncan R, Peat G, Thomas E, *et al.* Symptoms and radiographic osteoarthritis: not as discordant as they are made out to be? *Annals of the Rheumatic Diseases* 2007; **66(1)**: 86–91.

3 • Neogi T, Felson D, Niu J, *et al.* Association between radiographic features of knee osteoarthritis and pain: results from two cohort studies *British Medical Journal* 2009; **339**: b62844.

4 • Mackenzie R, Dixon AK, Keene GS, *et al.* Magnetic resonance imaging of the knee: assessment of effectiveness *Clinical Radiology* 1996; **51(4)**: 245–50.

5 • Warwick DJ *et al.* Influence of magnetic resonance imaging on a knee arthroscopy waiting list *Injury* 1993; **24(6)**: 380–2.

6 • Chan WP, Peterfy C, Fritz RC, *et al.* MR diagnosis of complete tears of the anterior cruciate ligament of the knee: importance of anterior subluxation of the tibia *American Journal of Roentgenology* 1994; **162**: 355–60.

7 • Trieshmann HW Jr, Mosure JC. The impact of magnetic resonance imaging of the knee on surgical decision making *Arthroscopy* 1996; **12(5)**: 550–5.

8 • Barry KP, Mesgarzadeh M, Triolo J, *et al.* Accuracy of MRI patterns in evaluating anterior cruciate ligament tears *Skeletal Radiology* 1996; **25(4)**: 365–70.

9 • Carmichael IW, MacLeod AM, Travlos J, *et al.* MRI can prevent unnecessary arthroscopy *Journal of Bone and Joint Surgery* 1997; **79(4)**: 624–5.

10 • Weinstabl R, Muellner T, Vecsei V, *et al.* Economic considerations for the diagnosis and therapy of meniscal lesions: can magnetic resonance imaging help reduce the expense? *World Journal of Surgery* 1997: **21(4)**: 363–8.

11 • DAMASK (Direct Access to Magnetic Resonance Imaging: Assessment for Suspect Knees) Trial Team. Influence of magnetic resonance imaging of the knee on GPs' decisions: a randomised trial *British Journal of General Practice* 2007; **57(541)**: 622–9.

12 • Gough-Palmer AL, Burnett C, Gedroyc WM. Open access to MRI for general practitioners: 12 years' experience at one institution – a retrospective analysis *British Journal of Radiology* 2009; **82(980)**: 687–90.

13 • National Collaborating Centre for Chronic Conditions. *Osteoarthritis: national clinical guideline for care and management in adults* London: Royal College of Physicians, 2008, www.nice.org.uk/CG59 [accessed October 2011].

14 • Tortolani PJ, Carbone JJ, Quartararo LG. Greater trochanteric pain syndrome in patients referred to orthopedic spine specialists *Spine Journal* 2002: **2(4)**: 251–4.

15 • Lievense A, Bierma-Zeinstra S, Schouten B, *et al*. Prognosis of trochanteric pain in primary care *British Journal of General Practice* 2005; **55(512)**: 199–204.

16 • Bahr R, Khan K. Management of lateral hip pain [editorial] *British Medical Journal* 2009; **338(7701)**.

17 • Cohen SP, Strassels SA, Foster L, *et al*. Comparison of fluoroscopically guided and blind corticosteroid injections for greater trochanteric pain syndrome: multicentre randomised controlled trial *British Medical Journal* 2009; **338**: b1088.

18 • Andres BM, Murrell GA. Treatment of tendinopathy: what works, what does not, and what is on the horizon *Clinical Orthopaedics and Related Research* 2008; **466(7)**: 1539–54.

19 • Neuman M, Cui Q, Siebenrock KA, *et al*. Impingement free hip motion: the normal alpha angle after chondroplasty *Clinical Orthopaedics and Related Research* 2008; **469(7)**: 699–703.

20 • Tobin S, Robinson G. The effect of McConnell's vastus lateralis inhibition taping technique on vastus lateralis and vastus medialis obliquus activity *Physiotherapy* 2000; **86(4)**: 173–83.

21 • Hinman RS, Crossley KM, McConnell J, *et al*. Efficacy of knee tape in the management of osteoarthritis of the knee: blinded randomised controlled trial *British Medical Journal* 2003; **327(7407)**: 135–8.

22 • Powell A, Teichtahl A, Wluka A, *et al*. Obesity: a preventable risk factor for large joint osteoarthritis which may act through biomechanical factors *British Journal of Sports Medicine* 2005; **39(1)**: 4–5.

23 • Hinman RS, Crossley KM. Patellofemoral joint osteoarthritis: an important subgroup of knee osteoarthritis *Rheumatology* 2007; **46(7)**: 1057–62.

24 • Fagan V, Delahunt E. Patellofemoral pain syndrome; a review on the associated neuromuscular deficits and the current treatment options *British Journal of Sports Medicine* 2008; **42(10)**: 789–95.

25 • Collins N, Crossley K, Beller E, *et al*. Foot orthoses and physiotherapy in the treatment of patellofemoral pain syndrome: randomised clinical trial *British Journal of Sports Medicine* 2009; **43(3)**: 169–71.

26 • Lau EM, Symmons DP, Croft P. The epidemiology of hip osteoarthritis and rheumatoid arthritis in the Orient *Clinical Orthopaedics and Related Research* 1996; **323**: 81–90.

27 • Bird PA, Oakley SP, Shnier R, *et al*. Prospective evaluation of magnetic resonance imaging and physical examination findings in patients with greater trochanteric pain syndrome *Arthritis and Rheumatology* 2001; **44(9)**: 2138–45.

28 • Blankenbaker DG, Ullrick SR, Davis KW, *et al*. Correlation of MRI findings with clinical findings of trochanteric pain syndrome *Skeletal Radiology* 2008; **37(10)**: 903–9.

29 • Kingzett-Taylor A, Tirman PF, Feller J, *et al*. Tendinosis and tears of gluteus medius and minimus muscles as a cause of hip pain: MRI imaging findings *American Journal of Roentgenology* 1999; **173(4)**: 1123–6.

## Appendix: Oxford Knee Score

| **Clinician's name (or ref.)** ........................................................ | **Patient's name (or ref.)** ........................................... |

*Please answer the following 12 multiple-choice questions*

During the past four weeks ...

**1** How would you describe the pain you usually have in your knee?

☐ None
☐ Very mild
☐ Mild
☐ Moderate
☐ Severe

**2** Have you had any trouble washing and drying yourself (all over) because of your knee?

☐ No trouble at all
☐ Very little trouble
☐ Moderate trouble
☐ Extreme difficulty
☐ Impossible to do

**3** Have you had any trouble getting in and out of the car or using public transport because of your knee? (With or without a stick)

☐ No trouble at all
☐ Very little trouble
☐ Moderate trouble
☐ Extreme difficulty
☐ Impossible to do

**4** For how long are you able to walk before the pain in your knee becomes severe? (With or without a stick)

☐ No pain >60 minutes
☐ 16–60 minutes
☐ 5–15 minutes
☐ Around the house only
☐ Not at all – severe on walking

**5** After a meal (sat at a table), how painful has it been for you to stand up from a chair because of your knee?

☐ Not at all painful
☐ Slightly painful
☐ Moderately pain
☐ Very painful
☐ Unbearable

**6** Have you been limping when walking, because of your knee?

☐ Rarely/never
☐ Sometimes or just at first
☐ Often, not just at first
☐ Most of the time
☐ All of the time

**7** Could you kneel down and get up again afterwards?

☐ Yes, easily
☐ With little difficulty
☐ With moderate difficulty
☐ With extreme difficulty
☐ No, impossible

**8** Are you troubled by pain in your knee at night in bed?

☐ Not at all
☐ Only one or two nights
☐ Some nights
☐ Most nights
☐ Every night

**9** How much has pain from your knee interfered with your usual work? (Including housework)

☐ Not at all
☐ A little bit
☐ Moderately
☐ Greatly
☐ Totally

**10** Have you felt that your knee might suddenly 'give away' or let you down?

☐ Rarely/never
☐ Sometimes or just at first
☐ Often, not at first
☐ Most of the time
☐ All the time

**11** Could you do household shopping on your own?

☐ Yes, easily

☐ With little difficulty

☐ With moderate difficulty

☐ With extreme difficulty

☐ No, impossible

**12** Could you walk down a flight of stairs?

☐ Yes, easily
☐ With little difficulty
☐ With moderate difficulty
☐ With extreme difficulty
☐ No, impossible

The Oxford
Knee Score ☐

## Grading for the Oxford Knee Score

| | |
|---|---|
| Score 0 to 19 | May indicate severe knee arthritis. It is highly likely that you may well require some form of surgical intervention. Contact your family physician for a consultation with an orthopaedic surgeon |
| Score 20 to 29 | May indicate moderate to severe knee arthritis. See your family physician for an assessment and X-ray. Consider a consultation with an orthopaedic surgeon |
| Score 30 to 39 | May indicate mild to moderate knee arthritis. Consider seeing your family physician for an assessment and possible X-ray. You may benefit from non-surgical treatment, such as exercise, weight loss, and/or anti-inflammatory medication |
| Score 40 to 48 | May indicate satisfactory joint function. May not require any formal treatment |

# Foot problems

6

*Anthony Redmond and Anne-Maree Keenan*

## Key learning points

▶ Foot problems are common in primary care but are missed if the foot is not assessed.

▶ The foot is a common site for the manifestation of systemic disease.

▶ The mechanical demands on the foot can cause local symptoms and will often exacerbate the symptoms of systemic disease.

▶ Mechanical therapies are often helpful either alone or in combination with pharmacological and other conventional treatments.

▶ Many of the best treatments for musculoskeletal foot problems can be mediated by the patient him or herself and do not require intensive intervention or referral.

## Introduction to foot problems

Foot pain is common with about 1 in 10 of all adults reporting significant foot pain at any one time. The incidence increases with age, with half of over-fifties reporting foot pain [1,2] and foot problems are as much as five times more common in females than males. [2–7] When present, foot pain impacts significantly on the patient, compromising function and impairing daily activities. [5,6,8–10] It is useful to remember also that foot problems are often concomitant with other musculoskeletal problems such as knee or hip pain [4,5,11,12] and this should be considered in assessment and treatment planning.

The importance of musculoskeletal pain in the foot has been well recognised in the systemic diseases such as rheumatoid arthritis, but most cases of foot pain occur in otherwise healthy people. [13–16] It is important to consider foot pathology in terms of both general health and local function.

This chapter aims to introduce the GP to the fundamentals of assessing the foot and its problems, to introduce the foot problems most commonly seen in primary care and to provide guidance on treatment and referral options.

## Assessing the foot

### *General approach to assessment*

It goes without saying that the foot should not be examined in isolation from the rest of the body, but the extent to which the foot is interdependent with proximal structures is easily underestimated. Deformity in neighbouring joints such as knees and hips can increase demands on the foot. Also, systemic problems, for example neuropathy, can manifest with specific signs in the feet. It is essential therefore to preface any musculoskeletal assessment of the foot with some consideration of the structures to which it is attached. As a minimum this should include:

▷ systemic disorders with a well-recognised effect on the structure and function of the foot (such as diabetes mellitus, peripheral neuropathy and inflammatory arthritis)
▷ spinal deformity (including neural tube defects, scoliosis, kyphosis and lordosis)
▷ hip alignment (ad/abduction and rotation)
▷ knee alignment (especially ad/abduction)
▷ muscle power reduction or imbalance (secondary to disease or trauma)
▷ neuropathy.

### *Assessment schema*

#### GALS / REMS

The GALS screen (gait, arms, legs and spine), if included as part of the routine musculoskeletal work-up, should have led to some assessment of the foot, although it is assumed that the reader of this chapter is interested in a more detailed local assessment. The foot components within the GALS screen are limited to a squeeze test across the metatarsals and a check for callosities.

The more recent Regional Examination of the Musculoskeletal System (REMS) proposed by Coady *et al.*[17] employs a more thorough lower-limb examination than the preliminary GALS screen (Box 6.1). It is a good starting point for the more detailed assessment of the foot described in this chapter.

The Leeds foot assessment protocol, which has now been well described,[18,19] is a much more comprehensive assessment of foot problems. However, it still employs a standard sequential approach of History → Observation → Examination, as represented in Figure 6.1 (or more precisely History + Look–Feel–Move).

---

Box 6.1 ○ *Regional Examination of the Musculoskeletal System*

---

- ▶ Examine sole of patient's feet.
- ▶ Recognize hallux valgus, claw and hammer toes.
- ▶ Assess the patient's feet in standing.
- ▶ Assess for flat feet (including patient standing on tiptoe).
- ▶ Recognise hindfoot/heel pathologies.
- ▶ Assess plantar- and dorsiflexion of the ankle.
- ▶ Assess movements of inversion and eversion of the foot.
- ▶ Assess the subtalar joint.
- ▶ Perform a lateral squeeze across the metatarsophalangeal (MTP) joints.
- ▶ Assess flexion/extension of the big toe.
- ▶ Examine the patient's footwear.

---

Figure 6.1 ○ *The Leeds foot assessment protocol*

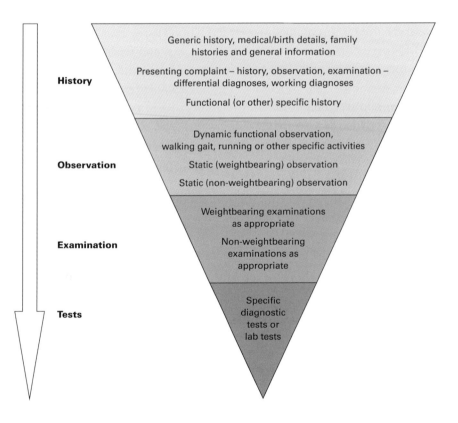

## Relevant history

The person-centred history-taking process starts with the usual medical, pharmacological and social history. In the absence of significant systemic factors, this will then be supplemented by relevant questions to assist with understanding of the local nature of the presenting foot problem. The presenting symptoms should be localised through a combination of description, direct indication by the patient if appropriate and, although not strictly history taking, by palpation or movement of the affected part. The characteristic features of the presenting symptoms should be determined as usual, along with any exacerbating or relieving factors. The past history of the symptoms including onset, change in character and any previous treatments should be noted.

## Look

The observation component will use the same sequential approach as employed by the whole assessment scheme, i.e. working from broad to narrow. Observations are made on the effect of both weightbearing and non-weightbearing. The most logical overview is provided by a general assessment of walking followed by observation of the legs and feet with the patient standing still. This is followed by observations made with the patient seated or lying supine (i.e. non-weightbearing). It is helpful to observe the transition between non-weightbearing and weightbearing to note any changes that occur as the limb accepts weight.

### Gait and weightbearing assessment

Observation of the patient walking and standing is essential to understand how the foot and lower limb function together. Watching the patient as he or she walks in to a consultation is an ideal way to commence. If possible, get the patient to walk along an unencumbered area, noting symmetry and general fluidity of walking.

### Observation of gait and still standing

The overall gait should be evaluated, noting the following:

▷ presence/absence of major gait abnormality, e.g. festination, Rombergism, Trendelenburg gait, foot drop
▷ presence of limp
▷ general fluidity and symmetry of walking.

Top-down evaluation should then be carried out (conducted first with the patient walking and again in still standing), as follows:

▷ **head** ▶ carriage/tilt
▷ **shoulders** ▶ level
▷ **arms** ▶ swing and carriage
▷ **spine** ▶ curvature
▷ **pelvis/hips** ▶ level, ad/abduction, rotation
▷ **knees** ▶ rotation/patellar position and varus/valgus
▷ **ankles** ▶ varus/valgus
▷ **feet** ▶ planus/cavus (see later section).

The patient can be directed to undertake a range of specific gait 'tests' such as heel–toe walking, stair climbing, sit-to-stand and others but these are beyond the remit of this chapter.

## Non-weightbearing observations

The following should be observed:

▷ **bones – proximal to distal**
  ▶ check overall limb alignment
  ▶ look for fixed deformity in the leg/ankle
  ▶ foot deformity – varus/valgus heels, midfoot deformity, bunions and clawing of the digits
▷ **joints – proximal to distal**
  ▶ swelling (including osteophytes) and/or discolouration of the joints of: ankle/hindfoot/midfoot/forefoot
▷ **soft tissue – proximal to distal**
  ▶ evaluate for swellings over joints and prominences (oedema or bursae), thickened tendons (tenosynovitis)
▷ **skin – proximal to distal**
  ▶ general appearance, oedema, contracture and presence of callosities.

---

Box 6.2 ○ *Clinical note – weightbearing versus non-weightbearing assessment*

The majority of musculoskeletal foot disorders presenting in primary care relate to weightbearing function or the consequences of weightbearing function. While the assessment process includes elements of both weightbearing and non-weightbearing structure and function, this is for clinical convenience only and care must be taken that the interpretation of the results includes consideration of the *actual function* of the limbs during normal activities.

## Feel

Assuming that the presenting symptoms have been evaluated thoroughly, the palpation component of the general assessment is really just an extension of the observations. Using the same proximal to distal approach coupled with systematic and sequential refinement, i.e. bone, joint, soft tissue, skin, the examiner can palpate joints for swelling, temperature and tenderness to palpation.

## Move

The final part of the regional assessment is to evaluate the movements of the ankle and foot. The patient should be encouraged to move the part him or herself first (i.e. active motion) while the examiner can place a hand over the joints to feel for crepitus without assisting the patient. Only once the patient has indicated his or her potential range of movement should the examiner conduct an assessment of passive movement.

Problems with quality of movement may manifest as pain, crepitus, clicks and clunks or unevenness in speed of rotation. The direction of movement should be consistent with anatomical function, as even minor deviations in position or tracking can be problematic when repeated over millions of gait cycles. The amount of movement in each joint will vary according to site and function. Restriction in some joints can be compensated for readily elsewhere, while minor deviations from normal in others lead to significant impairment. Rules of thumb for adequate motion in foot joints are given in Box 6.3. The end of the available range will be limited by bony block, limits of soft-tissue extension, or abutment to neighbouring structures.

## Other investigations

### X-ray

Plain films will differentiate gross radiographic features such as joint space narrowing, osteophyte formation or periarticular erosion. However, the images are limited to two dimensions and visualisation of soft tissues – often the cause of foot pain – is poor. The most usual sequence request is for an antero-posterior view (AP) combined with a lateral view. Other views will help visualise specific aspects of foot anatomy but the complexity of the structures of the foot often renders X-ray inconclusive. The more subtle mus-

---

**Box 6.3 ○ *Rules of thumb for normal joint motions in the ankle and foot***

---

**Ankle:**

▶ max. dorsiflexion = ±10°
▶ max. plantarflexion = ±30°

**Hindfoot:**

▶ total inversion/eversion = ±30°
  (distributed either equally or slightly in favour of inversion)

**Midfoot:**

▶ inversion/eversion/circumduction (no ranges *per se* but movement
  should be free and of adequate quality)

**Toe joints (especially 1st toe):**

▶ max. dorsiflexion = ±40°
▶ max. plantarflexion N/A

---

culoskeletal foot pathologies will often require more sophisticated imaging approaches such as MRI, CT or ultrasound, as detailed below.

## MRI/CT

Magnetic resonance imaging (MRI) allows good visualisation of soft-tissue structures such as ligaments, tendons and synovium. Standard sequences (T1W, T2W, proton density and STIR), particularly when enhanced with a contrast agent, provide good differentiation of healthy and inflamed soft tissues, and early identification of bone lesions.[20,21] MRI remains relatively expensive and difficult to access, and is rarely available as a first resort. For high-resolution imaging of bony structures in the foot, computed tomography (CT) remains the modality of choice for visualising subtle fractures or small bone lesions.

## HRUS

High-resolution ultrasound (HRUS) is increasingly used in primary and secondary care settings as it requires no exposure to ionisation radiation, it visualises soft tissues structures well and is relatively inexpensive.[21,22] HRUS can differentiate inflamed and healthy soft tissues readily, and importantly can investigate structures dynamically.[23,24] Where features of interest lie deep to the surface, or lie in the ultrasound shadow of structures that form a barrier to the imaging signal, HRUS is more limited. This can be a problem in imaging hips and knees but is less of an issue for structures of the foot and ankle.

## General foot problems

### Structural problems

#### FLAT FEET AND CAVUS FEET

One of the more common foot complaints presenting in primary care is so-called 'flat feet'. Crucially, many 'flat feet' are asymptomatic and many primary care consultations, particularly for flat feet in children, are for reassurance rather than to address specific pain or impairment.

While some feet do indeed present with marked and significant flattening of the medial arch, most so-called flat feet are a rather more complex entity than may first appear. First, it must be appreciated that the range of foot postures forms a continuum from cavoid (or highly arched), through normal, to flat (or planus). This continuum is roughly normally distributed, as one would expect of most anatomical variants. At the extremes of this continuum are features that are clearly pathological (such as the frank cavus foot of inherited neuropathy or the plano-valgus foot of established rheumatoid arthritis). Between these extremes, however, care must be exercised to avoid medicalising normal variants while acknowledging that abnormal foot posture can predispose to mechanical foot pain. Obviously the further towards the margin of the normal distribution a given foot lies, the greater the likelihood that presenting local foot pain may be linked to the foot type. Pathologies associated with flat and high arched feet are discussed subsequently.

While many primary care practitioners need only to recognise the basic features, a degree of quantification is helpful sometimes, for instance to provide a baseline prior to surgical referral or if the foot is changing shape. Many measures can be used but a simple rating scale, such as the Foot Posture Index[25] (www.leeds.ac.uk/medicine/FASTER/fpi.htm), can be helpful in quantifying foot posture quickly in the clinical setting (see Table 6.1).

#### CONDITIONS ASSOCIATED WITH FLAT FEET

'Flat feet' is a rather colloquial label and there is no specific validated definition as the presentation can vary. A useful working definition would describe a *weightbearing* foot posture where three characteristics are observable each to a greater or lesser extent: 1) the heel is in a valgus position, 2) the medial arch is flattened and 3) the foot is abducted away for the midline. It is important that the suspected flat or excessively pronated foot is assessed weightbearing. This is because the flattening is most often functional and the features will often disappear when the foot is non-weightbearing.

The heel raise test (Figure 6.2 on p. 142) should be performed whenever flat feet are being investigated to rule out fixed deformity, which can occur in

Table 6.1  ○  **Foot Posture Index**

| | | | Score 1 Date ........ Comment ........ | | Score 2 Date ........ Comment ........ | | Score 3 Date ........ Comment ........ | |
|---|---|---|---|---|---|---|---|---|
| **Factor** | **Plane** | | **Left** -2 to +2 | **Right** -2 to +2 | **Left** -2 to +2 | **Right** -2 to +2 | **Left** -2 to +2 | **Right** -2 to +2 |
| Rearfoot | Talar head palpation | Transverse | | | | | | |
| | Curves above and below the lateral malleolus | Frontal/transverse | | | | | | |
| | Inversion/eversion of the calcaneus | Frontal | | | | | | |
| Forefoot | Prominence in the region of the TNJ | Transverse | | | | | | |
| | Congruence of the medial longitudinal arch | Sagittal | | | | | | |
| | Abd/adduction forefoot on rearfront | Transverse | | | | | | |
| | Total | | | | | | | |

Reference values: Normal = 0 to +5 | Pronated = +6 to +9, highly pronated 10+ | Supinated = –1 to –4, highly supinated –5 to –12

*Source:* copyright © Anthony Redmond 1998. www.leeds.ac.uk/medicine/FASTER/.
(May be copied for clinical use and adapted with the permission of the copyright holder.)

Figure 6.2 ○ *A flexible pronated foot demonstrating inversion of the heel when raised on to tiptoe*

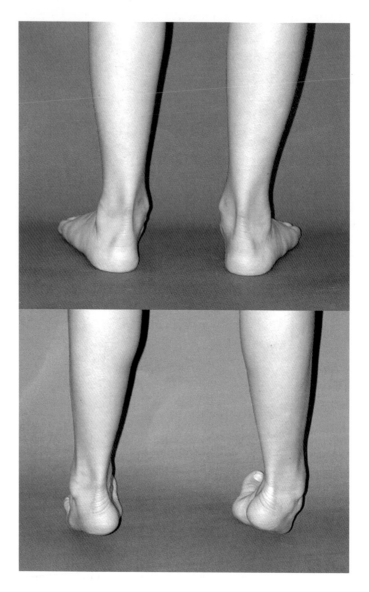

the presence of, for instance, tarsal coalitions. In the flexible flat foot, standing on tiptoe will restore the medial arch and invert the heels.

### ASYMPTOMATIC FLAT FEET

These are a common presentation, particularly in childhood where concerned parents have worries over a child's normal development and a sympathetic, person-centred approach to reassurance or action is important.

Normal values for the Foot Posture Index have been published[26] and these can be used as a reference for asymptomatic flat feet. As a rule, a child's foot posture will be significantly more flattened at first walking, with a more adult foot posture developing over the first seven years of life. There is no evidence that early functional treatment in asymptomatic cases will improve long-term outcomes, although *fixed* flat-foot posture warrants early referral. Markedly flat feet that persist into the teens probably warrants further consideration, although formal criteria are difficult to apply. Treatment of adult flat foot, unless fixed, should be predicated on pain not posture.

### SYMPTOMATIC FLAT FEET

Foot pain of mechanical origin may arise through a variety of mechanisms, most of which are not particularly well understood. Links have been postulated between pronated foot function and a range of musculoskeletal conditions either in the foot (heel and arch pain and forefoot problems such as bunions)[27,28] or proximally in the leg (e.g. patellofemoral or other knee pain and shin splints).[29,30] In most cases the evidence supporting these theoretical links are not strong. However, as with any pain of musculoskeletal origin, consideration of any potential causal relationships between function, anatomy and symptoms is appropriate.

Key features that will increase the index of suspicion for a causal link between foot posture and a patient's presenting pain are: the severity of flat-footedness, proximity of the symptom to the hindfoot (i.e. arch pain is more likely than hip pain to arise from abnormal foot posture), presence of systemic pathology such as joint hypermobility (Figure 6.3 on p. 474), the relationship with specific activities such as walking or running, and either the total amount of activity or relative change in activity levels (such as longer mileages or increasing mileages in recreational runners). The assessing practitioner can use generic problem-solving skills to establish whether the posture and symptoms are linked. If the foot posture is thought a risk factor for foot pain then other mechanical factors should also be considered including body mass and suitability of footwear.

Treatment of the flexible flat foot is aimed at improving posture and can include exercises, insoles and footwear advice as discussed later in this chapter.

### CAVUS / CAVOID FEET

The cavus or cavoid foot is characterised by a high medial arch and contracture of the lesser toes. The most extreme example is the club-foot or *talipes equino-varus* deformity, but more subtle variants may present in primary care. Frank pes cavus is usually observed in adults and is almost always of neurogenic origin (Figure 6.4 on p. 474). However, even the most obvious cavus foot may take time to develop. In childhood the foot may make a subtle transition from a fairly normal posture, through increasing degrees of cavoid features, before reaching a frankly pathological posture. Many more feet will demonstrate some but not all features of the pes cavus foot type and these are often termed 'cavoid'. In orthopaedics, the peek-a-boo heel sign, where the heel is visible on the medial side of the ankle when looking at the foot from directly in front of the patient, is used as a useful rule of thumb for identifying the cavoid foot.

In many cases there is a specific, if latent, underlying neurological condition and these cases are termed 'neurogenic' cavoid feet. Others will present with cavoid foot features in the absence of known neurological deficit and these are termed 'idiopathic' cavoid feet.

The presence of cavoid foot postures in children up to the age of ten or so should never be considered normal, and the child presenting with a cavoid foot type should be referred promptly for a comprehensive orthopaedic and/or neurological assessment. Conditions that could be considered include undiagnosed talipes, inherited peripheral neuropathy and neural tube defects. In adults presenting with symptomatic cavoid features, differentiation between neurogenic and idiopathic cases can be quite difficult, with minor neurological deficits often not readily detectable in the primary care setting.

Whatever the underlying pathology the characteristic consequences of the cavoid foot are: poor shock absorbency leading to risk of lower back, knee and heel pain; strain on flexor soft tissues, particularly the tendo Achilles and plantar fascia, increasing risk of calf and arch pain; and forefoot pain associated with higher than normal plantar pressures.[31] Treatments for the cavoid foot are aimed at improving shock absorbency and stretching tight soft tissues. Treatments will include cushioning insoles, change in footwear and stretching exercises, as discussed later in the chapter (see pp. 160–3).

## Arthritis

### OSTEOARTHRITIS

While considerable attention has been given to the impact and management of knee and hip osteoarthritis (OA), the foot and ankle are common sites for OA. Symptomatic foot OA prevalence may be as high as 1 in 5 in people aged between 24 and 75[32] and in the older population this could be as high as 4 in 5 adults.[33] The first MTP joint is the most common site of OA within the foot,[34] with the midtarsal and tarsometatarsal joint also affected commonly (Figure 6.5 on p. 474). OA is not usually seen in the ankle unless secondary to major trauma (e.g. complex ankle fracture), repeated minor trauma (e.g. recurrent ankle sprains) or following inflammatory arthritis. The typical clinical features are pain, particularly on weightbearing, swelling due to osteophyte formation or synovitis, limitation of movement and difficulty walking. Other joints in the foot are affected more sporadically, most commonly following trauma.[34]

On plain X-ray there will usually be osteophytic change evident as well as joint space narrowing. However, the importance of radiographic confirmation in OA has been recently questioned.[35,36] The diagnosis of foot OA is adequately made on the basis of the presence of joint pain, limitation of joint range of movement and palpable osteophytes.

Risk factors that have been associated with OA include genetic predisposition,[37] obesity,[38,39] diminished bone mineral density,[40] female gender[39] and insufficient nutrition.[41] In addition to these factors localised joint or direct mechanical influences, especially important considerations in the foot, include joint overloading (including occupational[42] and sporting participation[43]), joint malalignment,[39,44,45] previous joint trauma[46] and existing joint pathology, such as ligament damage.[47] OA in the ankle and foot is rarely seen in isolation: the most common combination of sites with foot OA are, perhaps unsurprisingly, the knee and hip.[48] Treatment should take the impact of other sites of pain into account.

The most common presentation of OA in the foot is as hallux limitus, hallux rigidus or hallux valgus. In these presentations degenerative changes at the first MTP joint lead to functional limitation.[49] Midfoot OA is also common, although is typically fairly silent clinically. It has been suggested that midfoot degenerative disease is associated with pes planus,[50] although the extent of any systematic relationship between foot function and OA at specific sites is yet to be established.

OA can be well managed in primary care. Pain is the most important symptom to both patient and physician alike:[51] It is the major impetus for people with OA to seek treatment[52] and is the general focus of most therapies. Treatment of OA should involve a holistic approach and individualised self-management strategies. The NICE guidance for treating OA (www.nice.org.uk/CG059)[53] is presented in Figure 6.6. The core treatments of education, exercise and weight loss if appropriate are represented in the middle of the circle, with consideration given to the second ring, which contains relatively safe pharmaceutical options. The NICE guidance principles are as relevant for foot OA as for arthritis in other joints.

Footwear change is a first option for many people with foot OA and this is discussed later in the chapter. Referral to a podiatrist for a functional assessment and relevant treatment is warranted in intractable cases, although direct referral for surgery can be considered.

Figure 6.6 ○ *Targeting treatment in OA – recommendations from the NICE OA guideline*

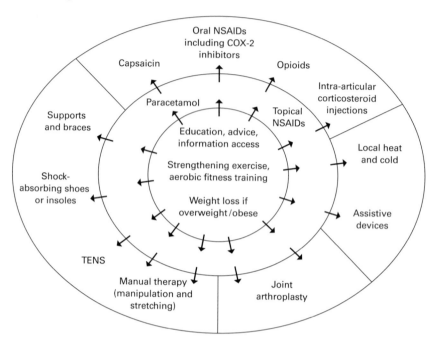

## RHEUMATOID ARTHRITIS

In primary care the two areas of main concern are in the diagnosis of new cases and community-based management of existing cases. The foot is the first site of involvement in about 1 in 8 cases of RA, and some 20% of patients report foot pain before any other manifestation of the disease.[54] GPs have an important role in the early recognition of as yet undiagnosed inflammatory arthritis.[55]

A European consensus statement identified referral recommendations on the basis of:[56]

▷ three or more swollen joints
▷ pain on lateral compression of the metacarpo- or metatarso-phalangeal joints (a positive squeeze test)
▷ morning stiffness of ≥ 30 minutes' duration.

More recently this has been summarised in a public awareness campaign endorsed by the Royal College of General Practitioners under the banner 'Have you got the S factor?' encouraging recognition of the triumvirate of Swelling, Stiffness and Squeeze test.

Patients with an existing diagnosis of rheumatoid or other inflammatory arthritis will usually be under the ongoing care of a hospital consultant. Some will be managed using a comprehensive approach with both the consultant and GP working under formal shared-care arrangements. For other patients, care will be more *ad hoc*, combining hospital-based care with other areas (such as foot care) often provided in a primary care setting. Guidelines for the management of foot problems for people with RA are set out in NICE guidance.[57] The NICE guideline recommends referral to a podiatrist for all people with RA and foot problems. The governing principles are for disease control to be stabilised by the consultant (in conjunction with the GP) while the mechanical consequences of the disease in the foot need to be addressed by a relevant specialist (podiatrist, nurse, physio, OT or orthopaedic surgeon) in either primary or secondary care, depending on local resources. Recent advances in biologic therapies have improved the prognosis for new cases of RA markedly.

### Seronegative inflammatory arthritis (psoriatic arthritis, ankylosing spondylitis, reactive arthritis)

The seronegative arthritides are a diverse group of conditions with a number of common features, the most obvious of which are an association with the HLA-B27 antigen, spinal involvement and inflammation of the entheses.[24] The foot is often involved because of the combined effect of systemic disease and local mechanical demands. Common sites for enthesopathy in the foot are the heel at the insertion of the tendo Achilles or the plantar fascia, and the forefoot.[24,58] In the toes the enthesitis and synovitis can present as marked dactylitis or 'sausage digits' and this is an important sign in undiagnosed seronegative arthritis. Imaging findings in the foot include periarticular proliferation of periosteum and bone on X-ray, and inflammation at the entheses on MRI or ultrasound.

Foot involvement is common in psoriatic arthritis, relatively uncommon (about 20% of cases) in ankylosing spondylitis and is often the first sign in reactive arthritis. Involvement of the foot in ankylosing spondylitis is usually transient and tends not to progress to severe degenerative joint disease.[24,59] Psoriatic arthritis will often present initially in the digits[60] and inflammation at the entheses results in bony erosions.[59] Forefoot involvement can be very severe while the midfoot is not often involved in psoriatic arthritis. Hindfoot involvement is similar to that of other seronegative arthropathies causing insertional heel pain.[24,61] Bony proliferation of the entheses and spur formation may cause deformity and discomfort around the heel.[59,60]

In reactive arthritis, multiple tendon involvement can cause diffuse swelling around the ankle.[59] Forefoot involvement is usually confined to the interphalangeal joint of the hallux.[59,60] For all of the seronegative diseases, once the diagnosis is made and the systemic disease reasonably well controlled, the local symptoms in the foot can be managed by local corticosteroid injection, appropriate footwear and provision of padding or orthoses to provide mechanical relief.[62]

### Systemic sclerosis/scleroderma

The foot will be affected during the course of the disease in about 90% of patients with systemic sclerosis, although foot involvement is less common and less severe than in the hands.[63] Disorders of the skin and vascular system are the most common but the skeletal structures of the foot are involved in three quarters of patients with progressive systemic sclerosis. With improvement in the management of the systemic effects (pulmonary artery hypertension, renal fibrosis, etc.) there is greater awareness of the peripheral complications. Raynaud's syndrome occurs in the feet of about 90% of sufferers, the incidence increasing with disease duration.[63] Localised vasculitic lesions and ulcers, typically on the dorsum of the forefoot and apices of toes, are common and can be long-lasting. The combination of skin and subcutaneous fibrosis, along with the changes in the underlying skeletal structures, lead to difficulties with shoes,[64] and these patients may require assistance with sourcing adequate footwear. It is desirable that all patients with systemic sclerosis undergo regular checks of their foot health and have ready access to foot health services where follow-up is needed.

### Gout

Gout occurs in around 1% of men and 0.3–0.6% of women.[65,66] In the foot, the first MTP joint is most commonly affected. The initial presentation is typically a severe and acute monoarthritis, often of the first MTP joint and lasting a few days. More diffuse swelling can result if more than one joint is involved.[67] Onset of gout will occur in the first MTP joint in about half of cases, although it is also seen in other sites in the foot including the lesser MTP joints, the first interphalangeal joint, midfoot joints, the subtalar joint and the ankle.[68,69] Pseudogout presents with a less severe synovitis and affects larger joints such as the ankle and knee.[69] In the chronically gouty joint,

Figure 6.7 ○ *T2W MRI of a navicular stress fracture with cortical breach*

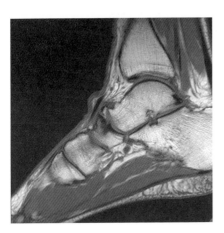

*Source*: Redmond AC, Helliwell PS, Robinson P. Investigating foot and ankle problems.[70]

Figure 6.8 ○ *T2W MRI of a grade 3 metatarsal stress reaction demonstrating intense bony oedema in the intermediate cuneiform and 2nd metatarsal bones*

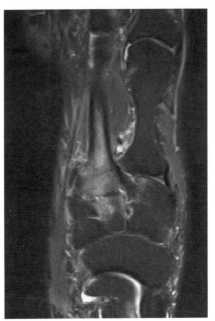

149

there will be considerable joint damage, which in the later stages may require excision or replacement to resolve symptoms.[66] In addition to systemic treatment (high-dose non-steroidal anti-inflammatory drugs (NSAIDs), allopurinol, febuxostat), footwear and orthotics may assist with symptoms in the chronic stage through off-loading the damaged joint.

### Bone stress reactions and stress fractures

Stress fractures are a partial or complete fracture resulting from repeated, low-grade application of a stress. Bone stress reaction is an alteration to the physiology of bone that can be symptomatic but is not associated with a loss of continuity of the cortex. There are two main classifications of stress fracture: overuse stress fractures, in which relatively healthy bone is exposed to an increased repetitive trauma, such as those seen in athletes who have changed their training regimen; and insufficiency stress fractures, which are associated with an underlying deficiency in bone stock, such as with osteoporosis.

The navicular is a common site for stress reaction and fracture in the foot, especially in highly active people (see Figure 6.7). They are characterised by a history of high or rapidly increased activity, diffuse pain in the mid-foot, exacerbation on activity and increasing intensity and localisation of pain. Diagnosis is tricky clinically and even plain film radiography does not show these fractures well; MRI or CT is preferred. Stress fractures or 'march fractures' of the shaft of the metatarsal (most commonly the 2nd, 3rd and 5th) are also common and occur in response to repetitive excessive loading or activity or as insufficiency fractures if bone density is reduced. The clinical presentation is again a diffuse pain in the affected region exacerbated by activity. Palpation of the affected bone reveals focal tenderness, but in some areas, such as the navicular, the fracture site is intra-articular and therefore difficult to assess. Stress fracture is often preceded by intense and painful bony oedema visible on MRI or scintigraphy (see Figure 6.8).

If the cause is addressed, most overuse stress fractures will heal without complications within a relatively short timeframe. Rest or modification of activity to reduce pain is indicated. For overuse stress fractures, particular attention should be given to changes in activity level or training, new activity or poor footwear. For insufficiency stress fractures, treatment of the underlying bone stock fragility (e.g. with bisphosphonates) is indicated. There is, however, a tension in treating insufficiency stress fractures within the lower limb: while rest is generally indicated, weightbearing activities are also important to maximise bone stock. Appropriate footwear and/or orthoses, which off-load the affected area, may help.

There are a number of sites in the foot that are prone to complications, including delayed or non-union. These include the talus, navicular and the fifth metatarsal. These should be treated with non-weightbearing cast immobilisation and onward referral is the best option.

### Nerve entrapments

Due to the sheer number of bones and bony prominences, the foot and ankle are common sites for nerve entrapments. Symptoms generally begin as sharp pain, numbness and/or tingling, radiating distally from the site of entrapment and exacerbated by activity. If left untreated, symptoms can radiate proximally, and may result in constant discomfort. Where the entrapment is superficial, a reproduction of symptoms can be elicited by percussion of the site. For deeper impingements, imaging may assist with diagnosis. The general principles of treatment centre on identification and removal of the cause, which may include surgical excision.

## Morton's neuroma

Morton's neuroma is a common nerve entrapment of the plantar digital nerve just proximal to the metatarsal heads. It is commonly seen in the third and fourth metatarsal space, but can occur between any digits. Several theories exist as to why this area is commonly affected, none of which is definitive. Morton's neuroma is not a true neuroma but a fibrotic enlargement of the perineureum and it is unclear whether the fibrosis is the cause of the pain or simply the result of ongoing tissue irritation. Tight footwear and high-heeled shoes often exacerbate symptoms. Clinical diagnosis can be made by squeezing the forefoot at the metatarsal area, while exerting a downward pressure between the digits of the affected area, which will often result in reproduction of symptoms. Ultrasound investigation suggests, though, that there is over-diagnosis of neuroma using clinical assessment alone. Treatment involves identification of the cause and removal, and may include footwear advice (wider fittings), local injection of steroid, orthoses or oral NSAIDs. In severe or chronic cases, surgical referral is indicated.

## Tarsal tunnel syndrome

As the tibial nerve passes around the medial aspect of the ankle where it is closely associated with the tendons under the flexor retinaculae, the nerve may become compressed. Symptoms of tingling, numbness and pain are generally felt in the arch area, but may also extend to the plantar area and medial aspect of the ankle. Tarsal tunnel syndrome may be caused by chronic inflammation of the tendons, such as seen with tibialis posterior syndrome, or compression secondary to severe valgus position of the ankle, such as seen in rheumatoid arthritis. Clinical diagnosis is made by reproduction of symptoms through percussion of the area (Tinel's sign). For positional compressions, short-term reduction of symptoms can be achieved by splinting or taping the ankle into a neutral or slight varus position, and orthoses may help in the longer term. In severe cases, referral for surgical assessment is required. Where the compression arises from local inflammation (e.g. tenosynovitis) local injection of steroid may be helpful.

## Impingement syndromes and accessory bones

Ankle impingement syndromes can occur due to overgrowth of bone or the presence of accessory ossicles at the joint margin. Impingement may occur posteriorly, anteriorly or antero-laterally. Posterior impingement is characterised by tenderness in the posterior ankle margin, not associated with the tendo-Achilles and develops secondarily to repeated or forced ankle plantar-flexion, e.g. in ballet dancers, jumping athletes, squash and football players.

Anterior impingement arises due to repeated supination/inversion injury or repeated dorsiflexion of the ankle. Chronic damage to the chondral margins ultimately causes enchondral ossification resulting in the formation of bone spurs. In all types of suspected impingement syndromes only imaging is diagnostic, with plain films and MRI the preferred modalities.

---

## Regional foot problems

### Ankle pain

#### ANKLE SPRAINS

Acute ankle injuries can present in primary care and care must be taken to ensure that more severe soft-tissue injuries and fractures are not missed. The Ottawa ankle rules for X-ray requirement are a useful triage for suitability of a presenting acute ankle sprain for local primary care management.

**The Ottawa ankle rules** – X-rays are only required if there is pain in the malleolar zone and any one of the following is present:

▷ bone tenderness along the distal 6 cm of the posterior edge of the tibia or tip of the medial malleolus, **or**
▷ bone tenderness along the distal 6 cm of the posterior edge of the fibula or tip of the lateral malleolus, **or**
▷ an inability to bear weight both immediately and in the clinic for four steps.

The most common site of ankle sprain is the lateral ankle. This is due to the shape of the ankle mortise, the motions encountered and the relative weakness of the composite lateral ligaments. Table 6.2 shows the site, mechanism and assessment of ankle sprains.

#### COMPLICATIONS OF ANKLE SPRAINS

Severe ankle sprain and chronic ankle instability can lead to osteochondral defects in the articular surface of the talus and the tibia. If ankle pain is chronic following sprain injury, osteochondral lesions should be considered. Fractures of the talar dome or the styloid process of the fifth metatarsal should also be considered, particularly with inversion and plantar flexion injuries. With severe sprains, such as shown in Figure 6.9 (see p. 474), imaging (typically MRI or CT) is required and surgical referral may be needed.

Table 6.2 ○ *Site, mechanism of injury and clinical assessment of ankle sprains*

| Ligament | Mechanism of injury | Clinical assessment |
| --- | --- | --- |
| Anterior talotibial ligament* | Plantar flexion and inversion injury | Pain on inversion and dorsiflexion of the foot while stabilising the ankle |
| Posterior talotibial | Dorsiflexion and inversion injury | Pain on inversion and plantarflexion of the foot while stabilising the ankle |
| Talofibular ligament* | Inversion injury | Pain on inversion of the foot while stabilising the ankle |
| Medial collateral ligament | Severe eversion force | Given the anatomy of the area, this is unusual. Pain on eversion, but other complications, such as fracture of the tibial or navicular tuberosity, should also be excluded on imaging |
| Interosseous tibiofibular ligament | Lateral ankle sprain with twisting and significant loading | Difficult to assess clinically; MR will confirm the diagnosis |

* Commonly occur together.

### Chronic ankle instability

Chronic ankle instability is a syndrome that is characterised by a sensation of the ankle 'giving way', when the foot in placed in even a mild amount of weightbearing inversion. While this may not result in any other symptoms, some patients report persistent swelling and discomfort. Chronic ankle instability is thought to be a complication of an inadequately rehabilitated ankle sprain. Given the dynamic nature of the condition, diagnosis is made generally on patient history and clinical signs and symptoms.

Non-surgical treatment for chronic ankle instability centres on physiotherapy, strengthening the peroneal muscles and improving proprioception. Bracing or taping will assist, particularly when used during activities where there is a risk of ankle sprain. If there is a lack of response to non-surgical treatments, referral for surgical evaluation with a view to stabilisation may be necessary.

## Achilles tendonopathy

The Achilles tendon is often a site for traumatic or degenerative damage. The regions most often affected are the myotendinous junction and the insertion into the calcaneus. The Achilles tendon is not invested in a synovial sheath so tenosynovitis cannot occur; however, the relatively poor blood supply to the tendon increases the risk of intrasubstance tendonopathy.

The Achilles tendon may be damaged as a result of either repetitive overload or an acute injury. Traumatic tears usually occur during rapid, unexpected dorsiflexion, such as tripping, or during unaccustomed activity, such as a sudden return to sporting activities. Full-thickness tears are obvious on clinical examination with absent plantar flexion power on the affected side. This requires urgent surgical intervention.

Diagnosis of partial tear is often made solely on clinical examination with symptoms of pain and swelling over the tendon exacerbated by weightbearing and dorsiflexion of the foot. In the latter, chronic state there is a thickening of the tendon body proximal to the insertion, where the bloody supply is poor. A fusiform swelling may be palpable and confirmed on MR or ultrasound imaging, where small longitudinal or, less commonly, transverse tears may be evident (Figure 6.10 on p. 475). Risk factors for chronic Achilles tendinosis include previous injury and older age.

While the evidence for the treatment for Achilles tendonitis remains sparse, Alfredson and Cook[71] have recently proposed a treatment algorithm based on the best evidence available (Figure 6.11, overleaf). The initial treatment includes RICER (Rest, Ice, Compression, Elevation and Rehabilitation); off-loading of the Achilles (through either taping or a heel lift) and careful eccentric strengthening exercises for the calf muscles are recommended. Physiotherapy referral should be considered and where there is a suspected significant rupture, surgical advice should be sought.

## Tibialis posterior tendon dysfunction

Tibialis posterior dysfunction (TPD) is a syndrome in which progressive tendonopathy of the tibialis posterior tendon causes an acquired flat foot in adults. Patients (typically post-menopausal females) present with pain and swelling on the medial aspect of the ankle, extending into the dorsum and arch area. There is often concern over the changing shape of the foot, particularly a progressive flattening of the arch. As the tendon deteriorates, the foot develops into a marked and progressively valgus position, with a flattened arch and an abducted forefoot. The patient is unable to single-limb stand on

Figure 6.11  ○  ***Treatment algorithm for the management of Achilles tendonitis***

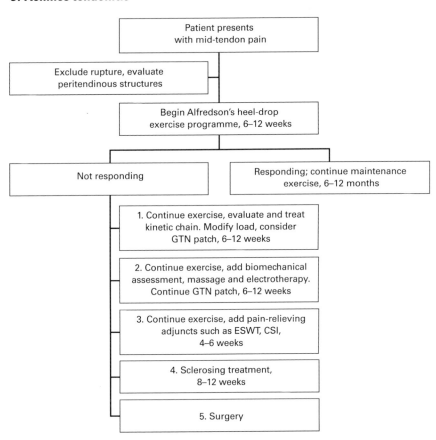

*Source*: adapted from Alfredson and Cook.[71]

*Abbreviations*: CSI = corticosteroid injection | ESWT = extracorporeal shock wave therapy | GTN = topical glyceryl trinitrate.

tip-toe on the affected side, unless counterbalanced by the contralateral limb. Stages of TPD are summarised in Table 6.3.

Diagnosis can now be made readily using ultrasound as a cost-effective alternative to MRI.[74] Early identification and treatment will help prevent progression, maintaining the integrity of the joints of the foot. Early non-surgical treatment is centred around reducing symptoms and off-loading the tendon and midfoot with orthoses, supportive footwear, high-Dye ankle taping and ankle bracing. Surgical treatment options include tendon transfer in the early stages, combined with rearfoot osteotomy. In severe cases reconstruction and arthrodesis of the rearfoot is necessary.

Table 6.3 ○ *Classification of TPD*

| Stage | Description |
|---|---|
| I | The arch is maintained but tibialis post-tendon is inflamed |
| II | The tendon is no longer functional and there is an acquired flat foot |
| III | There is an acquired flat foot and the subtalar joint valgus cannot be passively reduced |
| IV | There are arthritic changes in the ankle |

*Note*: based on Johnson and Strom,[72] with modification by Myerson.[73]

### Heel pain

#### PLANTAR HEEL PAIN

Plantar heel pain is one of the most common foot problems presenting in primary care, affecting 1 in 10 people at some stage in their lives.[75] Chronic pain under the heel most often arises due to pathology of the plantar fascia, irritation at the insertion of the fascia or bony spur formation. Bruising of the plantar fat pad can also cause discomfort, although is usually self-limiting.

The most common of the underlying pathologies is plantar fasciitis, characterised by thickening and, very occasionally, frank inflammation of the plantar fascia. The pathology may involve a length of the fascia or may be localised to the proximal attachment (enthesopathy). Heel spurs at the calcaneal attachment of the fascia can contribute to plantar heel pain but are a common incidental finding on plain film X-ray and are not necessarily causative.

The main symptom of plantar fasciitis is pain along the plantar surface of the foot during activity or weightbearing. The symptoms associated with enthesopathy or heel spur syndrome also include an exquisite focal tenderness at the proximal insertion, particularly evident first thing in the morning, or after a period of non-weightbearing. Rarely the fascia may rupture; this is generally associated with an acute, traumatic injury.

While the diagnosis is generally made on clinical signs and symptoms, MRI and ultrasound can be useful in assessing the confirmation of the diagnosis. Imaging will usually demonstrate thickening of the fascia, but inflammation is minimal. Physical therapies may be helpful, although patient-mediated treatments such as change of footwear and weight loss where appropriate should be the first resort. Although distressing to the patient, many cases of plantar heel pain will resolve spontaneously in the first 12 months following onset.

There is reasonable-quality evidence to suggest that both taping[76] and contoured foot orthoses[77] help further reduce symptoms in the short term. There is also some limited evidence for the short-term efficacy of injection therapy with corticosteroid,[75] although injections into the heel are painful and the long-term efficacy of injection is no greater than watchful waiting.

## BURSITIS

There are two bursae at the posterior aspect of the ankle, one deep to the Achilles tendon, the retrocalcaneal bursa, the other superficial to the tendon, the Achilles bursa. Inflammation of either bursa can result in pain at the posterior ankle region and is commonly caused by repetitive trauma. The more superficial Achilles bursa is particularly prone to aggravation associated with tight or ill-fitting footwear. Clinical diagnosis is made by reproduction of symptoms with palpation. This may be more difficult with the deeper, retrocalcaneal bursae, which is more often associated with systemic inflammatory disease. MR or ultrasound imaging is diagnostic.

Treatment of local, mechanical bursitis centres on physical therapies, RICER and NSAIDs. Modification to footwear is essential to prevent further irritation. Bursitis associated with inflammatory disease requires rheumatology referral.

## HAGLUND'S BUMPS

Haglund's deformity/bump (also referred to as pump bumps) is a large, bony prominence that develops at the back of the heel. It is thought to arise secondarily to irritation from footwear, although the initial predisposing factors are not clear. The bony prominence may be overlaid by a painful bursitis. Non-surgical treatment is the same as for Achilles bursitis. Surgical referral may be necessary when conservative treatment provides inadequate pain relief, although success is limited and should be considered only as a last resort for extreme and intractable cases.

## Midfoot and forefoot pain

### MECHANICAL FOREFOOT PAIN (METATARSALGIA)

Metatarsalgia is not in itself a diagnosis but is simply a descriptive term meaning pain in the metatarsal region. Where possible, the cause of the metatarsal pain should be investigated thoroughly using standard problem-solving skills and consideration of local anatomy. This is a complex area of anatomy, however, and there are many structures that can give rise to painful symptoms. The most common causes of midfoot pain proximal to the MTP joints are midtarsal joint degenerative disease or midshaft metatarsal stress reactions, both of which are discussed earlier in the chapter. At the level of the MTP joints themselves the most likely cause of symptoms is mechanical overload. This can be caused by a range of intrinsic factors (e.g. loss of the plantar fat pad, migration of the fat pad anteriorly, clawing/subluxation of the toes) or factors extrinsic to the foot (e.g. footwear with inadequate cushioning, excessive BMI, high levels of activity). The presenting features are of a chronic, usually low-grade discomfort, exacerbated by activity. Where loads over the MTP joints are excessive there may be associated physiological thickening of the skin, pathological thickening of the skin (callus and corn formation) or overlying bursitis. There will usually be a good response to off-loading treatments such as footwear change or provision of insoles, but patient compliance can be limited. In severe cases where both pain and deformity is significant, surgical opinion may be warranted.

The other common causes of forefoot joint pain are Morton's neuroma, which has been discussed earlier in this chapter and intermetatarsal bursitis (IMB). IMB is a common non-articular manifestation of inflammatory arthritis but can also be seen in otherwise healthy individuals. The symptoms are of an acute and varying forefoot pain, exacerbated by activity. Sharp pain will be elicited with a lateral squeeze test across the five metatarsal heads. Definitive clinical diagnosis is difficult and only imaging with MRI and ultrasound is confirmatory. Where IMB is strongly suspected and systematic inflammatory arthritis has been ruled out, the bursitis will respond well to local injection of corticosteroid into the IM space via the dorsal aspect of the foot. This can be undertaken in primary care as ultrasound guidance is not strictly necessary with such a clear target area.

### BUNIONS

Strictly speaking, bunions are osteophytic growths at the margins of the first MTP joint, often associated with an overlying adventitious bursa, which form after joint damage through chronic functional compromise. The term is often used more loosely to describe any pathology of the first MTP joint although there are specific sub-pathologies that should be considered. The most important of the specific pathologies are hallux valgus, hallux limitus and hallux rigidus.

Hallux valgus (syn. hallux abducto valgus or HAV) clinically presents where the big toe (hallux) is progressively deviated toward the mid-line of the foot, sometimes with associated axial rotation. In severe cases the hallux can overlie or underlie the 2nd – or even 3rd – lesser toe, causing significant pressure. Juvenile onset is not uncommon although most cases arise insidiously in adulthood. The deformity arises through a combination of intrinsic biomechanical factors and extrinsic factors such as footwear.[27] There is some evidence of an inherited tendency, especially in the juvenile form.[78] Non-surgical treatments are of limited efficacy. NSAIDs and footwear change can reduce symptoms and there is some evidence for the effectiveness of night splints, although compliance is generally poor. Evidence supporting the use of foot orthoses/insoles is lacking. Surgical treatments have improved significantly in the past 20 years and good outcomes can be expected with modern techniques. The indications for surgical referral in the NHS are pain and significant deformity rather than dissatisfaction with appearance.

Hallux limitus and hallux rigidus describe limitation of function at the first MTP joint without significant deviation of the hallux. There can be osteophyte formation at the joint margin and significant pain. The terms describe the progressive loss of function from initial limitation of dorsiflexion, through to fusion and rigidity. The cause is impaired biomechanical function of the foot, although the precise mechanism is not well understood.[79] If the joint progresses through to complete rigidity pain will often diminish. Some symptom relief will again be achieved with NSAIDs and physical therapies. Foot orthoses are also widely used and can benefit some people in the early stages, although effectiveness is patchy. Once the osteophyte is well developed, surgery is the only curative option, and again the indication for referral is severity of pain.

### Lesser toe deformities

Lesser toe deformities are a consequence of the combination of impaired foot mechanics and compression inside the shoe. There is a wide range of terminologies used, e.g. clawed, hammer, mallet, retracted toes, etc., but these are not of great relevance in most general practice situations. In summary, clawing of the toes is a useful sign of generally impaired foot mechanics but most attention should focus on the resulting symptoms.

The most common symptoms are pressure problems associated with:

▷ exposure of the metatarsal head
▷ anterior displacement of the plantar fat pad under the MTP joint
▷ pressure lesions (callus, corns) on the interphalangeal joints or the apices of the toes
▷ problems with shoe fitting.

Footwear change will help with symptoms but does not address the deformity once present. If footwear and lifestyle changes provide inadequate improvement and symptoms are significant then surgical opinion may be warranted. Toe straightening procedures are generally simple and effective.

---

## Treatment approaches

### *Self-management*

For many musculoskeletal foot problems, person-centred self-care is genuinely the best treatment option. Clinical interventions for foot problems are often supported poorly by evidence, and efficacy can be hit-and-miss. Innovative use of the first principles of minimising load and self-care of immediate symptoms is as likely to be helpful as many more comprehensive interventions. The two most practical self-management approaches for many foot problems are to encourage weight loss where appropriate, and provision of footwear/hosiery advice. Weight loss is a thorny issue for many patients, especially when they consider that their ability to exercise is compromised through their symptoms. However, reduction in body weight has a marked effect on reducing the loads in structures affected by mechanical disorders. Although difficult, every effort should be made to engage the patient with a comprehensive approach to encouraging weight loss.

Footwear and hosiery are discussed in the next section. In addition to these two basic principles, it is worth the GP bearing in mind that many patients with musculoskeletal foot disorders may need help or advice with basic foot care and hygiene tasks. Specific foot deformities may make these tasks difficult and concomitant conditions in the hands, back, etc. can compromise their ability to self-care.[80] There are many leaflets and self-care packs available from organisations such as Arthritis Research UK and Arthritis Care, and these can be a useful resource.

Finally, we have noted in this section that many of the musculoskeletal disorders affecting the feet can cause callus or cornified skin to form on areas of increased pressure. For patients who are otherwise well, self-removal of hard skin with a skin scraper or file is perfectly safe and is to be encouraged and facilitated in the person-centred model. For thicker areas of callus or where there is a cornified nucleus, filing or scraping is unlikely to be adequate. Caustic preparations (e.g. salicylic acid creams) can be helpful but must be used with caution and are contraindicated in patients with diabetes or other risk factors for ulceration. If self-management is not appropriate, patients can be referred to a podiatrist for assessment and relevant treatment. Depending on the availability of NHS services locally patients may prefer to try a private provider.

### Footwear (including hosiery)

Many of the footwear changes that would benefit the patient with musculoskeletal foot complaints could come under the auspices of person-centred care, as advice on the characteristics of good footwear is often all that is needed. Compliance with suggested changes can be limited, however, especially for women as footwear has such an important social role. It is important to engage with patients and to ensure that they understand that their choices have the potential to impact materially on their symptoms. Also, the extent to which they are prepared to compromise cosmesis for clinical benefit is, in many cases, as important as any clinical intervention that could be provided by the healthcare system.

The five basic characteristics of 'good' footwear are: a cushioned midsole, a flexible upper, adjustable fastenings, a non-slip outersole and a breathable upper. These characteristics are epitomised in modern trainer type shoes and so the choice to be made by the patient is the extent to which they, personally, are prepared to trade off these characteristics against the desired cosmetic appearance of their shoes. It can be helpful to point out that different shoes can be worn for different occasions with the extent of the trade-off varying with purpose. There are now high-street retailers that make shoes emphasising these characteristics and introducing other features such as extra forefoot depth that further improve the clinical benefits.

One under-estimated area of self-care in which benefit can be gained from footwear choice is that of hosiery. Retail hosiery made from terry-towelling or woven materials can provide significant levels of cushioning with little inconvenience. Again there may need to be recognition that certain hosiery is only compatible with certain occasions but the discussion about protecting the foot with socks or tights is worth having with patients. Therapeutic hosiery, strategically placed padding and cushioned inserts are also available from specialist outlets.

Once retail (including specialist retail) options have been exhausted, patients may need help with sourcing therapeutic footwear. Most NHS footwear is now 'modular', i.e. customised from a general specification. Traditional bespoke orthopaedic footwear is relatively rarely encountered. Mechanisms for access to modular or bespoke footwear vary locally but usually involve referral to an orthotic, podiatrist or orthopaedic department.

### Pharmacological treatments

As with most chronic musculoskeletal complaints, oral NSAIDs or analgesics may be helpful, as can topical NSAIDs. In general these should be used in conjunction with treatments aimed at addressing mechanical factors. Local injections of corticosteroid will often be of significant, if short-term, benefit. For many sites around the foot and ankle, the complex anatomy can make it difficult to inject the correct tissues accurately without ultrasound guidance, making this therapy logistically difficult in primary care unless imaging facilities are available locally. With few exceptions blind injections are notably less successful than guided injections.

### Physical therapies

The provision of physical therapies is beyond the scope of most GPs and, where mechanisms exist, referral to a podiatry or physiotherapy service is probably the best option.

The services offered by podiatrists and physiotherapists will usually include:

▷ comprehensive assessment of the underlying cause
▷ advice on stretching, particularly tight calf musculature and plantar fascia
▷ advice on footwear
▷ advice on the RICER approach and self-management
▷ electro therapies and other physical therapies
▷ insoles, orthoses and splints (see next section).

In many places extended-scope practitioners will also be able to access imaging technology and provide treatments such as joint injections.

### Orthoses

Foot orthoses are widely used by some specialties for managing musculoskeletal foot pain and warrant some separate discussion. Foot orthoses are insoles worn in the shoe that are intended to provide either symptom relief or to control the motion of distribution of force and pressure around the foot. The common types of in-shoe orthoses are, in order of sophistication and expense:

▷ **simple insoles** ▶ usually simple, cushioning insoles designed to reduce pressure under the foot
▷ **arch supports** ▶ D-shaped pads designed to fill the medial arch of the foot-aiding posture and redistributing load
▷ **contoured insoles** ▶ a modern evolution of the traditional arch support providing a contoured foot bed, which aids posture and

redistributes load. Sometimes these can be more comfortable to wear than a standard arch support

▷ **functional orthoses** ▶ insoles designed specifically to alter the function and loading of the foot. They are typically made of a relatively firm material and may be bought off the shelf or custom made to a patient-specific cast or model (Figure 6.12 on p. 475).

All four types can be bought off-the-shelf from pharmacies or sports shops and patients may be happy to try some of these approaches out of their own pocket (typical cost £15–£50). Better success would be expected if orthoses are prescribed by a specialist practitioner and referral is warranted if the patient is unable to buy his or her own or has failed to respond to off-the-shelf insoles. Podiatrists, orthotists and orthopaedic departments will all provide insole/orthotic treatments and referral guidance will be locally specific.

There is a growing body of evidence supporting the use of insoles in various conditions,[77,81,82] although in some quarters claims for benefit are overstated. In general, however, the use of orthoses as part of a comprehensive approach can be helpful in many musculoskeletal foot conditions.

**163**

---

## Summary

Foot problems are a common reason for primary care attendance, especially in older people. Many foot problems are poorly dealt with because they are not picked up or not assessed well. Adopting a simple assessment schema can allow the GP to evaluate foot problems systematically in just one or two minutes. This is especially important in the early detection of systemic disease where early recognition and referral is critical to the prognosis. The mechanical demands on the foot can be significant and lead to damage to local tissues and consequent symptoms. These are often perfectly well addressed in a primary care setting or through person-centred self-care. In addition, however, the mechanical demands on the foot may exacerbate the symptoms of systemic disease and this requires a more comprehensive approach. Standard pharmacological and other conventional treatments can address some of the symptoms, but mechanical therapies can be helpful in the lower limb and should be considered as part of the comprehensive approach. Finally, many of the best treatments for musculoskeletal foot problems can be mediated by the patient him or herself and do not require intensive intervention or referral.

**References**

1 • Peat G, Thomas E, Wilkie R, *et al*. Multiple joint pain and lower extremity disability in middle and old age *Disability and Rehabilitation* 2006; **28(24)**: 1543–9.

2 • Garrow A P, Silman A J, Macfarlane G J. The Cheshire Foot Pain and Disability Survey: a population survey assessing prevalence and associations *Pain* 2004; **110(1–2)**: 378–84.

3 • Dunn J E, Link C L, Felson D T, *et al*. Prevalence of foot and ankle conditions in a multiethnic community sample of older adults *American Journal of Epidemiology* 2004; **159(5)**: 491–8.

4 • Munro B J, Steele J R. Foot-care awareness. a survey of persons aged 65 years and older *Journal of the American Podiatric Medical Association* 1998; **88(5)**: 242–8.

5 • Leveille S G, Guralnik J M, Ferrucci L, *et al*. Foot pain and disability in older women *American Journal of Epidemiology* 1998; **148(7)**: 657–65.

6 • Benvenuti F, Ferrucci L, Guralnik J M, *et al*. Foot pain and disability in older persons: an epidemiologic survey *Journal of the American Geriatrics Society* 1995; **43(5)**: 479–84.

7 • Black J R, Hale W E. Prevalence of foot complaints in the elderly *Journal of the American Podiatric Medical Association* 1987; **77(6)**: 308–11.

8 • Chen J, Devine A, Dick I M, *et al*. Prevalence of lower extremity pain and its association with functionality and quality of life in elderly women in Australia *Journal of Rheumatology* 2003; **30(12)**: 2689–93.

9 • Thomas E, Peat G, Harris L, *et al*. The prevalence of pain and pain interference in a general population of older adults: cross-sectional findings from the North Staffordshire Osteoarthritis Project (NorStOP) *Pain* 2004; **110(1–2)**: 361–8.

10 • Gorter K, Kuyvenhoven M, de Melker R. Health care utilisation by older people with non-traumatic foot complaints. What makes the difference? *Scandinavian Journal of Primary Health Care* 2001; **19(3)**: 191–3.

11 • Gorter K J, Kuyvenhoven M M, de Melker R A. Nontraumatic foot complaints in older people. A population-based survey of risk factors, mobility, and well-being *Journal of the American Podiatric Medical Association* 2000; **90(8)**: 397–402.

12 • Odding E, Valkenburg H A, Algra D, *et al*. Association of locomotor complaints and disability in the Rotterdam study *Annals of the Rheumatic Diseases* 1995; **54(9)**: 721–5.

13 • Dawson J, Thorogood M, Marks S A, *et al*. The prevalence of foot problems in older women: a cause for concern *Journal of Public Health Medicine* 2002; **24(2)**: 77–84.

14 • Thomas E, Wilkie R, Peat G, *et al*. The North Staffordshire Osteoarthritis Project – NorStOP: prospective, 3-year study of the epidemiology and management of clinical osteoarthritis in a general population of older adults *BMC Musculoskeletal Disorders* 2004; **5**: 2.

15 • O'Connor K, Bragdon G, Baumhauer J F. Sexual dimorphism of the foot and ankle *Orthopedic Clinics of North America* 2006; **37(4)** 569–74.

16 • Hooper M M, Stellatov T A, Hallowell P T, *et al*. Musculoskeletal findings in obese subjects before and after weight loss following bariatric surgery *International Journal of Obesity* 2007; **31(1)**: 114–20.

17 • Coady D, Walker D, Kay L. Regional Examination of the Musculoskeletal System (REMS): a core set of clinical skills for medical students *Rheumatology* 2004; **43(5)**: 633–9.

18 • Redmond A C, Helliwell P S. Musculoskeletal disorders. In: P Frowen, M O'Donnell, JG Burrow, *et al.* (eds). *Neale's Disorders of the Foot* (8th edn) Edinburgh: Churchill Livingstone, 2010.

19 • Helliwell P, Woodburn J, Redmond A, *et al. The Foot and Ankle in Rheumatoid Arthritis: a comprehensive guide* Edinburgh: Churchill Livingstone, 2006.

20 • Bouysset M, Tavernier T, Tebib J, *et al.* CT and MRI evaluation of tenosynovitis of the rheumatoid hindfoot *Clinical Rheumatology* 1995; **14(3)**: 303–7.

21 • Ostergaard M, Szkudlarek M. Imaging in rheumatoid arthritis – Why MRI and ultrasonography can no longer be ignored *Scandinavian Journal of Rheumatology* 2003; **32(2)**: 63–73.

22 • Wakefield R J, Gibbon W W, Conaghan P G, *et al.* The value of sonography in the detection of bone erosions in patients with rheumatoid arthritis: a comparison with conventional radiography *Arthritis and Rheumatism* 2000; **43(12)**: 2762–70.

23 • Szkudlarek M, Court-Payen M, Jacobsen S, *et al.* Interobserver agreement in ultrasonography of the finger and toe joints in rheumatoid arthritis *Arthritis and Rheumatism* 2003; **48(4)**: 955–62.

24 • Olivieri I, Barozzi L, Padula A. Enthesiopathy: clinical manifestations, imaging and treatment *Baillière's Clinical Rheumatology* 1998; **12(4)**: 665–81.

25 • Redmond A C, Crosbie J, Ouvrier R A. Development and validation of a novel rating system for scoring standing foot posture: the Foot Posture Index *Clinical Biomechanics* 2006; **21(1)**: 89–98.

26 • Redmond A, Crane Y, Menz H. Normative values for the Foot Posture Index *Journal of Foot and Ankle Research* 2008; **1(1)**: 6.

27 • Eustace S, Byrne J O, Beausang O, *et al.* Hallux valgus, first metatarsal pronation and collapse of the medial longitudinal arch – a radiological correlation *Skeletal Radiology* 1994; **23(3)**: 191–4.

28 • Martin R L, Irrgang J J, Conti S F. Outcome study of subjects with insertional plantar fasciitis *Foot and Ankle International* 1998; **19(12)**: 803–11.

29 • Cowan D N, Jones B H, Frykman P N, *et al.* Lower limb morphology and risk of overuse injury among male infantry trainees *Medicine and Science in Sports and Exercise* 1996; **28(8)**: 945–52.

30 • Yates B, White S. The incidence and risk factors in the development of medial tibial stress syndrome among naval recruits *American Journal of Sports Medicine* 2004; **32(3)**: 772–80.

31 • Burns J, Crosbie J, Hunt A, *et al.* The effect of pes cavus on foot pain and plantar pressure *Clinical Biomechanics* 2005; **20(9)**: 877–82.

32 • Lawrence R, Helmick C G, Arnett F C, *et al.* Estimates of the prevalence of arthritis and selected musculoskeletal disorders in the United States *Arthritis and Rheumatism* 1998; **41(5)**: 778–99.

33 • Muehleman C, Bareither D, Huch K, *et al.* Prevalence of degenerative morphological changes in the joints of the lower extremity *Osteoarthritis and Cartilage* 1997; **5(1)**: 23–37.

34 • Chen B X. Arthritis of the foot and ankle *Current Opinion in Orthopedics* 1996; **7(3)**: 87–91.

35 • Birrell F, Croft P, Cooper C, *et al.* Health impact of pain in the hip region with and without radiographic evidence of osteoarthritis: a study of new attenders to primary care. The P C R Hip Study Group *Annals of the Rheumatic Diseases* 2000; **59(11)**: 857–63.

36 • McAlindon T E, Snow S, Cooper C, *et al*. Radiographic patterns of osteoarthritis of the knee joint in the community: the importance of the patellofemoral joint *Annals of the Rheumatic Diseases* 1992; **51(7)**: 844–9.

37 • Spector T D, Cicuttini F, Baker J, *et al*. Genetic influences on osteoarthritis in women: a twin study *British Medical Journal* 1996; **312(7036)**: 940–3.

38 • Lau E C, Cooper C, Lam D, *et al*. Factors associated with osteoarthritis of the hip and knee in Hong Kong Chinese: obesity, joint injury, and occupational activities *American Journal of Epidemiology* 2000; **152(9)**: 855–62.

39 • Sharma L, Cahue S, Song J, *et al*. Physical functioning over three years in knee osteoarthritis: role of psychosocial, local mechanical, and neuromuscular factors *Arthritis and Rheumatism* 2003; **48(12)**: 3359–70.

40 • Hannan M T, Anderson J J, Zhang Y, *et al*. Bone mineral density and knee osteoarthritis in elderly men and women. The Framingham Study *Arthritis and Rheumatism* 1993; **36(12)**: 1671–80.

41 • Felson D T, Lawrence R C, Dieppe P A, *et al*. Osteoarthritis: new insights. Part 1: The disease and its risk factors *Annals of Internal Medicine* 2000; **133(8)**: 635–46.

42 • Felson D T, Hannan M T, Naimark A, *et al*. Occupational physical demands, knee bending, and knee osteoarthritis: results from the Framingham Study *Journal of Rheumatology* 1991; **18(10)**: 1587–92.

43 • Buckwalter J A, Lane N E. Athletics and osteoarthritis *American Journal of Sports Medicine* 1997; **25(6)**: 873–81.

44 • Sharma L, Hurwitz D E, Thonar E J, *et al*. Knee adduction moment, serum hyaluronan level, and disease severity in medial tibiofemoral osteoarthritis *Arthritis and Rheumatism* 1998; **41(7)**: 1233–40.

45 • Brouwer G M, van Tol A W, Bergink A P, *et al*. Association between valgus and varus alignment and the development and progression of radiographic osteoarthritis of the knee *Arthritis and Rheumatism* 2007; **56(4)**: 1204–11.

46 • Honkonen S E. Degenerative arthritis after tibial plateau fractures *Journal of Orthopaedic Trauma* 1995; **9(4)**: 273–7.

47 • Tan A L, Grainger A J, Tanner S F, *et al*. High-resolution magnetic resonance imaging for the assessment of hand osteoarthritis *Arthritis and Rheumatism* 2005; **52(8)**: 2355–65.

48 • Keenan A M, Tennant A, Fear J, *et al*. Impact of multiple joint problems on daily living tasks in people in the community over age fifty-five *Arthritis and Rheumatism* 2006; **55(5)**: 757–64.

49 • Weinfeld S B, Schon L C. Hallux metatarsophalangeal arthritis *Clinical Orthopaedics and Related Research* 1998; **349**: 9–19.

50 • Greisberg J, Hansen S T Jr, Sangeorzan B. Deformity and degeneration in the hindfoot and midfoot joints of the adult acquired flatfoot *Foot and Ankle International* 2003; **24(7)**: 530–4.

51 • Dieppe P A, Lohmander S. Pathogenesis and management of pain in osteoarthritis *Lancet* 2005; **365(9463)**: 965–73.

52 • Dominick K L, Ahern F M, Gold C H, *et al*. Health-related quality of life and health service use among older adults with osteoarthritis *Arthritis and Rheumatism* 2004; **51(3)**: 326–31.

53 • National Collaborating Centre for Chronic Conditions. *Clinical Guideline 59, Osteoarthritis: national clinical guideline for care and management in adults* London: Royal College of Physicians, 2008, www.nice.org.uk/CG59 [accessed October 2011].

54 • O'Brien TS, Hart TS, Gould JS. Extraosseous manifestations of rheumatoid arthritis in the foot and ankle *Clinical Orthopaedics and Related Research* 1997; **340**: 26–33.

55 • American College of Rheumatology Subcommittee on Rheumatoid Arthritis. Guidelines for the management of rheumatoid arthritis: 2002 update *Arthritis and Rheumatism* 2002; **46(2)**: 328–46.

56 • Emery P, Breedveld FC, Dougados M, *et al.* Early referral recommendation for newly diagnosed rheumatoid arthritis: evidence based development of a clinical guide *Annals of the Rheumatic Diseases* 2002; **61(4)**: 290–7.

57 • National Institute for Health and Clinical Excellence. *Clinical Guideline 79, Rheumatoid Arthritis: the management of rheumatoid arthritis in adults* London: NICE, 2009, www.nice.org.uk/Guidance/CG79 [accessed October 2011].

58 • McGonagle D, Marzo-Ortega H, O'Connor P, *et al.* The role of biomechanical factors and HLA-B27 in magnetic resonance imaging-determined bone changes in plantar fascia enthesopathy *Arthritis and Rheumatism* 2002; **46(2)**: 489–93.

59 • Kumar R, Madewell JE. Rheumatoid and seronegative arthropathies of the foot *Radiologic Clinics of North America* 1987; **25(6)**: 1263–88.

60 • Gold RH, Bassett LW, Seeger LL. The other arthritides. Roentgenologic features of osteoarthritis, erosive osteoarthritis, ankylosing spondylitis, psoriatic arthritis, Reiter's disease, multicentric reticulohistiocytosis, and progressive systemic sclerosis *Radiologic Clinics of North America* 1988; **26(6)**: 1195–212.

61 • Galluzzo E, Lischi DM, Taglione E, *et al.* Sonographic analysis of the ankle in patients with psoriatic arthritis *Scandinavian Journal of Rheumatology* 2000; **29(1)**: 52–5.

62 • Gerster JC, Vischer TL, Bennani A, *et al.* The painful heel. Comparative study in rheumatoid arthritis, ankylosing spondylitis, Reiter's syndrome, and generalized osteoarthrosis *Annals of the Rheumatic Diseases* 1977; **36(4)**: 343–8.

63 • La Montagna G, Baruffo A, Tirri R, *et al.* Foot involvement in systemic sclerosis: a longitudinal study of 100 patients *Seminars in Arthritis and Rheumatism* 2002; **31(4)**: 248–55.

64 • Sari-Kouzel H, Hutchinson CE, Middleton A, *et al.* Foot problems in patients with systemic sclerosis *Rheumatology* 2001; **40(4)**: 410–13.

65 • Harris MD, Siegel LB, Alloway JA. Gout hyperuricemia *American Family Physician* 1999; **59(4)**: 925–34.

66 • McGuire JB. Arthritis and related diseases of the foot and ankle: rehabilitation and biomechanical considerations *Clinics in Podiatric Medicine and Surgery* 2003; **20(3)**: 469–85, ix.

67 • Chen LX, Schumacher HR. Gout and gout mimickers: 20 clinical pearls: a bigger diagnostic and management challenge than it may seem *Journal of Musculoskeletal Medicine* 2003; **20(5)**: 254–8.

68 • Egan R, Sartoris DJ, Resnick D. Radiographic features of gout in the foot *Journal of Foot Surgery* 1987; **26(5)**: 434–9.

69 • Kerr LD. Arthritis of the forefoot. A review from a rheumatologic and medical perspective *Clinical Orthopaedics and Related Research* 1998; **349**: 20–7.

70 • Redmond AC, Helliwell PS, Robinson P. Investigating foot and ankle problems. In: PG Conaghan, P O'Connor, D Isenberg (eds). *Oxford Specialist Handbook in Radiology: musculoskeletal imaging* Oxford: Oxford University Press, 2010.

71 • Alfredson H, Cook J. A treatment algorithm for managing Achilles tendinopathy: new treatment options *British Journal of Sports Medicine* 2007; **41(4)**: 211–16.

72 • Johnson K A, Strom D E. Tibialis posterior tendon dysfunction *Clinical Orthopaedics and Related Research* 1989; **239**: 196–206.

73 • Myerson M S. Adult acquired flatfoot deformity *Journal of Bone and Joint Surgery – American Volume* 1996; **78A**: 780–92.

74 • Miller S D, Van Holsbeeck M, Boruta PM, *et al*. Ultrasound in the diagnosis of posterior tibial tendon pathology *Foot and Ankle International* 1996; **17(9)**: 555–8.

75 • Crawford F, Atkins D, Edwards J. Interventions for treating plantar heel pain (Cochrane review) *Cochrane Database of Systematic Reviews* 2001; **3**: CD000416.

76 • Radford J A, Landorf K B, Buchbinder R, *et al*. Effectiveness of low-Dye taping for the short-term treatment of plantar heel pain: a randomised trial *BMC Musculoskeletal Disorders* 2006; **7(64)**.

77 • Landorf K B, Keenan A M, Herbert R D. Effectiveness of foot orthoses to treat plantar fasciitis: a randomized trial *Archives of Internal Medicine* 2006; **166(12)**: 1305–10.

78 • Kilmartin T E, Wallace W A. The significance of pes planus in juvenile hallux valgus *Foot and Ankle* 1992; **13(2)**: 53–6.

79 • Camasta C A. Hallux limitus and hallux rigidus. Clinical examination, radiographic findings, and natural history *Clinics in Podiatric Medicine and Surgery* 1996; **13(3)**: 423–48.

80 • Mann R A, Horton G A. Management of the foot and ankle in rheumatoid arthritis *Rheumatic Diseases Clinics of North America* 1996; **22(3)**: 457–76.

81 • Woodburn J, Barker S, Helliwell PS. A randomised controlled trial of foot orthoses in R A *Journal of Rheumatology* 2002; **29(7)**: 137–83.

82 • Clark H, Rome K, Plant M, *et al*. A critical review of foot orthoses in the rheumatoid arthritic foot *Rheumatology* 2006; **45(2)**: 139–45.

# Tendonopathy

*Adrian Dunbar and Daniel Wardleworth*

## 7

## Introduction

Patients presenting with painful, sore tendons are an everyday primary care occurrence. GPs will be very familiar with patients with sore lateral elbows (tennis elbow), sore Achilles tendons and shoulder pain suggestive of rotator cuff disease. They will have used terms to describe these problems – supraspinatus tendonitis, Achilles tendonitis and lateral epicondylitis.

Frequently affected sites include the:

▷ rotator cuff tendon
▷ common extensor origin on the lateral epicondyle of the elbow
▷ hip adductor tendon
▷ lateral hip tendons
▷ patella tendon
▷ tibialis posterior tendon
▷ Achilles tendon.

Having used a term implying inflammatory pathology, they will have been prescribed anti-inflammatory treatments. These problems can be remarkably persistent and, until recently, treatment of tendon pain was of limited effectiveness and carried a poor evidence base. This was largely because the prevailing understanding of the condition was incorrect.

Previously, tendon pain was attributed to an inflammatory process, the term tendonitis was used and anti-inflammatory treatments offered. Significant progress in the understanding of tendon disorders has been achieved in the last decade as follows:

▷ first, we now know from studies of tendon histopathology that inflammatory change (inflammatory cells and mediators) is conspicuously absent from symptomatic tendons
▷ second, we now know that the pathological process is one of mucoid degeneration with inadequate repair and remodelling. There is loss of the tightly bundled collagen structure and increased proteoglycan ground substance within the affected tendon

▷ third, we now know that symptomatic tendons show evidence of neovascularisation – the development of new blood vessels growing into the tendon. New vessel formation is also accompanied by the growth of nerve fibres into the tendon. It is thought that it is this process that results in degenerative tendons becoming symptomatic.

The terms tendonitis or tendinitis have been replaced by tendonopathy, tendinopathy or tendinosis. Modern treatments of tendon pain aim to reverse the neovascularisation of the tendon and encourage healing and remodelling. New treatments and more effective treatments are emerging – but, as yet, the evidence base remains rather small. Tendonopathy is often a complex problem to manage and recovery is slow.[1]

---

**Box 7.1 ○ *Old and new thinking***

**Old think**

▶ *Tendonitis (tendinitis).*

▶ Inflammatory condition.

▶ Anti-inflammatory treatments.

▶ Steroid injections.

▶ Surgery?

**New think**

▶ *Tendonopathy (tendinosis or tendinopathy).*

▶ Degenerative condition.

▶ Inadequate healing.

▶ Neovascularisation of the tendon.

▶ Treatments to accelerate healing.

▶ And reduce neovascularisation.

▶ Non-steroidal inflammatory drugs (NSAIDs) not appropriate.

▶ Slow recovery – takes several months.

---

**So how does it happen?**

There are a number of theories. The following may or may not occur in combination, including: mechanical stresses on the tendon with repetitive loading on the tendon; impingement of the tendon between adjacent structures – bone and ligaments; and impaired blood supply. Discussion of the competing theories is beyond the scope of this chapter and would probably be out of date by the time of printing – such is the current rapid progress in the understanding of tendon disorders.

However, it is probably safe to say that development of tendonopathy is probably multi-factorial and both intrinsic and extrinsic factors are now described.

## Intrinsic factors

### AGE

The incidence of tendonopathy increases with ageing. Sadly, more 'mature' tissues heal less efficiently than younger tissues.

### CHRONIC DISEASE

The presence of chronic disease, notably diabetes, rheumatoid arthritis and connective tissue disease, is also associated with increased incidence of tendonopathy.

### BIOMECHANICS

Adverse mechanical stresses may lead to tendon breakdown. Examples are impingement of the rotator cuff tendon in the subacromial space or shear forces on the Achilles tendon due to pronation at the subtalar joint.

## Extrinsic factors

Repetitive activity in work, sport and leisure can lead to the development of symptomatic tendonopathy. Work-related problems are particularly common, for example in repetitive upper-limb activity involving extension of the wrist and gripping tightly.

Tendon pain in the upper limb occurring as a result of repetitive overuse activity in an occupational context is referred to as work-related upper-limb disorder (WRULD).

Repetitive sporting activity – e.g. running or jumping – is often associated with upper-and lower-limb tendonopathy, and described by terms such as tennis elbow, runner's knee or jumper's knee.

Very often a sudden burst of intensive DIY activity – gardening on the first fine weekend of spring or a weekend spent redecorating the dining room – can lead to tendonopathy presenting more acutely, as in the cases described below (see pp. 176 and 179).

Sport-related symptoms can follow sudden increases in training or competitive intensity, changes in equipment (e.g. new shoes or a new racket), or environmental change (from training on grass to hard court). Work-related symptoms may follow longer shifts on a production line or increased speed of working.

Often a combination of these intrinsic and extrinsic factors combine, increasing the stresses on tendons and diminishing the opportunity for healing and remodelling.

## Presentation

Pain is the commonest presenting symptom. Pain is usually linked to activity but is often present at rest. This is particularly true of rotator cuff tendonopathy, where night pain is a common feature.

Pain is often felt after activity – or during prolonged activity – and can limit the ability to sustain activity, thus reducing performance at work or in sport.

In the early stages there can be a 'warming up' with symptoms easing within a short period of activity. Symptoms return later, limiting or curtailing activity.

Weakness of the affected part and loss of function often accompany pain. Sometimes there is overt swelling of the symptomatic tendon. Obviously this will only be visible if the involved tendon is a subcutaneous structure.

Occasionally, an acute tendon rupture may be the presentation of degenerative tendonopathy. This is most common in load-bearing tendons such as the Achilles and the long head of the biceps.

## Assessment

When taking a history the GP will need to enquire about the nature of the activity that preceded the development of symptoms. Sudden increase in activity volume or intensity will be relevant. Changes in equipment or environment should be sought.

Previous similar symptoms or injury affecting the same area will be important.

### Physical examination

Often there is little to see. Perhaps a little swelling may be evident and the tendon will be tender to the touch and during a stretch. A reduced range of motion may be evident, limited by tightness in the muscle tendon unit. It is important to try to reproduce the patient's pain with activity or special tests (see cases below on pp. 176 and 179). Impingement of the involved tendon between adjacent structures may elicit the patient's pain.

### Imaging – diagnostic ultrasound

Imaging is not usually required to make the diagnosis in most cases. However, it can be used to confirm the clinical suspicion and exclude other pathology.

Tendons are best imaged using diagnostic ultrasound. Ultrasound scanning is a dynamic investigation. The patient can be asked to move the affected part whilst being scanned. Often impingement of a swollen tendon can be observed. The tendon itself has a specific appearance on ultrasound scanning. It will often be observed to be thicker and hypoechoic – darker due to reduced reflection of the ultrasound beam. This is due to increased fluid within the tendon matrix. Neovascularisation can be visualised on the scan using colour doppler, where blood flow in new vessels can be shown as pulsations of colour. Calcification within affected tendons is sometimes demonstrated. This is also visible on a plain X-ray, but otherwise X-ray imaging is of very little use in patients with sore tendons.

At some sites, for example the subacromial space, the tendonopathy can be associated with a bursitis. Ultrasound imaging will demonstrate this.

Finally, ultrasound can demonstrate full or partial tears of the tendon. Partial tears are quite a common finding, sometimes in asymptomatic tendons. They occur more often in older patients. Knowledge of a significant tear in the affected tendon may have an influence on the treatment regimes described below.

---

### Treatments

At initial presentation the most pressing need for the patient is pain relief. Simple analgesics and other pain-relieving measures such as the regular application of ice, acupuncture and rest are appropriate here.

There is no evidence base to support the prescription of NSAIDs. This is not an inflammatory problem and there is therefore no additional benefit over simple analgesia. They are also much more expensive and potentially toxic, especially in the older patient and those with multiple co-morbidities.

Steroid injections have been used for many years to treat many tendon problems. The evidence suggests that they provide short- to medium-term pain relief but provide no long-term benefits. Evidence with respect to shoulder and elbow tendon problems suggests that patients sent to physiotherapy have greater long term-benefits. Where steroid injections do have a role is in treatment of any associated bursitis. In addition to the subacromial space, this may occur around the greater trochanter of the hip, the patella tendon and the insertion of the Achilles tendon on the posterior calcaneum.

Electrotherapies including therapeutic ultrasound, extra-corporeal shock-wave treatment and low-level (or cold) laser have, as yet, no good evidence base to support their use.

For some tendon problems the use of orthotic devices may be useful, but again there is little evidence to support widespread use. This includes devices placed in footwear to correct biomechanical abnormalities of the feet – relevant to Achilles and tibialis posterior tendonopathy (see the case study below, on p. 176).

Acute tendon ruptures should be referred as an emergency for an orthopaedic opinion with the exception of the long head of biceps, where function is usually maintained by an intact short head tendon.

### *Novel treatments*

Perhaps the most significant 'breakthrough' in the management of tendonopathy was the discovery of the effect of progressive eccentric loading on degenerative tendons and the development of a regime of exercise that reverses the neovascularisation and facilitates healing and remodelling of the tendon.

The term eccentric loading refers to the accompanying muscle activity. Muscles contract and shorten 'concentrically', they contract and lengthen 'eccentrically' and they contract at a constant length isometrically. Thinking of the Achilles tendon, a concentric contraction shortens the calf musculature and plantar flexes the ankle. In standing this raises the heel (and the entire body) off the ground – a calf raise. An eccentric contraction of the calf muscle then lowers the heel (and the body) to the ground again – a heel drop.

Eccentric loading focuses on slowly lowering the body weight after a calf raise. Extra range of movement is added by standing with the forefoot on the edge of a step and lowering the heel below the level of the step. Adding extra weight to the body – by holding increasingly heavy weights in the hands – or loading a backpack provides the progressive loading. These exercises are painful and, unusually in physiotherapy practice, the patients are encouraged to exercise into pain. It seems these exercises are much less effective if they are less painful. They also have to be continued for many months – gradually increasing the loading of the tendon. They should be done twice daily with three sets of 15 heel drops. The regime has become known as painful heel drops. Other regimes of progressive eccentric loading have been developed for other tendons. Limited evidence suggests that regimes of progressive eccentric loading will allow up to 90% of tendons to become asymptomatic.

However, recovery is slow and adherence to the exercise regime will be required for several months. For this reason the patient's expectations will need to be managed carefully.[2]

For the GP all this indicates the need for a referral to physiotherapy.

### Further treatments

A number of other novel treatments have been used to try to accelerate healing and treat tendons that respond incompletely to the progressive eccentric loading regime. These include the use of sclerosant injections, the application of a glyceryl trinitrate (GTN) patch over the affected tendon and the injection of autologous blood or platelet-rich plasma. At present there is only limited evidence of effectiveness from small clinical trials to support these treatments.

Discussion about the possible modes of action of these treatments is beyond the scope of this chapter.

## Specific regional problems

### Achilles tendonopathy

Pain in the mid-portion of the Achilles tendon is one of the commonest presentations of tendon pain, often but not exclusively occurring in athletic individuals. Assessment will need to cover the nature of the activity that led to the development of symptoms, any biomechanical issues (e.g. pronation of the foot), the equipment used (e.g. footwear), and any environmental factors (e.g. the underfoot surfaces). Management should start in the physiotherapy department and focus on the 'painful heel drop exercises' described above.

Sometimes patients present with pain at the insertion of the Achilles tendon on the calcaneum – the enthesis. This may be associated with swelling due to an accompanying bursitis. Insertional tendonopathy is often related to a combination of footwear issues and over-activity.

A modified regime of eccentric loading has been developed for insertional tendonopathy. The accompanying bursitis may be helped by a local steroid injection. Referral to physiotherapy and/or podiatry should be considered.[3]

Bilateral insertional Achilles tendon pain should raise suspicions of an underlying inflammatory disorder, the need for investigations and a possible rheumatology referral.

---

Box 7.2 ○ *Case study – the Achilles tendon*

---

Mr Richards presented to his GP with a sore Achilles tendon. He was training to run the London Marathon for a medical charity in memory of a family friend who had recently died.

Examination revealed marked over-pronation of his left foot. The heel raise and drop reproduced his pain. There was a visible swelling in the mid-substance of the left Achilles that was tender on palpation.

He was referred to physiotherapy and podiatry. He was advised to try cycling or swimming during his rehabilitation to maintain his aerobic fitness. He started on a progressive eccentric loading programme of heel drops. Podiatry produced some individually made insoles for his shoes and trainers to correct his pronation.

He was reviewed three months later. He had worked hard at the heel drop programme. On assessment he could perform multiple hops and heel raises without any pain. He had started running again and was planning to enter an ironman triathlon!

## COMMENT

The human body was designed by millions of years of evolution to run. However, a few hundred years of progressive inactivity since the Industrial Revolution have got most of us out of the habit! Often when taking up running, or a sport that involves running, there is always temptation or pressure to do too much too soon – before the body has had time to adapt to the activity. The older the body in question the longer this adaptation process takes. We do not know how old Mr Richards is but we do know that his mission to run a marathon has been inspired by a significant event – the death of a family friend and the desire to raise money for a medical charity. This adds to the pressures and can reduce the ability to listen to the body when it indicates that the training is a little too much just now. On the positive side those with athletic tendencies are highly motivated to do whatever it takes to recover and return to their sport. On the other hand they often need restraining from trying to return to sport too soon.

The 'advice to rest and the prescription for anti-inflammatory drugs' management plan is doomed to fail in this scenario! The role of the GP involves advice that resolution of the problem will take some time and that activities will need to be modified whilst healing takes place. It is possible that the patient may be quite upset to hear this advice. How patients express their distress is very individual and varies considerably from floods of tears to angrily demanding a second opinion. However, adherence to the exercise regime is vital and if the patient returns reporting a lack of progress the first three things that need checking are adherence, adherence and adherence!

Goals will need resetting as it is unlikely that recovery will occur in time to allow sufficient training to be done before the target event. It is often interesting to find that what appears to be a relatively simple musculoskeletal problem requires high-level consultation skills to manage effectively.

### Tibialis posterior tendonopathy

Pain in the medial longitudinal arch of the foot should suggest tendonopathy of the tibialis posterior tendon, which travels around the medial malleolus where it is contained by a synovial sheath within the tarsal tunnel. It then courses distally to insert into the undersurface of the navicular with slips to the cuneiforms. The tibialis posterior raises and supports the arch of the foot. Symptoms occur in people who spend prolonged periods of time on their feet, often in footwear that does not support the arch of the foot, and especially in the pronated foot. Sporting or occupational activity may be implicated and needs to be explored. Optimal management is probably by referral to podiatry. Treatment will involve eccentric loading exercise and support to the medial longitudinal arch, either with arch-supporting footwear or orthotic inserts.

### Patellar tendonopathy

Pain in the patella tendon is less common than other lower-limb tendon problems and tends to occur as a result of more 'explosive' athletic activity – jumping and sprinting. Once again there may be an associated bursitis causing local swelling. The eccentric loading regime for this problem is optimally performed on a decline board.

### Lateral hip tendonopathy

In the past, pain around the greater trochanter of the hip has been attributed to trochanteric bursitis. We now know that this is much less common than gluteal tendonopathy, which may or may not be accompanied by a bursitis. This may occur in athletic individuals but often occurs in the more sedentary and in association with degenerative change in the hip joint. A more acute presentation with a tender, palpable swelling might suggest a bursitis. Simple tendonopathy is perhaps more likely to present with more chronic low-level pain. At this site ultrasound is less helpful in demonstrating pathology and an MRI scan may be preferred. A bursitis may be treated effectively with a steroid injection or therapeutic ultrasound in addition to the eccentric loading regime.[4]

### Hip adductor tendonopathy

Pain deep in the groin can be difficult to assess and diagnose. Multiple pathology may coexist. Specialist expertise will usually be required to establish the diagnosis. Potential causes include hip joint pathology (degenerative change or labral tears) and abdominal wall pathology (hernias) and referred pain from the lumbar spine or viscera in addition to adductor tendonopathy. The 'groin strain' so common in football and other sports that involve side to side movements – 'cutting and weaving' – may be due to adductor tendonopathy, but can require multiple investigations before the diagnosis is established. Treatment and rehabilitation is often protracted and can involve significant time out of competitive sport.

A referral to a musculoskeletal specialist or an extended-scope physiotherapy practitioner with an interest in groin pain would be appropriate.[5]

### Rotator cuff tendonopathy

Shoulder pain is very common in primary care and has been reported to comprise up to 7% of primary care consultations. Most shoulder pain is due to rotator cuff tendonopathy. Rotator cuff pain is experienced in the lateral upper arm – in the C5 dermatome. Patients usually indicate the area of pain with a flat hand and fingers, although sometimes they may point at the deltoid insertion.

Assessment and management of rotator cuff disorders is complex and could involve a whole chapter in itself. Rotator cuff tendonopathy is common in the older patient and those whose sport, occupation or leisure involves repetitive activity where the hand is used above head height. A complex interplay of intrinsic and extrinsic factors may be involved including previous shoulder injury, notably dislocation (leading to instability), or a fall on to the outstretched hand (traumatising the cuff), muscle imbalance, biomechanical factors, posture, excessive volume of activity and equipment issues. The complexity of the problem means that rotator cuff tendonopathy is unlikely to respond to single, simple interventions such as a steroid injection, although an injection may be helpful if there is an accompanying subacromial bursitis. Referral to a musculoskeletal service is appropriate.

Use of the term supraspinatus tendinitis should be discontinued. The individual rotator cuff tendons fuse into a single structure that is complex and interweaving. Although the superior portion of the cuff is most often involved in rotator cuff injury fibres from more than one muscle may be involved and it is often not possible to link symptoms to the activity of a single muscle. In addition, this is not an inflammatory condition.[6]

## Lateral elbow tendonopathy – or epicondylopathy

Tennis elbow is a very common problem in primary care. It is usually an overuse injury due to excessive repetitive activity with poor technique, inappropriate equipment or a combination of these factors. Despite the name, most GPs will not see an abundance of tennis players with sore elbows. More often it is related to occupational activity, although different activities may combine to cause tissue overload and the onset of symptoms.

Once again an assessment of equipment, activity, technique and biomechanical factors is required. Reduction of activity overload and the modification of both techniques and equipment are likely to be more important than medical interventions in the long-term management of this problem.

A steroid injection can produce short- to medium-term pain relief but is not usually curative. Once again referral to physiotherapy for a progressive eccentric loading programme is recommended.

---

Box 7.3 ○ *Case study – lateral elbow pain*

Mrs Collins was a 35-year-old medical secretary. She presented to her GP with right lateral elbow pain. Several months ago she had returned to playing tennis now that both her children were attending school. She had found her form again and was doing well in the local league. Her symptoms started following a weekend when she played two matches on the Saturday and spent Sunday stripping wallpaper from the dining room walls.

Her GP prescribed some anti-inflammatory drugs and offered her a steroid injection. She declined the injection and asked if she could be referred to physiotherapy. The physiotherapist was relieved to hear that all the wallpaper had been removed and advised a rest from tennis for six weeks. He gave her an eccentric loading programme using therabands. He advised a graded return to tennis starting with 15 minutes twice a week and increasing by another 5 minutes each week. He gave her a tennis elbow clasp to wear whilst playing but she found it uncomfortable and soon dispensed with it.

For the future she was advised to consider hiring a decorator!

---

**COMMENT**

Mrs Collins's elbow problem may have arisen due to a number of factors or combinations thereof.

Her work involves use of a computer keyboard and mouse. Her sporting activity was greater than usual on the Saturday. However, on Sunday, as is often the case with DIY activity, she launched into the decorating activity with great enthusiasm but probably not a great deal of skill. She had not 'trained' for the activity and did not take the usual breaks that a professional decorator would have done. We cannot know whether she had any tendonopathy before the decorating marathon but she had no symptoms. If she experienced recurrence of symptoms without DIY overload it may be appropriate to suggests she gets a coach to look at her technique and racket grip. However, it is most likely that the onset of symptoms was largely due to her decorating.

Therabands are lengths of latex rubber of graded thickness that can be used to provide resistance to muscle action – such as wrist extension in Mrs Collins's case. They are very useful for rehabilitation regimes. Weights can be used but therabands are much more portable in the pocket or the kitbag and can be taken anywhere – so there are no excuses for not doing the exercises.

Epicondylar (or tennis elbow) clasps are popular but do not have good evidence of effectiveness. They are however cheap and safe so worth trying before more invasive interventions.[7,8]

### Other causes of tendon pain

Where tendons are encased in a synovial sheath there is the potential for tenosynovitis with overuse activity and adverse biomechanics. An underlying systemic inflammatory disorder should always be considered and investigated with tenosynovitis at multiple sites or in the presence of inflamed joints.

Tenosynovitis most commonly affects the tendon sheaths around the wrist and ankle. Signs of inflammation will be present with warmth, swelling and crepitus. Anti-inflammatory treatments are appropriate for tenosynovitis in addition to attention to activity and any biomechanical issues. Sometimes splinting to immobilise the painful structures is very helpful. A supervised rehabilitation programme from physiotherapy may reduce the risk of recurrence.

Finally it should be remembered that certain drugs can be associated with tendon pain. These include statins and fluoroquinolone antibiotics. It is probably worthwhile checking and stopping medication before embarking on a tendonopathy treatment regime.

### Work-related upper-limb disorder

This is a term used to classify painful conditions of the upper limb occurring in an occupational context. There are two types. In Type 1 WRULD, symptoms are well localised to a specific site and there is an easily identified pathological process. Included under this heading are lateral epicondylopathy, nerve entrapment syndromes and tenosynovitis at the wrist.

In Type 2 WRULD, symptoms are more diffusely experienced and it is impossible to identify a specific pathological process with currently available investigations. Other terms previously used to describe these conditions include reflex sympathetic dystrophy and repetitive strain injury. They are complex and challenging problems to manage. These problems do not respond to simple, single, biomedical interventions. Type 2 WRULD is an example of a complex regional pain syndrome.

WRULD is unlikely to be satisfactorily managed in a medical setting alone.

The most important management strategies should occur in the workplace and this means occupational health involvement. Type 2 WRULD may require referral to a chronic pain service.

---

Box 7.4 ○ *Complex regional pain syndrome*

Mary presented to her GP with a six-month history of lateral elbow pain. She was 59 years old and worked as a cleaner in a busy hotel kitchen. Her pain seemed to start when her workload increased when a colleague left and was not replaced. She had protested to her supervisor about her workload and was unhappy that the situation has not been resolved. She described the pain as severe, with simple analgesia bringing no relief. Her past medical history included lower-back pain and depression.

She was initially referred to physiotherapy. Mary's pain was elicited by provocative tests for extensor tendonopathy. She was supplied with an elbow clasp and started on a programme of eccentric loading exercises.

Unfortunately, Mary's pain failed to improve and she returned to her GP. She was issued with a sick note for one month and given a steroid injection to the lateral elbow.

Six months later she consulted again. Her pain had reappeared but was more diffusely experienced in the elbow and forearm. She had given up her job and been to Citizens Advice to discuss a claim for constructive dismissal. Her GP referred her to the musculoskeletal clinic. The GP specialist found evidence of allodynia (where an innocuous stimulus produces pain) and hyperalgesia (where a given stimulus produces increased pain perception) on local palpation. He made a diagnosis of complex regional pain syndrome and referred her for chronic pain management.

---

**COMMENT**

This much more complex case is an example of how socioeconomic issues can impact on health. When organisations and businesses are looking to save money (cost improvement!) employees are often not replaced when they leave, leading to increased workload for those remaining. What seems initially to be straightforward pathology, a lateral elbow tendonopathy (in this case a Type 1 WRULD) can subsequently become a more complex chronic pain problem – Type 2 WRULD.

It is possible that Mary may have been 'vulnerable' to this kind of problem – note her history of low-back pain and depression. We do not know how happy she was in her work previously or indeed how much she was looking forward to retirement, but these issues may be relevant. Relationships with others at work also have relevance in these challenging problems. It is unlikely that the GP would be able to manage this problem with simple medical interventions and without involving other services such as occupational health. Compensation seeking is often associated with poorer outcomes. Multidisciplinary interventions from a pain management team have the strongest evidence of effectiveness in these problems.

### Not to be forgotten – referred pain

Pain from neural compromise in the neck can sometimes refer to the lateral elbow, wrist or base of the thumb, and lure the physician into a misdiagnosis. Neurological examination should always be considered if symptoms and signs are atypical.

### Summary

We now have a completely new understanding of tendon pathology that requires a total revision of the assessment and management of these common problems. We now know that tendon pathology (as distinct from tendon sheath pathology) is not an inflammatory condition and that anti-inflammatory treatments are inappropriate.

New treatments are emerging for tendonopathy but as yet the evidence base of effectiveness is less than strong. At present the best evidence supports the use of progressive eccentric loading regimes to encourage tendon healing.

The assessment and management of tendon problems is more complex and multifaceted than previously thought. Tendonopathy is unlikely to resolve satisfactorily with single, simple interventions.

Referral to specialist services such as sports injury clinics, musculoskeletal clinics, occupational health, physiotherapy and podiatry is recommended.

Even with the best currently available treatments these problems are slow to resolve. Diligent adherence to treatment regimes is vital.

### References

1 • Khan KM, Cook JL, Kannus P, *et al.* Time to abandon the 'tendinitis myth' *British Medical Journal* 2002; **324(7338)**: 626–7.

2 • Rees JD, Wolman RL, Wilson A. Eccentric exercises: why do they work, what are the problems and how can we improve them? *British Journal of Sports Medicine* 2009; **43(4)**: 242–6.

3 • Alfredson H, Cook J. A treatment algorithm for managing Achilles tendinopathy: new treatment options *British Journal of Sports Medicine* 2007; **41(4)**: 211–16.

4 • Bahr R, Khan K. Management of lateral hip pain *British Medical Journal* 2009; **338**: b713. doi: 10.1136/bmj.b713.

5 • Holmich P. Long-standing groin pain in sportspeople falls into three primary patterns, a 'clinical entity' approach: a prospective study of 207 patients *British Journal of Sports Medicine* 2007; **41(4)**: 247–52.

6 • Lewis J S. Rotator cuff tendinopathy *British Journal of Sports Medicine* 2009; **43(4)**: 236–41.

7 • Stasinopoulos D, Stasinopoulos I, Pantelis M, *et al*. Comparison of effects of a home exercise programme and a supervised exercise programme for the management of lateral elbow tendinopathy *British Journal of Sports Medicine* 2010; **44(8)**: 579–83.

8 • Smidt N, van der Windt D A. Tennis elbow in primary care *British Medical Journal* 2006; **333(7575)**: 927–8.

# Osteoarthritis

**8**

*Claire Y J Wenham and Philip G Conaghan*

## Aims of this chapter

- To understand the pathology of osteoarthritis (OA) and the risk factors for its development.
- To be able to assess a person with suspected OA, make a diagnosis and refer for appropriate investigations if required.
- To manage OA symptoms using both pharmacological and non-pharmacological treatments.
- To consider the effect of pain and disability on a person's work and home life.
- To understand when to refer to secondary care/specialists.

## Introduction

OA is the most common form of arthritis worldwide. It is a major cause of joint pain and disability, and the most common reason for total hip and knee replacement. It places a large burden on primary care, with 3 million GP consultations for OA taking place in the UK in 2000[1] and, as a greater part of the population live longer, these figures are likely to increase. There are over 8 million people in the UK living with OA and the 2003 OA Nation survey (a survey of almost 2000 people with OA) found that 81% are in constant pain or are limited in their scope to perform everyday tasks. Despite this high prevalence of OA, many people will have had symptoms for months before they seek medical help and may never seek help, which may reflect a negative community outlook on OA treatment.[2] GPs have the potential to help reverse this rather pessimistic outlook.

## The role of primary care

The GP should be able to:

▷ confidently diagnose OA and also identify patients with an inflammatory arthritis who need early referral to rheumatology
▷ provide patient education and encourage self-help techniques as part of a holistic assessment of each person with OA
▷ address the potentially reversible risk factors for OA where possible
▷ initiate an appropriate management plan for OA, including the recommended National Institute for Health and Clinical Excellence (NICE) 'core' treatments
▷ use resources sensibly, avoiding investigations that do not change management and treatments that have no good evidence
▷ make appropriate referrals to secondary care.

---

## Pathogenesis of OA

Traditionally thought of as 'wear and tear' arthritis, we now recognise that the pathology of OA is far more complicated. The term 'wear and tear' also has negative connotations as it may imply to patients that nothing can be done to help them, hence this term is best avoided. The OA joint is best seen as a functional unit, so a person's gait, the strength of the supporting muscles and ligaments, and the alignment of the joint all play an important part in trying to maintain the joint's normal function. The joint damage that occurs in OA is, at least in part, the result of active joint remodelling. It involves all the joint structures and should be considered as failure of the joint's normal function.

The pathology of OA is characterised by thinning and focal changes of the articular cartilage with loss of joint space, the formation of bony outgrowths (osteophytes), increased bony sclerosis, cysts and deformity.[3] There is often associated meniscal damage, cruciate ligament tears and weakness of the muscles bridging the joint.

Imaging has played a crucial role in improving insight into the pathology of OA. With the more widespread use of magnetic resonance imaging (MRI) and ultrasound, it is now understood that inflammation of the synovium (synovitis) is common in the OA joint, despite the traditional belief that OA is non-inflammatory.[4] Frequent changes within the subchondral bone (bone underlying the cartilage) have also been demonstrated on MRI. These abnormalities are usually called 'bone marrow lesions' and represent areas of high signal on T2-weighted MRI.[5] Histology of these bone marrow lesions has suggested that they represent areas of altered trabecular bone structure.[6]

Both synovitis and bone marrow lesions have been associated with pain in large cohort studies. These structures are currently areas of research interest as potential treatment targets, as bone marrow lesions have also been associated with OA progression.[7]

At a structural level, there is increased local subchondral bone turnover, resulting in younger, less highly mineralised bone, with a subsequent decrease in subchondral bone stiffness and altered trabecular structure. Increased subchondral bone turnover, measured both by bone scans (scintigraphy) and urine/serum markers, may predict subsequent OA cartilage loss.[8,9]

---

## Defining OA

Definition of OA can be confusing because it can be classified pathologically, clinically or radiographically. Classification criteria are available from the American College of Rheumatology (see Box 8.1, Table 8.1 and Box 8.2) based on clinical, laboratory and radiographic features.

| Box 8.1 ○ *American College of Rheumatology classification criteria for OA of the hand* |
| --- |
| Hand pain, aching or stiffness, and three or four of the following:<br>▶ hard-tissue enlargement of two or more of ten selected joints*<br>▶ hard-tissue enlargement of two or more distal interphalangeal (DIP) joints<br>▶ fewer than three swollen MCP joints<br>▶ deformity of at least one of ten selected joints.*<br><br>(Both hands should be assessed.) |
| * The ten selected joints are the second and third DIP, the second and third proximal interphalangeal, and the first carpometacarpal joints of both hands. |

Table 8.1 ○ *American College of Rheumatology classification criteria for OA of the knee*

| Clinical and laboratory | Clinical and radiographic | Clinical |
|---|---|---|
| Knee pain | Knee pain | Knee pain |
| + at least 5 of 9: | + at least 1 of 3: | + at least 3 of 6: |
| Age >50 years<br>Stiffness <30 minutes<br>Crepitus<br>Bony tenderness<br>Bony enlargement<br>No palpable warmth<br>ESR <40 mm/hour<br>RF <1:40<br>SF OA | Age >50 years<br>Stiffness <30 minutes<br>Crepitus<br>+ osteophytes | Age >50 years<br>Stiffness <30 minutes<br>Crepitus<br>Bony tenderness<br>Bony enlargement<br>No palpable warmth |
| 92% sensitive | 91% sensitive | 95% sensitive |
| 75% specific | 86% specific | 69% specific |

*Notes*: ESR = erythrocyte sedimentation rate (Westergren) | RF = rheumatoid factor | SF OA = synovial fluid signs of OA (clear, viscous, or white blood cell count <2000/mm³).

---

Box 8.2 ○ *American College of Rheumatology classification criteria for OA of the hip*

**Hip pain and:**

▶ hip internal rotation <15°

▶ ESR ≤45 mm per hour (if ESR not available, substitute hip flexion ≤115°)

*or*

**hip pain and:**

▶ hip internal rotation ≥15°

▶ pain on hip internal rotation

▶ morning stiffness of the hip ≤60 minutes

▶ age >50 years.

This classification method yields a sensitivity of 86% and a specificity of 75%.

*Note*: ESR = erythrocyte sedimentation rate (Westergren).

## Radiographic OA

Radiographic OA is more common than symptomatic OA, but it is important to note that *radiographic changes of OA do not necessarily equate to the symptoms of OA*. Indeed, about half of those with radiographic OA report no symptoms.[10] Likewise, a 2008 review reported that the proportion of patients with knee pain found to have radiographic OA ranged from 15–76%.[11] This variability might be due to studies not using X-ray views of all three compartments of the knee. However, even when all compartments are imaged, the highest proportion of people with pain who have radiographic knee OA is 76%. MRI studies show a high prevalence of joint pathologies in people with little radiological change. Hence, the diagnosis of OA should be largely clinical and imaging should be limited to when there is diagnostic difficulty.

## Symptomatic OA

Recognised clinically is a syndrome of joint pain with associated structural joint pathology. For patients, the syndrome of OA is joint pain and stiffness with an inability to participate in usual daily activities, and subsequent reduced quality of life. While joint pain is common, not all joint pain is attributable to OA (depending on the definition of OA and extra-articular causes of pain such as tendonitis). Women report more pain than men, and symptoms differ according to the joints affected.

It is important to realise that, unlike in clinical trial scenarios, many people have multiple joint pains, with a recent study in people over the age of 55 suggesting a median number of four painful joints. The most common combinations of joint pain are knee and foot pain, knee and back pain, and knee and hand pain.[12] These may well be biomechanically interrelated, e.g. limping due to a painful knee aggravates the lower back, or poor quadriceps strength associated with knee pain means increased reliance on upper limbs for everyday tasks such as climbing stairs or getting out of chairs.

## Which joints are affected by OA?

The joints most commonly affected by OA are as follows.

### *Hands: base of thumb, distal and proximal interphalangeal joints*

About a third of all adults have radiographic OA of the hands.[13] A recent study of over 1500 people over the age of 50 reported an incidence of hand pain of 20–24% over a period of three years, with a subsequent detrimental effect on global physical function.[14] Twenty-six per cent of women and 13% of men over the age of 70 have symptomatic OA in at least one hand joint. They commonly have difficulty in day-to-day activities such as gripping, writing and picking up small objects.[15]

### Hips

The prevalence of radiographic hip OA has been reported at around 8% in men and 6% in women. Symptoms are more common in the older age group, with 17% of men over 65 and 32% of women reporting hip pain.[16]

### Knees

The prevalence of disabling knee pain from OA has been estimated at 10% (in the over-55s).[2] Interestingly, the level of disability experienced by people with knee OA has been shown to correlate more accurately with their age and psychological involvement than with their radiographic scores.[17] This emphasises the importance of addressing mood, sleep patterns and coping skills when assessing a person with OA. Nonetheless, in a 2007 study of over 700 patients with knee pain, the presence of radiographic OA was consistently associated with the severity of pain, stiffness and physical function.[18]

### Spine: cervical and lumbosacral

Facet joint OA is very common, with a prevalence of approximately 60% in men and 67% in women. Prevalence increases with age but there is no clear correlation between low-back pain and the presence of facet joint OA on computerised tomography (CT) imaging.[19]

### First metatarsophalangeal joint

The presence of radiographic OA at the 1st metatarsophalangeal (MTP) joint has been associated with radiographic OA at both the hand and knee.

## Risk factors and prognostic factors for OA

Several risk factors for knee and hip OA are recognised. These can be divided into risk factors for development of OA and factors for its progression. Less evidence is available for hand OA. However, for a patient with Heberden's nodes, the mother is twice as likely, and the sister three times as likely, to demonstrate the same OA changes.

Table 8.2 ○ *Factors associated with the development and progression of hip OA*

| Factors associated with the development of hip OA | Factors associated with the progression of hip OA |
|---|---|
| Increasing age[20] | Superolateral migration of the femoral head[21] |
| Obesity[3] | Atrophic bone response (as defined on X-ray; an atrophic bone response can be associated with progression of hip OA, as opposed to a hypertrophic response)[21] |
| Occupational factors (heavy physical labour, e.g. farming)[22] | Age and female sex (conflicting evidence) |
| Physical sporting activity (highest risk in high-intensity sports)[21] | Reduced joint space width on first X-ray (conflicting evidence) |
| Hip dysplasia (weaker evidence) | |
| Oestrogen therapy may have a protective effect (weaker evidence) | |
| Lower levels of vitamin D (conflicting evidence) | |

## Preventing OA: the role of primary care

Most of the current therapies for OA target symptom control, as there are, as yet, no therapies that have been shown to have definite structure-modifying effects. The best current advice for the prevention of OA relates to lifestyle changes and includes:

▷ weight loss if overweight (with the aim of maintaining a BMI within the normal range)
▷ avoiding joint trauma
▷ avoiding high-impact loading of the joints (e.g. sports or occupation) – farming/construction workers are at higher risk of OA and these people would benefit from early joint protection advice
▷ maintaining aerobic fitness, which helps with weight control and periarticular muscle strength.

Table 8.3 ○ *Factors associated with the development and progression of knee OA*

| Factors associated with the development of knee OA | Factors associated with the progression of knee OA |
| --- | --- |
| Age[20] | Generalised OA |
| Occupational factors (physical workload), e.g. farmers, construction workers[22] | Varus alignment of the knee (bow-legged) and medial-compartment knee OA (four times the risk of radiographic progression) |
| Physical sporting activity (highest risk in high-intensity sports) | Valgus alignment of the knee (knock-kneed) and lateral-compartment knee OA (four times the risk of radiographic progression)[23] |
| Joint trauma (e.g. fracture through the joint line, meniscectomy,[24] anterior cruciate ligament rupture)[25] | Obesity[3] (conflicting results). Obesity increases progression in knees with normal alignment[26] |
| Obesity[3] | Low bone density, age, presence of Heberden's nodes (conflicting evidence)[27, 28] |
| Oestrogen therapy may have a protective effect (weaker evidence) | Lower levels of vitamin D (conflicting evidence).[29, 30] Routine testing not recommended |

## Person-centred care: the impact on the individual

### Symptoms

When OA is symptomatic, the most common complaint is *pain*. Patients vary in their description of pain, but pain is often felt when weightbearing through the joint. People with OA often feel worse at the end of the day, with symptoms worsening after repetitive weightbearing after a walk or after going up and down stairs.

Importantly, the cause of joint pain in OA is not clear. Recent MRI studies have suggested the synovium, subchondral bone, osteophytes and menisci as potential sources of pain.

Other symptoms include:

▷ **stiffness** ▶ usually after a period of inactivity – prolonged early morning stiffness (greater than 30 minutes) should make the GP suspicious of an inflammatory arthritis

▷ **gelling** ▶ (stiffening of the joint with inactivity, e.g. with prolonged sitting) is common in OA and is often mistaken for locking of the joint
▷ **swelling** ▶ or a feeling of fullness in the joint
▷ a **grinding** ▶ or clicking sensation with movement (may be painful)
▷ the knee **'giving way'** ▶ which usually represents weak quadriceps muscles.

### Impaired participation in activities

The OA Nation survey of 2003 demonstrated that 81% of people with OA had constant pain or were limited in performing everyday tasks. When their OA pain was 'bad', over half struggled to get out of bed. Although each painful joint has a considerable effect on a person's functional ability, the overall effect is substantially increased when more than one joint is involved.[12]

### Impaired quality of life

The psychological effect of OA should not be underestimated. People with OA report loss of self-esteem, loss of independence and feeling old before their time. Depression is common and should be looked for and treated appropriately.[31]

### Assessing the patient: a comprehensive approach

A holistic assessment of people with OA is the key to their successful management. The consultation should take into account a person's existing concerns and expectations, and their available support network.

Any assessment of joint pain should assess the:

▷ number of joints involved and their pattern (OA commonly involves multiple joints in the over-fifties)
▷ current pain symptoms
▷ current medical and self-help treatments being used
▷ consequences on participation in important daily activities and hobbies
▷ effects on the patient's ability to perform his or her job (are adjustments in the workplace necessary?)
▷ associated sleep and mood disturbance.

For busy primary care clinicians, this initial evaluation may need to take place over more than one consultation.

### History

▷ The most important differential to exclude is an inflammatory arthritis. Symmetrical joint pain, especially with *prolonged* early morning stiffness (more than 30 minutes) and raised inflammatory markers, should raise suspicion and warrants early rheumatology referral.
▷ Ask about diseases that are associated with an inflammatory arthritis such as diarrhoeal illnesses, sexually transmitted infections, inflammatory bowel disease and psoriasis.
▷ Ask about features that may be associated with a connective tissue disease, including photosensitivity, mouth ulcers or a rash.
▷ Ask about a family history of inflammatory arthritis (remember gout).

### Examination

Examination findings in OA may include:

▷ tenderness (most marked over the joint line)
▷ swelling (synovial or bony)
▷ crepitus
▷ reduced range of movement
▷ reduced muscle strength.

#### HANDS

Examination findings range from minimal tenderness to marked bony deformity, with Heberden's nodes at the distal interphalangeal joints and Bouchard's nodes at the proximal interphalangeal joints (see Figure 8.1 on p. 475). OA of the 1st carpometacarpal (CMC) joint, or thumb base, is common, with resulting tenderness at the anatomical snuff box or marked squaring.

Weakened grip strength, with associated weak forearm muscles, may result from prolonged hand pain.

#### KNEE

There may be a flexion deformity, which may be reversible early in the disease and fixed later on. Note any varus or valgus deformity (risk factors for OA progression) and examine for the presence of a knee effusion, bony enlargement or tenderness, and crepitus. Examine for a swelling posteriorly, which may be a popliteal (Baker's) cyst; these are quite common in moderate to severe knee OA. It is also important to check for ligament stability of the collateral and cruciate ligaments.

## HIP

While patients may attribute lateral thigh pain to hip disease, true hip joint pain is usually felt in the groin or deep buttock and people may complain of difficulty in putting on shoes or socks.

In early hip OA there is usually loss of internal rotation with the patient lying on his or her back and the knee flexed to 90°. Symptoms can often be reproduced with active or passive movements of the hip joint.

## Investigations

### RADIOGRAPHY

The diagnosis of OA is mainly clinical. Radiographs are useful only if there is diagnostic uncertainty, or to assess the structural severity of the disease.

The typical radiographic findings of OA are:

▷ joint-space narrowing (the patient should be weightbearing for knee films)
▷ osteophytes (bony outgrowths)
▷ subchondral bone thickening or sclerosis
▷ cysts in the subchondral bone.

Figures 8.2 and 8.3 demonstrate radiographic findings. Figure 8.2 shows severe erosive OA. Note that predominantly the PIPs and DIPs are affected, as well as severe thumb base disease. The distal location, hypertrophic nature (note osteophytosis) and asymmetrical pattern favour the diagnosis of OA.

Figure 8.3 demonstrates severe OA, particularly of the medial tibiofemoral compartment, with flattening of the articular surfaces, florid osteophytes and marked medial-joint space loss.

Chondrocalcinosis (calcification of areas of the hyaline cartilage) is common in OA and may be secondary to the deposition of calcium pyrophosphate crystals. These crystals are commonly seen in patients with underlying OA (over 60% have calcium pyrophosphate crystals in knee synovial fluid).[32]

Small calcified foreign bodies may also be noted on X-rays and these are usually only of clinical significance if the patient complains of true knee locking.

### OTHER IMAGING TECHNIQUES

MRI has revolutionised knowledge of the pathology and potential sources of pain in OA. However, it has no current role in the routine investigation or management of OA and at present remains primarily a research tool.

Figure 8.2 ○ *Radiograph of osteoarthritic hands*

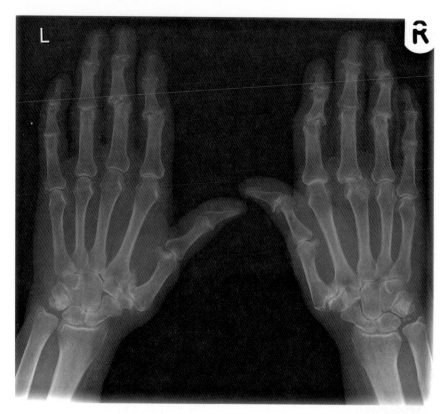

Ultrasound can accurately assess effusions and synovitis but as yet has no routine role in the investigation of a person with suspected OA. However, it can be useful for differentiating between inflammatory arthritides and OA, particularly in symptomatic hands.

**BLOOD TESTS**

There are no specific blood tests that exclude or diagnose OA. C-reactive protein (CRP) or rheumatoid factor should be checked only if inflammatory arthritis is suspected.

**SYNOVIAL FLUID**

Analysis of synovial fluid can be very useful, especially in diagnostic dilemmas. The detection of monosodium urate crystals along with inflammatory symptoms can help to confirm the diagnosis of gout. Calcium pyrophosphate crystals are commonly detected in the synovial fluid of OA knees, although

Figure 8.3 ○ *Radiograph of osteoarthritic knee*

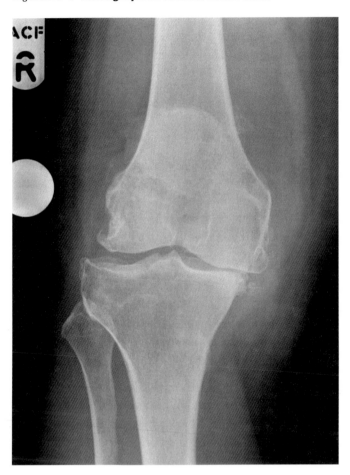

patients are often asymptomatic. However, their deposition within the joint can cause acute and painful inflammatory symptoms (pseudogout), commonly in the knee and wrist.

### The management of OA

Several key principles must be implemented:

#### EDUCATION

Education is essential. This involves providing information about the condition and the safety and range of treatment options available so that people can be involved in their own management. Patient information leaflets and helpful website addresses should be offered (see the online resources section at the end of this chapter).

## PHARMACOLOGICAL AND NON-PHARMACOLOGICAL THERAPIES

Management involves both pharmacological and non-pharmacological therapies. Therapies with moderate efficacy and minimal toxicity/side effects, e.g. exercise, should be used first.

## TAILORED MANAGEMENT

Management should be tailored according to each person's needs, risk factors and co-morbidities. The effects of treatments should be regularly reviewed for efficacy and side effects, and treatments should be altered if the desired therapeutic effect is not achieved.

**198**

## Current treatment guidelines

All current treatments for OA are based on symptom control, as there are currently no accepted structure-modifying drugs. Recommended treatment options are based on two recent (2008) evidence-based guidelines: the NICE guideline[33] and the Osteoarthritis Research Society International (OARSI) guideline.[34] The main difference between the two is that NICE includes a health economic analysis relevant to the UK.

NICE recommendations for management are divided into core therapies and additional treatment options (see Figure 8.4). This approach reflects the fact that most people with OA will need multiple treatment options, both pharmacological and non-pharmacological. The core options are safe and effective, and should be initiated as first-line treatment.

The OARSI guidelines are evidence based, with recommendations based on worldwide expert consensus. These recommendations may be adapted for use according to the availability of different treatment modalities. The subsequent discussion takes into account recommendations by both groups.

### First-line treatments

#### EXERCISE

Regular exercise must be a first-line recommendation for all people with OA and is recommended in all existing OA guidelines, supported by good evi-

Figure 8.4 ○ **_Targeting treatment in OA – recommendations from the NICE OA guideline_**

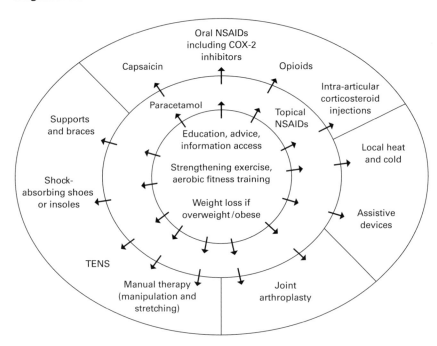

*Source*: reproduced from National Collaborating Centre for Chronic Conditions. *Osteoarthritis: national clinical guideline for care and management in adults* London: Royal College of Physicians, 2008. Copyright © 2008 Royal College of Physicians. Reproduced by permission.[33]

dence from systematic reviews and meta-analyses.[35] Exercise reduces pain, disability, medication intake and improves both physical functioning and mental health. Pain should not be a barrier to exercise and regular analgesia may be needed.

Exercise should be of two forms: aerobic and muscle strengthening, specific to the joints involved (for example forearm-strengthening exercises for hand OA and quadriceps exercises for knee OA). For patients with hip OA, exercise in water can be particularly helpful. Many council-run swimming pools run regular women-only or disabled swimming sessions, which those with particularly poor mobility, or who have a negative body image, may find easier to attend.

While basic exercise advice (general aerobic fitness, forearm and quadriceps exercises) should be initiated in primary care, referral to a physiotherapist is helpful for people with OA struggling with persistent symptoms.

The 'Exercise on Prescription' scheme is a partnership between Primary Care Trusts (PCTs) and local-authority leisure services, and is now widely available. For the cost of a prescription charge, suitable patients can be referred for a ten-week, individually tailored fitness programme at a nearby leisure centre.

### WEIGHT LOSS

Weight loss in those who are overweight or obese has been shown to improve function in hip and knee OA. The evidence for reduction of pain is less convincing,[36] but new trials are underway. Weight should be maintained within the normal BMI range (20–25).

PCTs may also fund local schemes for weight loss, for example the Weight Watchers or Slimming World programmes in which PCTs can purchase a course at a much reduced price, thereby allowing patients to attend at no cost to themselves.

## Pharmacological treatments

### PARACETAMOL AND / OR TOPICAL NSAIDS

After exercise and weight loss have been initiated, these are the recommended first treatments if additional analgesia is needed. Multiple daily applications of topical non-steroidal anti-inflammatory drugs (NSAIDs) may be needed for maximum analgesic effect, which can reduce compliance. However, they are effective, at least in the short term. A recent 12-month community study found equivalent pain-reducing benefits from advice to prescribe either oral or topical NSAIDs.[37] Paracetamol has been shown to be effective, particularly for knee OA, and it has a reassuring long-term safety profile. However, patients should be aware that infrequent dosing may reduce its efficacy.

### TOPICAL CAPSAICIN

This topical application is derived from chilli peppers and can give effective pain relief for knee or hand OA when applied up to four times a day. However, local redness or irritation can occur in 40% of patients, especially with the first few applications.

### OPIOIDS AND ORAL NSAID / COX-2 DRUGS

If insufficient pain relief is gained from paracetamol and topical NSAIDs then the additional use of an opioid or oral NSAID/COX-2 should be considered.

NSAID/COX-2 drugs should be used at the lowest effective dose for the shortest possible time period. Their potential gastrointestinal, cardio-renal and liver toxicity must be noted when prescribing, and these risk factors assessed at least on a yearly basis. NICE now recommends that all NSAIDs and COX-2 drugs should be co-prescribed with a proton pump inhibitor (PPI). This was based on a health economics analysis, driven by gastrointestinal side effects and the recent availability of generic PPIs.

The use of NSAIDs or COX-2 drugs in coexisting cardiovascular disease is problematic and often contraindicated. Potential interactions between NSAIDs and aspirin may interfere with the antiplatelet effects of aspirin.[38] NICE therefore recommends that people taking low-dose aspirin (usually a marker of significant cardiovascular disease or risk) should try alternative analgesics before considering an NSAID/COX-2 inhibitor.

A recent meta-analysis of the use of opioids in OA suggested reasonable analgesic efficacy, although there was less effect on function.[39] The evidence for the optimal dose or route of administration is less clear. Opioids have a high incidence of minor side effects (e.g. confusion and constipation), which may be more troublesome in older patients and therefore doses should be titrated.

## INTRA-ARTICULAR INJECTIONS

Corticosteroid injections can be used for the relief of moderate to severe pain in people with knee and base of thumb OA. Usually no more than three to four per year are recommended and the period of pain relief post-injection is a good time to promote muscle-strengthening exercises. Intra-articular steroid to the knee gives a modest but short-term benefit (usually two to four weeks) in approximately 70% of patients.[40]

## HYALURONAN INJECTION

Although there are many trials of hyaluronans, there is mixed data on their effectiveness. NICE does not recommend them (based on health economics analysis); however, the OARSI guideline notes that some preparations may be useful for knee and hip OA.[34] The difficulty is that there is no good current evidence to select subgroups who may have a better and therefore more cost-effective response to hyaluronans.

## GLUCOSAMINE AND/OR CHONDROITIN

The use of these agents is controversial due to differing trial results and available preparations. Recently one preparation of glucosamine hydrochloride has been licensed for use in the UK, but results from glucosamine hydrochloride trials have not suggested any benefit. There is some evidence for symptomatic relief of knee OA with the use of glucosamine sulphate (not licensed in the UK) at a dose of 1.5 g daily[34] and a short trial can be considered. Most PCTs will not support the prescription of glucosamine as it is not recommended by NICE; however, patients may be happy to buy these products over the counter. People could therefore be advised that a trial of glucosamine sulphate at a dose of 1.5 g per day is reasonable, and that pain should be evaluated before starting treatment and then at three to six months. If no benefit is noticed within six months then the treatment should be discontinued.

The evidence from systematic reviews of the efficacy of chondroitin is less convincing. As with glucosamine, chondroitin is not recommended by NICE.

### Non-pharmacological treatments

#### MANUAL THERAPY

Manual therapy includes mobilisation, soft-tissue massage, manipulation, and stretching and passive movements to the joints and soft tissue. In most studies, manual therapy was used in conjunction with other treatments such as exercise, reflecting current physiotherapy practice, in which manual therapy is used as part of a range of treatments. There is limited evidence that manual therapy may be of use in hip OA and specialist referral to physiotherapy should be considered for these patients.

#### AIDS AND DEVICES

Patients should be advised to wear appropriate footwear (shock-absorbing with arch support) for knee/hip OA. Lateral-wedged insoles can be of symptomatic benefit for patients with medial tibiofemoral-compartment OA (see below for podiatry referral). Walking aids can reduce pain in knee or hip OA, with the aid used in the contralateral hand.

A splint for base of thumb OA can give pain relief (in conjunction with forearm-strengthening exercises).

A knee brace can reduce pain and the risk of falls in knee OA and mild/moderate valgus or varus instability. However, for most patients with OA, this is not a substitute for quadriceps exercises. A referral to the local orthotics department would be required.

#### ELECTROTHERAPY (TENS)

TENS may give additional short-term pain relief for some people with hip or knee OA, although it cannot be predicted which patients may respond.

Proper training in the placing of pads and selection of stimulation intensity could make a difference to the benefit obtained. Patients should be encouraged to experiment with different intensities and length of application, and this encourages a self-management approach. No adverse events or toxicity have been reported with TENS and most people purchase their own TENS machine so the cost implication for the NHS is minimal. TENS is also recommended by NICE.

**THERMOTHERAPY**

Local cold or heat application can reduce symptoms and is a simple self-management technique. Although there is little evidence for the effectiveness of thermotherapy, NICE recommends this intervention as it is cheap and extremely safe.

**ACUPUNCTURE**

Acupuncture remains controversial due to mixed trial results and differing regimens and types of acupuncture interventions. There is some evidence for short-term (two to six weeks) symptomatic relief for knee OA.[34] Acupuncture is not currently recommended by NICE due to the mixed trial results.

Some NHS Trusts may offer acupuncture services via referral to the physiotherapy department. It should be noted that the benefit is often short lived, and a limited number of sessions are usually available on the NHS. However, some patients may be willing to pay for acupuncture in the community, if they find it beneficial.

203

---

## Facilitating self-help strategies

A range of strategies are available to improve the individual's ability to self-manage his or her OA symptoms.

▷ Regular and accurate information provision should be ensured.
   Numerous websites are available to support and advise people with
   OA (see the online resources section at the end of this chapter). Useful
   information leaflets are provided by Arthritis Research UK.
▷ The self-treatment measures described above, especially regular exercise
   and weight loss, should be regularly reviewed and encouraged.
▷ Local exercise programmes can help improve fitness and confidence
   (e.g. local swimming sessions).

▷ Support groups, for example Arthritis Care (see the online resources section at the end of this chapter), can be used by patients. Arthritis Care provides a UK-wide network of self-management training sessions; these courses are usually provided in partnership with local PCTs.

---

## When to refer?

### *Orthopaedics*

#### ARTHROPLASTY

Total hip arthroplasty (THA) and knee joint arthroplasty (TKA) are universally recommended in existing OA treatment guidelines. They are generally accepted as reliable and appropriate surgical procedures to restore function and improve quality of life in people with hip and knee OA who are not obtaining adequate pain relief and functional improvement with pharmacological and non-pharmacological treatments.[41,42] Unicompartmental knee replacement can be effective for knee OA limited to one compartment of the knee, which may represent a third of people with knee OA.[43] Osteotomy and joint-preserving procedures may be considered in young adults with symptomatic hip OA, especially in the presence of dysplasia, but are not frequently performed these days.[34]

There are a number of scoring systems that were used as a guide for surgical referral, but review of the literature has not demonstrated the validity or usefulness of these systems so they are no longer recommended. It is helpful to ask a few simple questions that can assess a patient's functional limitation: How far can the patient walk? Can the patient get round the supermarket and do his or her shopping? Does the patient work and is this affected by OA? Is sleep disturbed? Has the patient had to stop leisure activities?

There is limited evidence on the optimal timing for referral but NICE recommends that people should be referred *before* they have prolonged or established functional limitation or severe pain. NICE also recommends that, after discussion with surgical experts, individual features such as age, obesity or other co-morbidities should not deter health professionals from referring a patient with significant pain or limitation for a surgical opinion.

#### ARTHROSCOPY

A clear history of mechanical locking, which is an inability to move the flexed knee without physical manipulation, may represent a meniscal tear or loose body. It is an appropriate reason for referral for arthroscopy; however, loose bodies on plain X-ray do not warrant referral for arthroscopy unless there is associated locking. Arthroscopic knee washout alone has no demonstrated clinically useful benefit in the short or long term for knee OA.

## RHEUMATOLOGY

Referral to a rheumatologist should be considered if:

▷ an inflammatory arthritis is suspected
▷ there is diagnostic uncertainty and the patient or GP is concerned
▷ there is substantial impact of joint symptoms on quality of life.

## PHYSIOTHERAPY

There is time in a quick consultation to instruct a patient in simple quadriceps- or forearm-strengthening exercises. There should be a low threshold for referring a patient for physiotherapy if a patient has ongoing symptoms despite basic aerobic and local exercise (e.g. quadriceps exercises) initiation. Most people with OA will benefit from expert assessment and regular exercises.

## PODIATRY

A podiatry referral may be appropriate for patients with foot pain and abnormalities of the feet, for example a pronounced varus or valgus deformity or MTP pain, as specialised insoles may reduce pain and improve mobility.

---

Box 8.3 ○ *Case study*

Mrs Evans, a 76-year-old woman, is complaining of pain in her right knee when going up and down stairs. She is relatively fit for her age and has no other co-morbidities. Her only medication is paracetamol and glucosamine. Her 70-year-old husband has carcinoma of the prostate gland and senile macular degeneration; he is registered as blind. Her sleep is disturbed by pain from the knee.

On examination she had full range of movement in the right knee but there was a slight effusion. She was tender along the joint line. Tests for ligament weakness and cartilage problems were negative.

X-rays were requested (PA and lateral views to demonstrate the patello-femoral joint), which showed moderately severe OA of the medial compartment of the right knee and also in the patello-femoral compartment.

---

### Analysis of case study with respect to the six domains of Being a GP

What are the options for management? With reference to the core competences of general practice:

#### DOMAIN 1: PRIMARY CARE MANAGEMENT

▷ Clinical management: the medical condition here has been diagnosed as OA of the knee (medial and patello-femoral compartments).
▷ Onward referral may be an option; there may be a GP with specialist interest in musculoskeletal medicine within the practice team; referral to physiotherapy for quadriceps strengthening would be an option, or onward referral to an orthopaedic surgeon for operative management.
▷ Onward referral may involve referral systems such as 'choose and book'; the patient must be given a choice of referral destination.

#### DOMAIN 2: PERSON-CENTRED CARE

▷ During the consultation, Mrs Evans's concerns about her medical condition would be explored. Her worries about the future may have a bearing on why she has presented now. Her husband is dependent on her because of his visual impairment and now has carcinoma of the prostate gland; she may be worried about how she will cope with his illness if she is struggling with her own mobility.

#### DOMAIN 3: SPECIFIC PROBLEM-SOLVING SKILLS

▷ Data gathering and interpretation: the GP chose to undertake a knee examination, looking for signs of mechanical damage, inflammation or OA. On the basis of the examination an X ray was requested as the GP suspected that the main problem was OA.
▷ Making a decision: Mrs Evans was invited to return for a follow-up consultation to discuss the options for management and she chose to be referred on to an orthopaedic surgeon. Her analgesia was increased to co-codamol (8/500). Another option would have been to add amitryptiline at night to aid sleep and control the pain.

## DOMAIN 4: A COMPREHENSIVE APPROACH

▷ Thinking around Mrs Evans's problem knee, the GP could enlist help with the day-to-day care of her husband, by involving social services and asking for a home assessment of their care needs.

▷ The GP could review Mr Evans's notes and see if he has all the support that he can get regarding his visual impairment. The GP may need to contact his ophthalmic consultant who issued the certificate of visual impairment (GOS15).

▷ The GP could also review the stage of his prostate cancer and see how this was being managed; a review would be necessary if the practitioner was involved with his care or if he or she needed to discuss the situation with a GP colleague. Was Mr Evans on the Gold Standards Framework register and was he known to the local hospice team?

▷ The GP could review Mrs Evans's other possible co-morbidities such as hypertension and ensure that she has had a recent BP measurement and lipid check, and also a dental check, so that if she comes to surgery she will be fit to proceed.

## DOMAIN 5: COMMUNITY ORIENTATION

▷ The GP could enquire about support from relatives so that if Mrs Evans needs knee surgery then support networks are in place.

## DOMAIN 6: A HOLISTIC APPROACH

▷ The GP needs to consider if his or her management plan is acceptable to both Mr and Mrs Evans.

▷ Does the GP need consent to discuss Mr Evans with his or her colleagues or the hospital consultant?

▷ Does the GP know enough about what will happen when Mrs Evans attends the orthopaedic out-patients' department? Does the GP have any learning needs in this area? Can the GP advise her accordingly?

▷ Is the GP making the best use of local resources by complying with Mrs Evans's request to be referred straight away, or should he or she suggest a course of physiotherapy first?

So a simple case of OA knee may actually reveal a number of coexisting problems that must also be addressed in the management of Mrs Evans.

It is imperative that Mrs Evans's GP should explore each of these areas and consider their impact on her care plan.

## Summary

▷ OA is the most common type of arthritis and should be considered as failure of the joint. The pathology includes thinning of the articular cartilage, joint space loss, the formation of bony osteophytes and bony sclerosis. Synovitis and subchondral bone marrow change seen on MRI are frequent findings and have been associated with pain.

▷ The most common symptom of OA is pain, but depression, poor sleep and impaired participation in activities are common and these issues must also be addressed.

▷ The initial steps of education, exercise and weight loss should be offered to all. A range of pharmacological and non-pharmacological treatments can then be explored.

▷ Self-help strategies include repeated education, patient support groups and exercise classes, and should be promoted in all patients.

▷ Appropriate referrals to specialists, including orthopaedics, rheumatology and physiotherapy, allow good use of limited resources.

### Online resources

▷ Arthritis Research UK, **www.arthritisresearchuk.org**.
▷ Arthritis Care, **www.arthritiscare.org.uk**.
▷ National Institute for Health and Clinical Excellence, **www.nice.org.uk**.

### References

1 • Arthritis Research Campaign. *Arthritis: the big picture* Chesterfield: ARC, 2002, www.ipsos-mori.com/Assets/Docs/Archive/Polls/arthritis.pdf [accessed October 2011].

2 • Peat G, McCarney R, Croft P. Knee pain and osteoarthritis in older adults: a review of community burden and current use of primary health care *Annals of the Rheumatic Diseases* 2001; **60(2)**: 91–7.

3 • Felson D T, Lawrence R C, Dieppe P A, *et al*. Osteoarthritis: new insights. Part 1: the disease and its risk factors *Annals of Internal Medicine* 2000; **133(8)**: 635–46.

4 • Hill C L, Hunter D J, Niu J, *et al*. Synovitis detected on magnetic resonance imaging and its relation to pain and cartilage loss in knee osteoarthritis *Annals of the Rheumatic Diseases* 2007; **66(12)**: 1599–603.

5 • Felson D T, Chaisson C E, Hill C L, *et al*. The association of bone marrow lesions with pain in knee osteoarthritis *Annals of Internal Medicine* 2001; **134(7)**: 541–9.

6 • Hunter D J, Gerstenfeld L, Bishop G, *et al.* Bone marrow lesions from osteoarthritis knees are characterized by sclerotic bone that is less well mineralized *Arthritis Research and Therapy* 2009; **11(1)**: R11.

7 • Felson D T, McLaughlin S, Goggins J, *et al.* Bone marrow edema and its relation to progression of knee osteoarthritis *Annals of Internal Medicine* 2003; **139(5 Pt 1)**: 330–6.

8 • Dieppe P, Cushnaghan J, Young P, *et al.* Prediction of the progression of joint space narrowing in osteoarthritis of the knee by bone scintigraphy *Annals of the Rheumatic Diseases* 1993; **52(8)**: 557–63.

9 • Bailey A J, Buckland-Wright C, Metz D. The role of bone in osteoarthritis *Age and Ageing* 2001; **30(5)**: 374–8.

10 • Lanyon P, O'Reilly S, Jones A, *et al.* Radiographic assessment of symptomatic knee osteoarthritis in the community: definitions and normal joint space *Annals of the Rheumatic Diseases* 1998; **57(10)**: 595–601.

11 • Bedson J, Croft P R. The discordance between clinical and radiographic knee osteoarthritis: a systematic search and summary of the literature *BMC Musculoskeletal Disorders* 2008; **9**: 116.

12 • Keenan A M, Tennant A, Fear J, *et al.* Impact of multiple joint problems on daily living tasks in people in the community over age fifty-five *Arthritis and Rheumatism* 2006; **55(5)**: 757–64.

13 • Lawrence R C, Helmick C G, Arnett F C, *et al.* Estimates of the prevalence of arthritis and selected musculoskeletal disorders in the United States *Arthritis and Rheumatism* 1998; **41(5)**: 778–99.

14 • Thomas E, Croft P R, Dziedzic K S. Hand problems in community-dwelling older adults: onset and effect on global physical function over a 3-year period *Rheumatology* (Oxford) 2009; **48(2)**: 183–7.

15 • Zhang Y, Niu J, Kelly-Hayes M, *et al.* Prevalence of symptomatic hand osteoarthritis and its impact on functional status among the elderly: the Framingham Study *American Journal of Epidemiology* 2002; **156(11)**: 1021–7.

16 • Reijman M, Pols H A, Bergink A P, *et al.* Body mass index associated with onset and progression of osteoarthritis of the knee but not of the hip: the Rotterdam Study *Annals of the Rheumatic Diseases* 2007; **66(2)**: 158–62.

17 • Salaffi F, Cavalieri F, Nolli M, *et al.* Analysis of disability in knee osteoarthritis. Relationship with age and psychological variables but not with radiographic score *Journal of Rheumatology* 1991; **18(10)**: 1581–6.

18 • Duncan R, Peat G, Thomas E, *et al.* Symptoms and radiographic osteoarthritis: not as discordant as they are made out to be? *Annals of the Rheumatic Diseases* 2007; **66(1)**: 86–91.

19 • Kalichman L, Li L, Kim D H, *et al.* Facet joint osteoarthritis and low back pain in the community-based population *Spine* 2008; **33(23)**: 2560–5.

20 • Felson D T. Risk factors for osteoarthritis: understanding joint vulnerability *Clinical Orthopaedics and Related Research* 2004; **427(Suppl)**: S16–21.

21 • Bierma-Zeinstra S M, Koes B W. Risk factors and prognostic factors of hip and knee osteoarthritis *National Clinical Practice Rheumatology* 2007; **3(2)**: 78–85.

22 • Felson DT, Hannan MT, Naimark A, *et al.* Occupational physical demands, knee bending, and knee osteoarthritis: results from the Framingham Study *Journal of Rheumatology* 1991; **18(10)**: 1587–92.

23 • Sharma L, Song J, Felson D T, *et al*. The role of knee alignment in disease progression and functional decline in knee osteoarthritis *Journal of the American Medical Association* 2001; **286(2)**: 188–95.

24 • Roos E M, Ostenberg A, Roos H, *et al*. Long-term outcome of meniscectomy: symptoms, function, and performance tests in patients with or without radiographic osteoarthritis compared to matched controls *Osteoarthritis Cartilage* 2001; **9(4)**: 316–24.

25 • Lohmander L S, Ostenberg A, Englund M, *et al*. High prevalence of knee osteoarthritis, pain, and functional limitations in female soccer players twelve years after anterior cruciate ligament injury *Arthritis and Rheumatism* 2004; **50(10)**: 3145–52.

26 • Niu J, Zhang Y Q, Torner J, *et al*. Is obesity a risk factor for progressive radiographic knee osteoarthritis? *Arthritis and Rheumatism* 2009; **61(3)**: 329–35.

27 • Hannan M T, Anderson J J, Zhang Y, *et al*. Bone mineral density and knee osteoarthritis in elderly men and women. The Framingham Study *Arthritis and Rheumatism* 1993; **36(12)**: 1671–80.

28 • Nevitt M C, Lane N E, Scott J C, *et al*. Radiographic osteoarthritis of the hip and bone mineral density. The Study of Osteoporotic Fractures Research Group *Arthritis and Rheumatism* 1995; **38(7)**: 907–16.

29 • Lane N E, Gore L R, Cummings S R, *et al*. Serum vitamin D levels and incident changes of radiographic hip osteoarthritis: a longitudinal study. Study of Osteoporotic Fractures Research Group *Arthritis and Rheumatism* 1999; **42(5)**: 854–60.

30 • Felson D T, Niu J, Clancy M, *et al*. Low levels of vitamin D and worsening of knee osteoarthritis: results of two longitudinal studies *Arthritis and Rheumatism* 2007; **56(1)**: 129–36.

31 • Soares J J, Jablonska B. Psychosocial experiences among primary care patients with and without musculoskeletal pain *European Journal of Pain* 2004; **8(1)**: 79–89.

32 • Gibilisco P A, Schumacher H R, Jr, Hollander J L, *et al*. Synovial fluid crystals in osteoarthritis *Arthritis and Rheumatism* 1985; **28(5)**: 511–15.

33 • National Collaborating Centre for Chronic Conditions. *Osteoarthritis: national clinical guideline for care and management in adults* London: Royal College of Physicians, 2008, www.nice.org.uk/CG59 [accessed October 2011].

34 • Zhang W, Moskowitz R W, Nuki G, *et al*. OARSI recommendations for the management of hip and knee osteoarthritis, Part II: OARSI evidence-based, expert consensus guidelines *Osteoarthritis and Cartilage* 2008; **16(2)**: 137–62.

35 • Roddy E, Zhang W, Doherty M. Aerobic walking or strengthening exercise for osteoarthritis of the knee? A systematic review *Annals of the Rheumatic Diseases* 2005; **64(4)**: 544–8.

36 • Christensen R, Bartels E M, Astrup A, *et al*. Effect of weight reduction in obese patients diagnosed with knee osteoarthritis: a systematic review and meta-analysis *Annals of the Rheumatic Diseases* 2007; **66(4)**: 433–9.

37 • Underwood M, Ashby D, Cross P, *et al*. Advice to use topical or oral ibuprofen for chronic knee pain in older people: randomised controlled trial and patient preference study *British Medical Journal* 2008; **336(7636)**: 138–42.

38 • Gladding P A, Webster M W, Farrell H B, *et al*. The antiplatelet effect of six non-steroidal anti-inflammatory drugs and their pharmacodynamic interaction with aspirin in healthy volunteers *American Journal of Cardiology* 2008; **101(7)**: 1060–3.

210

39 • Avouac J, Gossec L, Dougados M. Efficacy and safety of opioids for osteoarthritis: a meta-analysis of randomized controlled trials *Osteoarthritis and Cartilage* 2007; **15(8)**: 957–65.

40 • Bellamy N, Campbell J, Robinson V, *et al*. Intraarticular corticosteroid for treatment of osteoarthritis of the knee *Cochrane Database of Systematic Reviews* 2006; **2**: CD005328.

41 • Harris WH, Sledge CB. Total hip and total knee replacement (2) *New England Journal of Medicine* 1990; **323(12)**: 801–7.

42 • Harris WH, Sledge CB. Total hip and total knee replacement (1) *New England Journal of Medicine* 1990; **323(11)**: 725–31.

43 • Ledingham J, Regan M, Jones A, *et al*. Radiographic patterns and associations of osteoarthritis of the knee in patients referred to hospital *Annals of the Rheumatic Diseases* 1993; **52(7)**: 520–6.

# Osteoporosis and metabolic bone disease

**9**

*Pam Brown*

## Aims of this chapter

▶ Improve understanding of the relationship between fractures and osteoporosis.
▶ Increase identification, investigation and initiation of therapy in those at high fracture risk.
▶ Foster appropriate use of dual-energy X-ray absorptiometry (DXA) and other investigations in patients with osteoporosis.
▶ Understand the role of patient education and empowerment in adherence and persistence with therapy.
▶ Understand how to diagnose and manage osteomalacia and Paget's disease of bone, and where to refer if necessary.

## Learning outcomes

### Primary care management of osteoporosis

▶ Explain the aetiology and pathogenesis of osteoporosis and the mechanism of action of common treatments.
▶ Describe the key national guidelines for managing patients with osteoporosis and fracture; critically evaluate any differences between these.
▶ Describe which patients need referral to a specialist service.
▶ Explain how the disease can be prevented.

### Patient-centred care

▶ Know how to communicate a diagnosis of osteoporosis and how to empower the patient to adhere to and persist with therapy.

### Specific problem-solving skills

▶ Decide which patients need a DXA scan to aid treatment decisions.
▶ Explore ways to encourage adherence and persistence with therapy.
▶ Manage patients who are intolerant of first-line therapy.

### A comprehensive approach

▶ Outline possible side effects of therapy and how these can be managed.
▶ Discuss the holistic management of patients with recent fracture.
▶ Understand the social and psychological impact of falls and fractures.

### Community orientation

▶ Understand the roles that different members of the primary healthcare team can play in managing a patient with osteoporosis.
▶ Explore the evidence base for use of acupuncture, transcutaneous electrical nerve stimulation (TENS) and hydrotherapy for fracture pain.

### Contextual aspects

▶ Describe the local referral pathways for patients with osteoporosis and fractures in your locality.
▶ Is there a fracture liaison service and, if so, what is the model of care?

### Attitudinal aspects

▶ Demonstrate empathy and compassion with frail elderly patients with osteoporotic fractures.

### Key learning points

▶ Osteoporosis is a common, chronic skeletal disease with fracture as the acute exacerbation. Most patients can be managed in primary care.
▶ DXA scanning is required to confirm osteoporosis. Patients at very high fracture risk may not need DXA; local units will provide guidance.
▶ Exclude secondary osteoporosis and other underlying disease before initiating therapy.
▶ National Institute for Health and Clinical Excellence (NICE) and the National Osteoporosis Guideline Group (NOGG) offer guidance on who to treat.

▶ Drug treatments are effective in reducing fracture risk in high-risk patients.

▶ Most treatments are suitable for use in primary care.

▶ Primary care teams have a key role in optimising adherence and persistence with therapy.

## Introduction

Osteoporosis is defined as 'a progressive, systemic skeletal disease characterised by low bone mass and microarchitectural deterioration of bone tissue, with consequent increase in bone fragility and susceptibility to fracture'.[1] Alternatively, osteoporosis can be framed as 'a chronic skeletal disease, with fracture as the acute exacerbation'[2] reinforcing the relationship between fracture and osteoporosis.

Post-myocardial infarction (MI) patients are always investigated and underlying risk factors managed to reduce risk of further MI. However, post-fracture, the underlying disease is often ignored and only 10–14% of high-risk women receive appropriate treatment to reduce future fracture risk.[3] It is hoped that this new paradigm will ensure all fracture patients are assessed and receive treatment for underlying osteoporosis where appropriate.

The RCGP curriculum includes osteoporosis as one of the important, common musculoskeletal diseases and hence it is likely to be included in the CSA and AKT examinations. Osteoporosis is important because of the fractures that it causes, and these in turn are responsible for huge morbidity, mortality and loss of independence. NICE and NOGG have issued guidance on who should be treated and how treatments should be used, and therefore most registrars feel it is an appropriate knowledge area to update during their training year.

## The role of primary care in osteoporosis and fracture prevention

There are several key roles and responsibilities that could be met by the primary care team. These include:

▷ identifying those with osteoporosis and those at highest risk of future fracture

▷ educating and empowering identified patients to make lifestyle changes to reduce fracture risk

▷ using DXA and other investigations appropriately

▷ initiating drug therapy and optimising adherence and persistence with therapy

▷ referring those patients who will benefit from secondary care assessment or management.

---

### Epidemiology of osteoporosis

Osteoporosis development is multifactorial, including genetic, environmental and hormonal influences. Changes in cell biology result in imbalance between osteoclastic bone resorption and osteoblastic bone formation, resulting in bone loss. Rapid decline in oestrogen at menopause influences bone loss in women.

Fractures result in mortality, morbidity and loss of independence, and cost £1.8 billion annually in the UK. Up to 20% die within six months of sustaining a hip fracture and a further 20% previously living independently end up in care homes. Two million bed days are utilised by fractures in the over-sixties in England annually, with an average stay of nearly 27 days (eight days average for all conditions). Fracture workload impacts on elective orthopaedic waiting lists as surgeons, beds and other resources are occupied with fracture patients. Yet cost-effective drugs are available that can reduce fracture rates by 30–50% over three years in patients at high risk of fracture.

Tackling osteoporosis and fracture prevention in primary care can make a large impact on future fracture burden.

---

### Pathogenesis

At thousands of individual sites throughout the skeleton, bones are continuously being broken down by osteoclasts and built up again by osteoblasts throughout life. In children and adolescents, the laying down of bone exceeds removal at each site, and the skeleton grows. Around the early twenties, peak bone mass is achieved – this is the point where bone mass is maximal. There is then a plateau for a few years but from the mid-thirties a slow decline in bone mass occurs, and this continues throughout life in men. A faster phase of bone loss lasting five to ten years occurs in women following the menopause, in response to lack of oestrogen. During these bone loss stages, more bone is resorbed by the osteoclasts than is added by the osteoblasts, impacting on quality and quantity of remaining bone.

## Patient-centred care

Primary care teams will want to empower their patients by providing education about osteoporosis, its relationship to fractures, and how fracture risk can be reduced. For patients who fracture, this education should start in the A&E department or the fracture clinic, where they can learn about the underlying disease process that has made their bones more fragile, resulting in their fracture. This education and empowerment should include adequate analgesia for fracture pain, choices about appropriate therapy, and understanding of how to take this to ensure optimal benefits, as well as holistic guidance on lifestyle changes that they can make to reduce future fracture risk. For those who have not yet sustained a fracture but who are at high risk of fracture, education will include lifestyle measures and drug treatment if appropriate to reduce the risk of first and subsequent fractures.

## Identifying high-risk patients

Active case-finding of people at high risk of fractures, and DXA used where it will change management, is recommended in the UK. Screening for osteoporosis is not recommended.

Four groups of patients at highest risk of future fracture should be prioritised for identification and management, with the first three groups being tackled in every practice:

▷ post-menopausal women and men over 50 with previous fragility fracture (see definition below)
▷ those committed to oral steroids for three months or more
▷ frail, housebound elderly without previous fracture
▷ those without fractures but with multiple risk factors for osteoporosis or fracture.

Tackling these groups will make the most impact on UK fracture burden. Fragility fractures result from a fall from standing height or less in a patient over 50, or a low-trauma vertebral fracture resulting from normal daily activities. Age is a major risk factor for fracture, so older patients are at increased risk compared with younger patients. Coding high-risk patients ensures they are identifiable in future searches. Some commonly used codes are shown in Table 9.1 (overleaf). Entering the terms into your computer should bring up a picking list of suitable codes. Agree a core set of codes for use in your practice, otherwise searches at a later date will be onerous. When coding individual fractures, add the fragility fracture code also, as this will simplify searches.

FRAX (see below) allows calculation of the ten-year absolute risk of hip fracture and major osteoporotic fracture in post-menopausal women and men over 50.

Table 9.1 ○ *Commonly used codes*

| Read code | Condition/investigation |
| --- | --- |
| N330. | Osteoporosis |
| 8HQA. | Referral for DXA |
| 58EG. | Hip DXA osteoporotic |
| 58EM. | Lumbar spine DXA osteoporotic |
| N331N. | Fragility fracture |
| 14G9. | History of fracture |
| 14G6. | History of fragility fracture |
| 14G8. | History of vertebral fracture |
| 38DC. | FRAX ten-year risk of major osteoporotic fracture |
| 38DB. | FRAX ten-year risk of hip fracture |
| 14OC. | At risk of falls |
| 8I7E. | Bisphosphonate not tolerated |
| 8I7H. | Strontium ranelate not tolerated |
| 8I7F. | Calcium and vitamin D not tolerated |

### Steroid-induced osteoporosis

Oral steroid therapy greatly increases fracture risk. Risk increases rapidly after treatment onset and declines when treatment is stopped. Bone mineral density (BMD) loss is greatest in the first few months of steroid therapy and continues in the long term; therefore, bone-sparing therapy should be started when steroid therapy starts. Fractures occur at higher BMD thresholds on steroids; therefore, the treatment threshold occurs at a T-score of -1.5, rather than the T-score of -2.5 used for diagnosing osteoporosis (see definition, Table 9.2). FRAX and the NOGG guideline also offer guidance on which patients need DXA and treatment. Although oral bisphosphonates are used to treat patients on steroids, not all are licensed for this indication. Practitioners should check the *British National Formulary* for guidance. Steroid dose and duration should be minimised, alternative immunosuppressives used when possible, and patients encouraged to optimise dietary calcium intake, increase physical activity, stop smoking and reduce alcohol intake to <2 units daily.

## Making the diagnosis of osteoporosis

Osteoporosis can only be diagnosed by DXA scan, usually of the lumbar spine and femoral neck/total hip (axial DXA). The World Health Organization (WHO) interpretation of DXA T-scores is shown in Table 9.2. Lumbar spine DXA should be used to monitor therapy only if it is likely to change therapy – intervals of at least 18–24 months are recommended. However, some have argued that there is no need for monitoring in patients receiving bisphosphonates.[4]

Table 9.2 ○ *WHO definitions of DXA T-scores*

| | |
|---|---|
| Normal T-score | > -1.0 |
| Osteopenia T-score | -1.0 to -2.5 |
| Osteoporosis T-score | < -2.5 |

*Source*: World Health Organization. *Assessment of Fracture Risk and its Application to Screening for Postmenopausal Osteoporosis.*[5]

*Notes*: T-scores are a standardised way of comparing a patient's BMD with that of an adult at his or her time of peak bone mass (usually around 20 years of age). The distribution of bone density in any population has a NORMAL distribution, with a bell-shaped curve on an incidence graph. T-scores give a value to the number of standard deviations away from the mean for any given BMD. A normal BMD (compared with a 20-year-old) would have a T-score of 0; a more dense bone would have scores of +1.5, for example, and an osteoporotic bone would have a T-score of -2.5 or below.

Z-scores (not shown in the table) compare the bone density to that of a *person of the same age* as the patient.

Every standard deviation decrease in BMD translates into a doubling of the fracture risk. DXA should only be undertaken if the result will influence clinical management.

The NICE osteoporosis guideline was planned to provide detailed guidance on who needs DXA, but NICE will now provide this in a different format. NOGG, NICE and local scanning units currently provide guidance. When following NICE primary prevention guidance, review risk factors first to assess whether the woman would qualify for treatment if she meets the DXA threshold. If she does not have the appropriate risk factors, undertaking a DXA scan is inappropriate.

X-rays are useful for diagnosing fractures but not for diagnosing osteoporosis since up to one third of bone mass must be lost before it is consistently visible on X-rays. Peripheral DXA scanning (pDXA) is used in some centres, but scanning at the site of major osteoporotic fractures is the gold standard.

## Investigations

It is important to identify secondary osteoporosis and exclude other underlying causes for fractures, and ensure renal function and bone profile are suitable for proposed treatments (see Box 9.1). Men, people with previous cancer, those under 65 and those with vertebral fractures need more detailed investigation.

Other diseases such as osteomalacia (deficiency of vitamin D or disturbance of its metabolism), Paget's disease and hyperparathyroidism should be considered and investigated where appropriate (see further information on osteomalacia and Paget's disease later in this chapter). If in doubt about the diagnosis, refer for expert advice. Patients with suspected renal bone disease need specialist assessment.

---

Box 9.1 ○ **Investigations to consider in patients with fragility fractures or osteoporosis**

▶ Full blood count and erythrocyte sedimentation rate or C-reactive protein.

▶ Renal and liver profile.

▶ Bone profile.

▶ Thyroid profile.

▶ TTG or other test for coeliac disease.

▶ Serum immunoglobulin electrophoresis/urinary Bence Jones protein.

▶ Testosterone/androgen screen for men.

▶ Vitamin D or PTH level (if osteomalacia suspected and no vitamin D supplements).

---

### Reflective learning cycle

Think back to the last consultation where you had to share a diagnosis of osteoporosis and run through a reflective cycle. Describe the case, reflect on your feelings during the consultation, analyse the adequacy of the information you provided to your patient and the likely impact this may have had on his or her adherence and persistence with treatment, and describe what you might choose to do differently the next time.

## Guidelines and guidance

Three pieces of guidance make recommendations for treatment use in the UK:

▷ NICE primary prevention guidance (*Alendronate, Etidronate, Risedronate, Raloxifene and Strontium Ranelate for the Primary Prevention of Osteoporotic Fragility Fractures in Postmenopausal Women* [TA 160])[6]
▷ NICE secondary prevention guidance (*Alendronate Alendronate, Etidronate, Risedronate, Raloxifene, Strontium Ranelate and Teriparatide for the Secondary Prevention of Osteoporotic Fragility Fractures in Postmenopausal Women* [TA 161])[1,8]
▷ NICE guidance on the use of denosumab (*Denosumab for the Prevention of Osteoporotic Fractures in Postmenopausal Women* [TA 204])[7]
▷ The NOGG guideline[8] for prevention and treatment, and the linked FRAX calculator.

Previous NICE guidance[9] recommended treatment for women with fragility fracture, but this was poorly implemented.[3] Women receiving treatment who no longer qualify can continue as long as they or their clinician feels it appropriate.[1]

TA 160 and 161 apply to post-menopausal women not taking steroids. The guidance has been challenged in a judicial review, but is currently still in force. The complexities of the guidance make them difficult to implement, and clinicians have challenged the differential treatment thresholds for different drugs on ethical grounds, as some women with osteoporosis and previous fracture would not qualify for other treatments if intolerant of alendronate. Individual primary care organisations, trusts and doctors need to make their own decision on how to manage such high-risk women.

FRAX and the NOGG guideline are designed to guide DXA and treatment decisions in post-menopausal women and men over 50, including those on steroids. Clinicians therefore need to decide between NICE and NOGG guideline use in post-menopausal women. The latter has been challenged for recommending treatment without DXA in women with previous fracture, as treatments may be most effective in those with T-scores < -2.5.

### *NICE TA 160 and 161*

NICE TA 160 and 161 are summarised in Box 9.2 and Box 9.3 (overleaf). TA 160, 161 and the Quick Reference Guides are available, respectively, at:

▷ www.nice.org.uk/nicemedia/pdf/TA161quickrefguide.pdf
▷ www.nice.org.uk/nicemedia/pdf/TA160quickrefguide.pdf.

The inclusion of etidronate has been challenged, as there is no randomised controlled trial (RCT) evidence for hip fracture reduction. Likewise, RCTs failed to demonstrate hip fracture reduction with raloxifene.

---

**Box 9.2**  ○  *Summary of NICE TA 160*

**Alendronate**

▶ BMD T-score ≤ -2.5 AND

▶ age ≥ 70 AND independent clinical risk factor OR indicator low BMD

   ▷ ≥ 75 AND two or more independent clinical risk factors or indicators low BMD, may not need DXA.

▶ Aged 65–9 AND independent clinical risk factor.

▶ Aged < 65 AND independent clinical risk factor AND additional indicator low BMD.

**Risedronate and etidronate**

▶ Unable to comply with alendronate dosing or C/I or intolerant.

▶ BMD ≤ -2.5 to -3.5 depending on age/number of independent clinical risk factors.

▶ ≥ 75 years and ≥ 2 independent clinical risk factors or indicators of low BMD may not need DXA.

**Strontium ranelate**

▶ Unable to comply with bisphosphonates dosing or C/I or intolerant to alendronate and either etidronate or risedronate.

▶ BMD ≤ -3.0 to -4.5 depending on age/number of clinical risk factors for fracture.

*Independent clinical risk factors for fracture* – parental hip fracture, ≥ 4 units alcohol/day, rheumatoid arthritis.[1]

*Indicators of low BMD* – BMI < 22, untreated premature menopause, prolonged immobility, AS, Crohn's.[1]

*Unsatisfactory response* – having another fragility fracture despite adhering fully to treatment for one year, and evidence of decline in BMD below pre-treatment levels.[1]

---

NICE recommends assessing whether women are calcium and vitamin D replete before starting treatment.[6] However, this is difficult so most will need adjuvant calcium (1000–1200 mg per day) and vitamin D (800 IU per day) supplements.

### NICE TA 204

Denosumab is recommended for primary prevention of osteoporosis fragility fractures only in postmenopausal women at increased risk of fracture who are unable to comply with alendronate and either risedronate or etidronate dosing or have an intolerance or C/I to those treatments and whose BMD T-score is between -3 and -4.5 depending on age/number of independent clinical risk factors.

Denosumab is recommended as a treatment option for secondary prevention of fragility fractures in women at increased risk of fractures who are unable to comply with alendronate and either risedronate or etidronate dosing or have an intolerance or C/I to those treatments. Pragmatically, 'at increased risk of fractures' is interpreted as having osteoporosis (T-score of ≤-2.5).

Patients currently receiving denosumab who do not meet these criteria may continue if their clinician feels it appropriate.

### FRAX calculator and National Osteoporosis Guideline

The FRAX calculator (see Figure 9.1) uses UK-specific epidemiological data to calculate ten-year absolute hip and major osteoporotic fracture risk in a

---

Box 9.3 ○ **Summary of NICE TA 161**

**Alendronate**

▶ BMD T-score ≤ -2.5.

▶ ≥75 may not need DXA.

**Risedronate and etidronate**

▶ Unable to comply with alendronate dosing or C/I or intolerant.

▶ BMD ≤ -2.5 to -3.0 depending on age/number of clinical risk factors for fracture.

▶ ≥75 years may not need DXA.

**Strontium ranelate and raloxifene**

▶ Unable to comply with bisphosphonate dosing or C/I or intolerant.

▶ BMD ≤ -2.5 to -4 depending on age/number of clinical risk factors for fracture (see Table 9.2 on p. 219).

▶ ≥75 with >1 clinical risk factor or indicators of low BMD may not need DXA.

**Teriparatide**

▶ Unable to comply with bisphosphonate dosing or C/I or intolerant alendronate and either risedronate or etidronate or strontium ranelate OR unsatisfactory response to bisphosphonates AND ≥65 with T-score ≤ -4.0 OR T-score ≤ -3.5 + >2 fractures OR 55–64 and T-score ≤ 4 + >2 fractures.

similar way to ten-year cardiovascular disease risk calculators. The risk can be calculated without DXA initially, and the link to the NOGG site plots risk graphically (see Figure 9.2 on p. 224) and makes recommendations for need for DXA or treatment. Once femoral neck BMD is available, ten-year risk can be recalculated and the recommendation will be to treat or reassure.

Figure 9.1 ○ *Front screen of FRAX calculator*

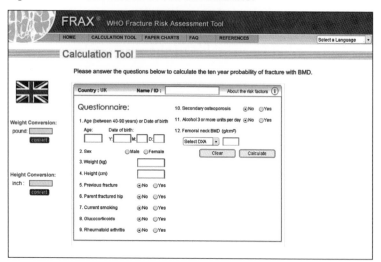

*Source*: copyright© World Health Organization Collaborating Centre for Metabolic Bone Diseases. University of Sheffield. Used with permission.

Figure 9.2 ○ *Management chart for osteoporosis*

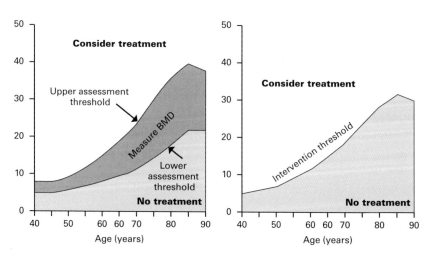

*Source*: Kanis J A, McCloskey E V, Johansson H, *et al*. Approaches to the targeting of treatment for osteoporosis.[10] Reprinted by permission from Macmillan Publishers Ltd: *Nature Reviews. Rheumatology*, copyright© 2009.

Table 9.3 ○ *Bone-sparing therapies*

| Drug | Administration | Frequency | Lumbar spine fracture reduction | Hip fracture reduction |
|------|----------------|-----------|----------------------------------|------------------------|
| Calcium and vitamin D | Oral | Daily | | Frail elderly |
| Alendronate | Oral | Daily/weekly | ✓ | ✓ |
| Etidronate | Oral | | ✓ | |
| Risedronate | Oral | Daily/weekly | ✓ | ✓ |
| Ibandronate | Oral/intravenous (IV) | Monthly/ 3-monthly | ✓ | |
| Zoledronate | IV | Annually | ✓ | ✓ |
| Denosumab | Subcutaneous injection | Twice yearly | ✓ | ✓ |
| Strontium ranelate | Oral | Daily | ✓ | ✓ |
| Raloxifene | Oral | Daily | ✓ | |
| Teriparatide | Subcutaneous injection | Daily | ✓ | |

## Management of osteoporosis

### Lifestyle advice

All patients at risk of osteoporosis or fracture should be counselled to stop smoking, eat a well-balanced diet containing at least 700 mg of calcium daily, and aim for 20 minutes of sun exposure to face and arms daily during summer months. Vigorous weightbearing physical activity or resistance gym work is appropriate for maintaining BMD in those at low fracture risk, while tai chi and balance work may reduce falls in the elderly. Heavy lifting should be avoided in those at vertebral fracture risk.

### Drug treatment

Currently available bone-sparing therapies and their key sites of fracture reduction are shown in Table 9.3 and discussed in Box 9.4 (see p. 226).

Unfortunately, NICE has sought to largely remove patient choice from therapy decisions for osteoporosis in post-menopausal women, as discussed above. Also, due to the cost-effectiveness of generic alendronate, most Primary Care Trusts and Local Health Boards will enforce the use of this as first-line therapy. Generic risedronate became available from 2010 when it went off-patent. All patients currently should therefore have generic alendronate as first-line therapy, unless they are unable to comply with directions for taking it, or have upper-gastrointestinal (GI) conditions in which therapy is contraindicated, e.g. oesophageal stricture.

High-dose calcium and vitamin D should be used as adjuvant therapy in all patients receiving bone-sparing therapy and in all those at risk of steroid-induced osteoporosis.

When initiating bone-sparing therapy it can be useful to initiate calcium and vitamin D alone for two weeks, giving the patient a choice of chewable, swallowable or liquid/soluble therapy. Then, if he or she is tolerating this, oral generic alendronic acid 70 mg weekly can be added. This prevents confusion over which drug has caused any side effects that occur.

Further information on all drugs can be found in the *British National Formulary*. Key practical information to allow effective use is included in Box 9.4 (overleaf). Note that all bisphosphonates are used for prevention and treatment of steroid-induced osteoporosis but only daily branded alendronate, risedronate and cyclical etidronate and teriparatide injections are currently actually licensed for steroid-induced osteoporosis.

---

**Box 9.4** ○ ***Bone-sparing drug therapy***

**Anti-resorptive therapies**

***High-dose calcium and vitamin D (1000–1200 mg and 800 IU daily)***

▶ Sole therapy in housebound elderly without previous fractures; reduces hip fracture risk.

▶ Patients receiving bone-sparing therapy should receive adjuvant calcium and vitamin D.

▶ Little evidence that calcium/vitamin D alone reduces fracture in other groups, although some studies using >700 IU vitamin D have been effective.

***Bisphosphonates***

▶ Weekly generic alendronate, followed by weekly risedronate if intolerant.[1]

▶ Daily bisphosphonates are difficult to take and are rarely used.

▶ Bisphosphonates must be taken first thing in the morning on an empty stomach with a full glass of tap water and no food, drink or medication for at least 30 minutes (alendronate and risedronate), 60 minutes (ibandronate) or two hours (etidronate).

▶ Upper-GI side effects are common; if severe, discontinue therapy.

▶ Short-duration flu-like symptoms are common after first infusion of ibandronate and zoledronate.

---

▶ There is a small risk of developing atrial fibrillation with zoledronate (and alendronate).

▶ High-dose IV bisphosphonates in cancer patients significantly increase osteonecrosis of the jaw, a non-healing area of exposed bone following dental treatment. Risk is very low with oral therapy (1 in 10,000 to 1 in 100,000).

### Raloxifene

▶ Daily therapy with no special dosing instructions.

▶ Reduces risk of vertebral fractures.

▶ Significantly reduces the risk of oestrogen-positive breast cancer.[11]

▶ Increased risk of deep-vein thrombosis (DVT), leg cramps and menopausal flushes.

### Denosumab

▶ For use in post-menopausal women.

▶ Twice-yearly subcutaneous therapy.

▶ Reduces risk of vertebral, non-vertebral and hip fractures.

▶ Small increased risk of some types of infection (skin, UTI, URTI).

### Effects on bone resorption and formation

### Strontium ranelate

▶ Sachet of granules made up with water and taken each evening.

▶ Taken at night at least two hours after food or calcium-containing drinks.

▶ May cause diarrhoea in the first three months – stop laxatives before initiating therapy.

▶ Small increased DVT risk and contraindicated if previous DVT.

▶ Very rarely causes drug rash with eosinophilia and systemic symptoms (DRESS); warn patients to stop therapy and seek medical advice if skin rash develops.

### Bone formation agents

### Teriparatide and 1-84 PTH

▶ Restricted to secondary care initiation and follow-up.

▶ Reserved on NHS for women ≥65 with severe osteoporosis and fractures who have not tolerated or responded to other therapies.

▶ 12–24 month treatment course of daily subcutaneous injections depending on the drug (patients trained to self-inject).

227

### Reflective learning cycle

Reflect on your last consultation with a patient who required therapy for osteoporosis. Describe the case, and your feelings as you made the treatment decision. When you analyse your treatment choice, was it supported by the

NICE guidance or use of FRAX and the NOGG guidance? Would your choice of guideline influence treatment decisions? Did you share the treatment decision with your patient in the most effective way? What did you learn and what will you do differently next time?

If you find reflection difficult, you may prefer to discuss the case with your trainer in a 'hot review' session.

### Adherence and persistence with therapy

Primary care teams have a vital role in improving adherence and persistence with all therapies but this is particularly important when managing people with osteoporosis, where the therapies need to be taken in a specific way and where persistence with therapy long term is vital. Many patients, particularly those in care homes, do not take or are not given their medication correctly, or do not persist with therapy, resulting in reduced BMD [12] and fracture reduction benefits. NICE has recently published guidance on improving adherence with all types of medicines,[13] and it is useful to refer to this for more detailed advice on how to improve these aspects of your prescribing.

Around 50% of patients will have discontinued bone-sparing therapy by six months, so effort is needed to help patients understand the need for long-term therapy, and the importance of returning for advice if the first drug does not suit. Whether you choose to adhere to the exact criteria in the NICE primary and secondary prevention guidance for post-menopausal women or not, ideally you will become familiar with the ways that all the common oral therapies are used so that you can counsel patients appropriately and improve adherence. Patients unable to tolerate any oral therapy should be referred to your local specialist service for consideration for IV or subcutaneous therapy depending on local guidance. Note that patients with an eGFR less than 30 ml/minute will not be suitable for IV therapy, but your specialist will be able to initiate other therapies such as calcitriol or alphacalcidol that are safe with very poor renal function.

It is important to help patients understand that their bone-sparing therapy will not help with any symptoms from previous fractures, as many patients stop therapy because they do not see any difference in their symptoms, for example chronic back pain. During this discussion you can also check that they are being prescribed appropriate analgesics, and are taking enough of them to control their pain. Many elderly patients are frightened that if they take full doses of analgesics the drugs will stop working, and they will then have intolerable pain. Equally, many restrict their use due to side effects, e.g. constipation, and offering appropriate medication to minimise their side effects may allow improved pain control. Remember that non-drug therapies such as acupuncture, TENS and hydrotherapy may be highly beneficial for pain associated with kyphosis or muscle spasm.

---

### Referral to secondary care

Consider referring:

▷ anyone where the diagnosis is uncertain
▷ patients with osteomalacia and other metabolic bone diseases
▷ men
▷ patients intolerant of oral therapy
▷ patients with severe osteoporosis for consideration of teriparatide
▷ young patients with underlying disease, e.g. inflammatory bowel disease.

---

### The way forward

#### *Fracture Liaison Services*

Several parts of the UK now have Fracture Liaison Services, which ensure all new patients sustaining fractures receive education and are referred for DXA scanning if appropriate. There are many different models: some initiate therapy, while others refer back to primary care for treatment and follow-up. These are an effective and efficient way to ensure reduction in fracture risk in new fracture patients.

#### *Reflective cycle*

Do you know whether there is a local Fracture Liaison Service in place? How does your practice handle fracture clinic letters notifying new fractures? Are these coded appropriately?

#### *New drugs*

Denosumab has recently been launched and is a licensed fully human monoclonal antibody to RANKL, a ligand that activates osteoclasts. Denosumab blocks osteoclast differentiation, proliferation and function, and in the FREEDOM randomised controlled trial[14] produced significant relative risk reduction in vertebral fractures (68%), non-vertebral fractures (20%) and hip fractures (40%)

over three years. Denosumab is given by subcutaneous injection twice yearly.

Four new anti-resorptive drugs may become licensed in the UK within the next few years.

Lasofoxifene and bazedoxifene are selective oestrogen receptor modulators (SERMs). Bazedoxifene reduces vertebral fractures and in high-risk women decreases non-vertebral fractures. Lasofoxifene decreases both vertebral and non-vertebral fractures in women with osteoporosis, with an 81% reduced risk of oestrogen-positive breast cancer, and 68% decreased risk of major coronary heart disease events, but increased venous thromboembolism risk similar to raloxifene.

Odanacatib and balicatib are also biological treatments, targeting cathepsin K, a cysteine protease enzyme in osteoclasts, which degrades Type 1 collagen in bone. Odanacatib is a once-weekly oral therapy without the dosing restrictions of bisphosphonates.

### Summary and conclusions

Osteoporosis and fracture prevention can be managed effectively in primary care, and this chapter has clarified the process for delivering such care. This is summarised below.

Start by reviewing highest-risk groups – those with previous fracture, oral steroids and frail housebound elderly. Once these groups are identified and treated, consider older patients with multiple risk factors who have not yet suffered a fracture. Code all patients identified so they are visible on future searches. Assess and investigate to exclude secondary osteoporosis and other conditions that may cause fractures. As a practice agree to follow national (NICE and NOGG) or local guidance on whom to refer for DXA. Use FRAX/NOGG and NICE to identify who needs treatment to prevent future fractures. Encourage patients to learn more about osteoporosis, and where possible provide patient choice of therapy (e.g. calcium and vitamin D). Ensure patients understand how to take their medication correctly to optimise absorption and provide support to encourage persistence long enough for fracture reduction benefits. Refer the following to secondary care: men, patients with diagnostic difficulties, patients intolerant of oral therapies if denosumab initiation is not available in primary care, and those who qualify for teriparatide.

Primary care teams can make a real and lasting difference to the fracture burden by diagnosing and treating osteoporosis.

## Paget's disease

Paget's disease is relatively common, affecting around 1–2% of white adults over 55 and the UK has the highest prevalence in the world. Prevalence increases with age. There is increased bone turnover with increased resorption, marrow fibrosis, increased vascularisation and greatly increased bone formation, with laying down of disorganised bone, which is weaker than normal bone and therefore more likely to fracture. The axial skeleton (pelvis, femur, lumbar spine) is preferentially affected,[15] and it has been postulated that this reflects sites of local mechanical loading.

The aetiology is unclear, but there appears to be a genetic component since around 15% of patients have a family history and relatives have a 7–10 times' greater risk of developing the disease than the general population.[15] Several environmental triggers have also been explored but none has been confirmed as definitely being involved.

Paget's may be asymptomatic, and be diagnosed incidentally by finding a raised alkaline phosphatase or by typical findings on X-rays carried out for another reason. Patients with only small areas of involvement may have normal alkaline phosphatases. Some patients develop bone pain or deformity, prompting X-rays to confirm or refute the diagnosis. It is often difficult to differentiate between pain due to osteoarthritis (which should be more localised to joints) and bone pain due to Paget's disease (which should respond to bisphosphonate treatment), and the two conditions commonly coexist, particularly around the hips, pelvis and lumbar spine. Complications of Paget's disease are shown in Box 9.5 below.

---

Box 9.5 ○ *Complications of Paget's disease of bone*[15]

▸ Bone pain.

▸ Bone deformity.

▸ Secondary osteoarthritis and need for hip and knee replacement.

▸ Pathological fracture.

▸ Deafness.

▸ Nerve compression syndromes.

▸ Spinal stenosis.

▸ High-output cardiac failure (rare).

▸ Osteosarcoma (rare).

Symptomatic patients, rather than all those with elevated alkaline phosphatase, should be treated with bisphosphonates and the symptoms managed with analgesics or NSAIDs (with proton pump inhibitor co-prescription if appropriate).[15] Risedronate 30 mg daily for two months is suitable for use in primary care, but ensure that this high dose is not continued longer term. Alternatively, patients can be referred into secondary care for 5 mg single dose of IV zoledronate. Alendronate is not licensed in the UK for treatment of Paget's disease. Many will not feel confident managing Paget's disease in primary care, and therefore referral may be appropriate for all patients where the diagnosis is considered and the patient symptomatic.

## Osteomalacia

Osteomalacia is a disease of defective mineralisation of bone due to deficiency of vitamin D or resistance to it. It is usually asymptomatic in the early stages, but can cause bone pain, proximal muscle weakness and increased risk of fractures.

Although there are several different types of osteomalacia, only the common type due to deficiency of vitamin D will be discussed here. The following groups are at risk of developing osteomalacia:

▷ housebound or institutionalised elderly
▷ those with diet low in vitamin D or high in phytates
▷ South Asians and others who stay indoors or wear clothing covering the face and body
▷ those with malabsorption, e.g. untreated coeliac disease
▷ those with liver or kidney disease
▷ pregnant women and those who breastfeed for prolonged periods.

Ninety per cent of vitamin D is made from the action of sunlight on skin and only 10% is obtained from the diet, from foods such as oily fish, egg yolks, liver and fortified foods, e.g. margarine and some breakfast cereals.

It is useful to review vitamin D metabolism in a textbook or an internet search. In summary, sunlight acts on 7-dehydrocholesterol in skin to produce cholecalciferol, which is then metabolised in the liver to 25-hydrocholecalciferol, and then further hydroxylation in the kidney produces 1,25-dihydroxycholecalciferol, the active form of vitamin D. In severe renal disease, there is an inability to complete the final step in this metabolism, so vitamin D deficiency occurs.

Lack of active vitamin D results in decreased absorption of calcium from the gut, and this in turn stimulates parathyroid hormone (PTH) secretion (secondary hyperparathyroidism) increasing calcium and phosphate loss from bone and defective mineralisation.

If osteomalacia is suspected renal function should be checked, as should calcium, phosphate, 25-hydroxyvitamin D and PTH levels. Low calcium and increased alkaline phosphatase are usually found, with low vitamin D levels and raised PTH.

X-rays are usually normal in the early stages, but later may show pseudofractures (Looser's zones), especially in the long bones, pelvis and ribs. In children the classical finding is of thickening and widening of the radial epiphyses, and rib ends, producing the classical 'rickety rosary'. Definitive diagnosis is made on bone biopsy but this is usually only used in those with renal bone disease, where it also provides further information about bone turnover. This will aid choice of treatment for renal osteodystrophy.

20,000–60,000 IU (Dekristol) vitamin D once weekly, together with 1000–1200 mg of calcium daily, usually results in rapid resolution of symptoms if these are present, and this dose is usually continued for two to three months until the vitamin D level returns to normal (although some laboratories refuse to do follow-up levels in patients on treatment). If there are difficulties accessing suitable products, active vitamin D metabolites such as one-alpha can be used. In either case, renal function, calcium and alkaline phosphatase should be monitored carefully during treatment, and it is important to ensure such high-dose therapy is not accidentally continued longer term. Alkaline phosphatase should return to normal when the osteomalacia is adequately treated. Thereafter a standard high-dose calcium and vitamin D preparation containing 800 IU vitamin D3 per day can be used as maintenance if recurrence of deficiency is likely.

Babies breastfed for more than six months may be at risk of vitamin D deficiency, especially if their mothers fall into high-risk categories, and should receive vitamin D supplements. In the UK these are best provided as Abidec drops, as vitamin D supplements alone are hard to access.

*AKT questions*

### EXTENDED MATCHING QUESTION

Option list:

▶ lifestyle advice only

▶ generic alendronate once-weekly first thing in the morning with a full glass of tap water, remain upright and no food, drinks or medication for at least 30 minutes

▶ strontium ranelate 150 mg sachet daily

▶ strontium ranelate 150 mg sachet at bedtime at least two hours after any food or drink containing milk

▶ referral for consideration of IV zoledronate annual infusion

▶ referral for consideration of IV zoledronate annual infusion and daily high-dose calcium with vitamin D supplement; renal function check.

For each patient select the **single most appropriate** therapy regimen. Each answer may be used once, more than once or not at all:

▷ a 75-year-old woman with previous wrist fracture and family history of parental hip fracture; never had previous DXA or treatment

▷ a 65-year-old woman with T-score of -3.0 at femoral neck, previous DVT and eGFR of 40; no previous treatment

▷ an 80-year-old woman with previous hip fracture, severe upper-GI symptoms and previous DVT; T-score -2.8 when measured two years ago

▷ a 70-year-old woman concerned regarding her risk of fracture. No previous fractures, smokes 20/day, drinks three units of alcohol most days, eGFR 72, femoral neck T-score -2.8. No maternal hip fracture or rheumatoid arthritis.

**AKT ANSWERS**

▷ Generic alendronate.

▷ Generic alendronate.

▷ Referral for consideration IV zoledronate and daily calcium and vitamin D; depends on eGFR/renal function being good enough.

▷ Under NICE would not qualify for treatment so lifestyle only. FRAX/ NOGG suggests consider treatment.

---

Box 9.6 ○ *Case study 1*

Mrs Carolyn Thomas is a 58-year-old woman who had her menopause aged 41 and took hormone-replacement therapy (HRT) only for a few months. Her current medication is citalopram 30 mg daily for long-term depression, bendroflumethiazide 2.5 mg daily for hypertension, simvastatin 10 mg at night for hyperlipidaemia, and lansoprazole 15 mg daily for reflux-type symptoms. She admits to consistently heavy alcohol intake over the last few months, averaging 4–5 units per day, and smokes 30 cigarettes daily. She does not enjoy milk but occasionally eats yoghurts. Her height is 161 cm with a weight of 50 kg. Her father had a hip fracture in his fifties, but also had severe asthma, drank and smoked heavily.

*What are Mrs Thomas's current risk factors for osteoporosis and fracture?*

These are: high alcohol use; smoker; low calcium intake; lowish BMI of 19.3; parental hip fracture; may have postural hypotension and increased risk of falls.

*Should Mrs Thomas have a DXA scan to measure her BMD?*

Yes. Under NICE she would qualify for treatment if her BMD is < -2.5 so appropriate to refer for DXA. Under FRAX her 10-year risk of major osteoporotic fracture is 20% and of hip fracture 5.9% (remember to add early menopause as secondary osteoporosis risk factor) and NOGG suggests considering treatment without DXA. However, this highlights one of the controversial areas of NOGG and most experts would suggest that she should have DXA to assess BMD before making a treatment decision.

*Assume Mrs Thomas had a DXA scan which showed a T-score of -2.2 at the lumbar spine and -2.0 at the femoral neck. Would you prescribe any treatment for her and, if so, what would you choose?*

**235**

Under NICE she would not qualify for treatment for primary prevention. Under NOGG addition of her femoral neck BMD reduces her ten-year risks to 14% and 3.2% respectively. However, she is still in the treatment recommended zone, and you should consider the use of generic alendronate and high-dose calcium and vitamin D.

---

Box 9.7 ○ **Case study 2**

Mrs Sinclair is 64 and presents with acute mid-thoracic back pain that started after moving heavy furniture. This is subsequently diagnosed as a vertebral fracture of T10. Her general health is now good, but she had a lumpectomy and radiotherapy ten years ago for breast cancer. On direct questioning you discover that her mother had a hip fracture aged 68 and has since been receiving treatment for osteoporosis.

Prior to her fracture Mrs Sinclair was very active, has never smoked, and has always eaten a healthy diet that included several portions of milk and dairy produce each day. She drinks three to four glasses of wine per week and had her menopause at the age of 52.

---

*What, if any, investigations would you carry out?*

FBC, ESR, CRP, myeloma screen – protein electrophoresis and urine for Bence Jones protein, bone profile. If there was any abnormality on the plain X-ray she may warrant a bone scan to exclude early bony secondaries.

*What treatment would you offer her at present?*

Adequate analgesia, e.g. co-codamol +/- NSAID if no contraindications; consider use of short-term nasal calcitonin in the acute phase for pain relief if severe; use of TENS machine and later hydrotherapy may be helpful for pain.

*Assume Mrs Sinclair has a DXA scan four weeks later and the results show a T-score of -2.8 at the lumbar spine and -2.3 at the femoral neck. What treatment would you provide and why?*

Treatment with alendronate is recommended by both NICE and NOGG. When Mrs Sinclair attends for medication review three months later you notice she has not requested any further repeats of either of her osteoporosis medications prescribed last time.

*What advice would you offer Mrs Sinclair this time?*

Explore her understanding of duration of treatment, and whether she had any side effects that encouraged her to discontinue. Many simply do not understand that this is long-term treatment to be repeated. If the medication was stopped due to upper-GI side effects, then restart calcium and vitamin D initially and counsel fully regarding alternative treatments.

*What treatment, if any, would you now offer?*

Mrs Sinclair is 64 with one clinical risk factor and osteoporosis on DXA at her lumbar spine (T -2.8). If she stopped her alendronate due to upper-GI intolerance, you need to consider her for further therapy. She does not qualify for risedronate or raloxifene according to current NICE guidance, but if you chose to follow NOGG you could offer a trial of either of these treatments since she is intolerant of alendronate. Alternatively, it is worth restarting her calcium and vitamin D preparation to see if she tolerates this. Then, if her upper-GP side effects were only mild, you may want to consider restarting alendronate, as many patients tolerate it on re-challenge.

---

Box 9.8 ○ **Case study 3**

Mrs Jones is 62, and has just been diagnosed with polymyalgia rheumatica and commenced on oral prednisolone 20 mg/day. She has not had any previous fractures, smokes ten per day, does not drink alcohol and has no other major health problems. Her mother had a hip fracture in her early 60s. Mrs Jones weighs 65 kg and her height is 165 cm.

*What lifestyle advice would you give her?*

Stop smoking, moderate alcohol intake to 1–2 units per day maximum, eat a well-balanced diet rich in fruit and vegetables, and containing around 600–1000 mg calcium daily. If no contraindications, expose hands, forearms and face to sunlight for 15–20 minutes daily in summer months to optimise vitamin D production without increasing risk.

*Should she have bone-sparing therapy, and, if so, what would you prescribe?*
*Explain how you reached your decision.*

NICE specifically states that its guidance in TA 160 is not for women receiving oral steroid therapy. Therefore it is appropriate to use FRAX and NOGG to aid in decision making. This demonstrates a ten-year risk of major osteoporotic fractures of 22% and of hip fracture 4.3%. As a result of this, NOGG recommends consideration of bone-sparing therapy. First-line therapy would be high-dose calcium and vitamin D supplements, and generic alendronate unless there were any contraindications.

*It is now two years later and Mrs Jones is about to stop oral steroid therapy. What advice would you give her at this stage?*

There is no hard and fast evidence for when bone-sparing therapy should be stopped when oral steroid therapy is discontinued. Since most patients reduce the dose gradually prior to stopping, and many are on 1–2 mg for some time before ceasing therapy, stopping the bone-sparing therapy at the same time is common practice. However, in the frail, housebound elderly, it is probably appropriate to continue the high-dose calcium and vitamin D long term if tolerated.

**References**

1 • National Institute for Health and Clinical Excellence. *Alendronate, Etidronate, Risedronate, Raloxifene, Strontium Ranelate and Teriparatide for the Secondary Prevention of Osteoporotic Fragility Fractures in Postmenopausal Women* [Technology Appraisal 161] London: NICE, 2008, http://guidance.nice.org.uk/TA161 [accessed October 2011].

2 • British Orthopaedic Society, British Geriatric Society. *The BOA-BSG Blue Book on the Care of Patients with Fragility Fracture* London: BOA, BGS, 2007.

3 • Hippisley-Cox J, Bayly J, Potter J, *et al. Evaluation of Standards of Care for Osteoporosis and Falls in Primary Care* London: QRESEARCH, the Information Centre for Health and Social Care, 2007.

4 • Compston J. Monitoring bone mineral density during antiresorptive treatment for osteoporosis *British Medical Journal* 2009; **338**: 1511–13.

5 • World Health Organization. *Assessment of Fracture Risk and its Application to Screening for Postmenopausal Osteoporosis: report of a WHO study group. Technical Report Series* Geneva: WHO, 1994.

6 • National Institute for Health and Clinical Excellence. *Alendronate, Etidronate, Risedronate, Raloxifene and Strontium Ranelate for the Primary Prevention of Osteoporotic Fragility Fractures in Postmenopausal Women* [Technology Appraisal 160] London: NICE, 2008.

7 • National Institute for Health and Clinical Excellence. *Denosumab for the Prevention of Osteoporotic Fractures in Postmenopausal Women* [Technology Appraisal 204] London: NICE, 2010.

8 • National Osteoporosis Guideline Group. *Osteoporosis Clinical Guideline for Prevention and Treatment* London: NOGG, 2008.

9 • National Institute for Health and Clinical Excellence. *Bisphosphonates (Alendronate, Etidronate, Risedronate), Selective Oestrogen Receptor Modulators (Raloxifene) and Parathyroid Hormone (Teriparatide) for the Secondary Prevention of Osteoporotic Fragility Fractures in Postmenopausal Women* [Technology Appraisal 87] London: NICE, 2005.

10 • Kanis J A, McCloskey E V, Johansson H, *et al*. Approaches to the targeting of treatment for osteoporosis *Nature Reviews. Rheumatology* 2009; **5(8)**: 425–31.

11 • Cranney A, Tugwell P, Zytaruk N, *et al*. IV. Meta-analysis of raloxifene for the prevention and treatment of postmenopausal osteoporosis *Endocrine Reviews* 2002; **23(4)**: 524–8.

12 • Yood R A, Emani S, Reed J I, *et al*. Compliance with pharmacologic therapy for osteoporosis *Osteoporosis International* 2003; **14(12)**: 965-8.

13 • National Institute for Health and Clinical Excellence. *Clinical Guideline 76, Medicines Adherence: involving patients in decisions about prescribed medicines and supporting adherence* London: RCGP, 2009, http://guidance.nice.org.uk/CG76/Guidance/pdf/English [accessed October 2011].

14 • Cummings S, McClung M R, Christiansen C, *et al*. A Phase III study of the effects of denosumab on vertebral, nonverterbral and hip fracture in women with osteoporosis: results from the FREEDOM trial *Journal of Bone and Mineral Research* 2008; **23**: S80.

15 • Ralston S, Langston A, Reid I. Pathogenesis and management of Paget's disease of bone *Lancet* 2008; **372(9633)**: 155–63.

# Fibromyalgia and allied syndromes

# 10

*Peter Glennon*

## Introduction

Originally described in the nineteenth century as 'rheumatism with hard and tender places', fibromyalgia is a common, chronic, controversial and often disabling illness that can present a severe challenge to the GP. Good management of this condition requires the full panoply of GP skills including a comprehensive and holistic approach. The aim of this chapter is to provide the reader with confidence in diagnosing and managing fibromyalgia but also, and perhaps more usefully, to provide a template for the management of a range of medically unexplained symptoms and related musculoskeletal disorders that collectively form a significant part of day-to-day general practice. Traditionally these conditions have been tentatively diagnosed, inadequately treated and often referred to secondary care where they have been subjected to narrow biomedical care. This has resulted in unhappy doctors, unhappy patients, unhappy carers and sometimes fruitless use of expensive resources. However, things can change, and confident use of a biopsychosocial* approach by GPs should lead to more patients being satisfactorily and appropriately treated in a primary care-led paradigm.

## Primary care management of fibromyalgia

Fibromyalgia is common in primary care. Its management requires a good understanding of aetiology and natural history, as well as common symptoms and signs, when to refer, investigate and how to treat. It is also helpful to view it as a paradigm for all medically unexplained symptoms and its management is really important as it falls squarely on a GP's shoulders – there are no real specialists in these generalist conditions except GPs!

Its prevalence depends on how closely the widely accepted American College of Rheumatology (ACR) criteria are adhered to. These are listed overleaf (Box 10.1).

---

*The biopsychosocial model, first proposed by Engel in 1977, states that biological, psychological and social factors all have an important part to play in the context of disease or illness.

Using the ACR criteria the prevalence in US primary care communities is estimated at 3.4%.[1] A recent survey in five European countries estimated overall prevalence at 4.7%. Studies have shown the prevalence to be similar in many countries, climate zones and ethnic groups. Women seem to be affected between five and ten times more frequently than men. The peak age of onset is between 30 and 50, and 7–8% of women will have the condition by age 70.

## Diagnosis

As there are no diagnostic tests, the diagnosis is made solely on clinical grounds. Box 10.1 lists the well-known ACR criteria, which are accepted as 'gold standard' and widely used in research.

---

**Box 10.1 ○ *The ACR 1990 criteria for the classification of fibromyalgia*[2]**

**History of widespread pain (i.e. all of the following):**

**a** ▶ Pain in left side of the body

**b** ▶ Pain in right side of the body

**c** ▶ Pain above the waist

**d** ▶ Pain below the waist

**e** ▶ Axial skeletal pain (cervical spine or anterior chest or thoracic spine or low back).

**Pain on digital palpation in at least 11 of the following 18 tender points:**

**a** ▶ Occiput: *bilateral*, at the suboccipital muscle insertion

**b** ▶ Low cervical: *bilateral*, at the anterior aspect of the intertransverse spaces at C5–7

**c** ▶ Trapezius: *bilateral*, at the midpoint of the upper border

**d** ▶ Supraspinatus: *bilateral*, at the origin, above the scapular spine near the medial border

**e** ▶ Second rib: *bilateral*, at the second costochondral junction, just lateral to the junction on the upper surface

**f** ▶ Lateral epicondyle: *bilateral*, 2 cm distal to the epicondyle

**g** ▶ Gluteal: *bilateral*, in the upper outer quadrant of the buttock

**h** ▶ Greater trochanter: *bilateral*, posterior to the trochanteric prominence

**i** ▶ Knee: *bilateral*, at the medial fat pad proximal to the joint line.

*Notes*: digital palpation should be performed with approximately 4 kg pressure (just enough pressure to blanch the examiner's fingernails) and the palpation should be deemed 'painful' by the patient. To satisfy the diagnosis both criteria 1 and 2 must have been present for at least three months. The ACR found that using this approach gave a sensitivity of 88% and a specificity of 81%.

In a general practice setting, patients with evolving fibromyalgia may present with more localised regional pain – 'myofascial pain syndrome'. In practice the diagnosis may be made with less rigid criteria, especially in the presence of other symptoms that are common in the syndrome (see below). Indeed the ACR has very recently proposed a more streamlined set of criteria for the diagnosis of FMS. These do not require the palpation of tender points and take into account both the severity and number of somatic symptoms.[3] These new criteria are more usable in primary care and are summarised in a modified format that could be used both for diagnosis and as a longitudinal scoring system (see the appendix to this chapter).

Most fibromyalgia can be managed in primary care and, like irritable bowel syndrome (IBS), should not need a specialist opinion to confirm the diagnosis – provided GPs use their normal 'red flag' safety-netting procedures (the skill to intervene urgently when necessary). Some of the specific problem-solving competences required of GPs include the use of incremental investigation, the tolerance of diagnostic uncertainty and the ability to handle undifferentiated illness. Diagnosing fibromyalgia correctly is likely to challenge all of these skills.

As well as the ACR criteria most fibromyalgia patients will have a range of other symptoms. Indeed, one of the key features of the condition is the large number of symptoms that are often diffuse and subjectively severe. These include muscle pain after exertion that is often described in graphic terms, morning stiffness, non-dermatomal peripheral numbness, joint pains and Raynaud's-like symptoms. Other symptoms include cold intolerance, fatigue, unrefreshed sleep, headaches, dizziness and lightheadedness, cognitive impairment, anxiety, low mood and subjective weakness. Most of the symptoms can be made worse by stress and anxiety, and may sometimes be triggered by infections and other physical illness. Fibromyalgia does occur in patients with other illnesses, particularly rheumatoid, lupus and other connective-tissue diseases (secondary fibromyalgia). This distinction between primary and secondary fibromyalgia is no longer thought to be useful. Part of the comprehensive approach to patients required of GPs involves the ability to simultaneously manage patients with multiple complaints and pathologies. This includes the skill of being able to synthesise information from multiple sources including the patient record and other information, not just the information gathered in the current consultation. Such skills are likely to be needed in the confident diagnosis of fibromyalgia.

## Taking a person-centred approach

Taking a person-centred approach to history-taking is particularly important in fibromyalgia. GPs will usually already have a good knowledge of the patient's medical and social history, and his or her previous consultation patterns. In making a diagnosis it is often worth arranging a slightly longer appointment and/or a notes review to bring all the relevant information together on a one-off basis, rather than resorting to multiple and possibly disparate appointments with different doctors over a protracted period. Fibromyalgia patients may sometimes elicit feelings of 'heartsink' in the consulting doctor. Such feelings (transference) should alert the doctor to the possibility that the patient may have complex biopsychosocial problems. The doctor should resist any temptation to curtail the consultation, for example by offering a potentially inappropriate referral or prescription. Rather, the opportunity should be taken to gather more psychological and social information to place the complaint in context. Sometimes the initial presenting complaint may be an opening 'gambit' by the patient to ascertain whether the doctor is interested and sympathetic.

## Pathophysiology

There have been numerous theories of the causation of fibromyalgia since Gower's original description in 1904 (he used the term 'fibrositis' to describe a group of patients with fatigue, poor sleep and sensitivity to touch). No single theory has gained the ascendancy. From a primary care perspective it is more useful to be familiar with a range of associations that increase the probability of diagnosis rather than seeking a unified theory. This situation is reflected in the fact that there is no specific 'test' for fibromyalgia and that, to date, all routine investigations have proven to be normal. Some of the theories that are currently favoured include disturbances of sleep, particularly stage 4 non-rapid eye movement (NREM) sleep. Disturbances of serotonin, growth hormone, substance P and cortisol have been demonstrated in various studies. Autonomic dysfunction has also been postulated as a cause of fibromyalgia.[4]

Psychological dysfunction has been observed in about 30% of cases of fibromyalgia. Depression, anxiety, somatisation disorders and hypochondriasis are frequently reported. Studies have also demonstrated a high incidence of sexual and physical abuse in childhood (odds ratio 6.9) as well as a significantly increased incidence of eating disorders.[5,6] In terms of prognosis it used to be thought that fibromyalgia was usually chronic and often lifelong.

However, more recent community studies have shown that after two years about one quarter of patients will be in remission and nearly half will no longer fit the ACR criteria for diagnosis.[7]

There has been debate about the effect of labelling itself on the prognosis of various fatigue syndromes, including fibromyalgia. There is a fine line between ascribing a fibromyalgia label too early, on the one hand, and leaving the patient in diagnostic 'limbo', on the other. Different doctors and patients will vary in their tolerance of diagnostic uncertainty, but a person-centred approach should allow a more comfortable and appropriate period of formulation. A person-centred approach to explaining the diagnosis to a patient and his or her family is crucially important and may determine whether or not a second opinion is requested.

Stone and colleagues have discussed the concept of 'number needed to offend' (NNO).[8] [Many diagnostic labels that are used for symptoms unexplained by disease have the potential to offend patients.] Their study showed that using pejorative explanations such as 'all in the mind' had an NNO of 2 whereas use of the word 'functional' was more acceptable with an NNO of around 9 (95% CI 5–21). It is important to take into account the patient's ideas, concerns and expectations (ICE), and to incorporate these into an explanation. Honesty is the best policy. It is also important to steer the patient in the direction of appropriate websites, such as Arthritis Research UK (www.arthritisresearchuk.org/), as there is otherwise a danger of being directed to one of the more controversial sites, which may not be in the patient's best interests.

---

## Fibromyalgia and allied syndromes – one disease or many?

One of the controversies surrounding fibromyalgia is whether or not it is a distinct condition. There is a significant overlap in symptom clusters with other conditions such as IBS, irritable bladder, dysmenorrhoea, headaches, premenstrual syndrome, temporomandibular joint pain, non-cardiac chest pain, and chronic fatigue syndrome (CFS). A substantial proportion of each of these conditions cannot currently be explained by disease-specific abnormalities. So-called 'splitters' would argue that they are separate entities, whereas 'lumpers' would say that they have more commonalities than differences. It is estimated, for example, that depression occurs in 40% of patients with fibromyalgia, anxiety in 45% and IBS-like symptoms in 70%. Historically, most of the research on these conditions has been specialist-led, resulting in the assertion that 'to a man with a hammer an awful lot of things look like nails'. The debate continues but it is clear that in primary care many patients have 'hybrids' of these conditions and it is often useful to classify them all as 'functional somatic disorders' as their pragmatic management in primary care is broadly very similar.

It is important to clarify the term *somatisation*. There are limitations with DSM-IV (*Diagnostic and Statistical Manual of Mental Disorders*, fourth edition) and its classification of somatisation, not least of which is where to draw the line between disease and normality. It is also debatable to what extent the proliferation of diagnoses around somatoform disorders is helpful for day-to-day management of real patients in primary care. Experts disagree on how to define somatisation. One definition simply maintains that it is the process whereby individuals experience and describe physical symptoms that, after appropriate investigation, cannot be explained by a known medical condition. Another definition requires, in addition, the presence of psychological factors that cause or at least contribute to the problem.

Fibromyalgia and these related functional somatic disorders form quantitatively a significant part of general practice. Studies have shown that at least one third, and maybe up to half, of all symptoms in primary care are medically unexplained. The term MUPS – 'medically unexplained physical symptoms' – is sometimes used.[9] One of the hallmarks of these conditions is the poor inter-observer agreement on diagnosis, which is often determined by the doctor's specialist background. The diagnostic heterogeneity often leads to over-investigation with the risk of 'false positive' results, so called 'incidentalomas' and mislabelling of patients – what Clifton Meador, a US physician renowned for his critical analyses of the excesses of medical practice, referred to as the 'art and science of non-disease'. Richard Smith gives a short and useful summary of this subject.[10] Functional somatic disorders and medically unexplained symptoms are, collectively, major consumers of healthcare resources. Many of these patients will have had multiple referrals, many investigations, inappropriate polypharmacy, lack of a diagnosis and information, with ongoing distress, disability and perhaps long-term sickness certification. Telling patients what they do not have does not work. The GP needs a 'toolkit' of skills that will serve well for the management of all these patients (see Box 10.4 on p. 251). The community orientation competences required of GPs include the ability to balance available resources. This may mean protecting the fibromyalgia patient from potentially unhelpful referrals while at the same time making available appropriate services and acting as an advocate for the patient.

## Specific problem-solving skills in fibromyalgia

While the diagnosis of fibromyalgia is clinical and the importance of not over-investigating has already been emphasised, some baseline investigations are useful. Some examples of specific problem-solving skills include the ability to exclude inflammatory rheumatic disorders and other more serious conditions that may need referral, understanding the risks of 'non-disease' and the positive predictive values of tests, and being able to positively and proactively assess for somatisation and psychological distress without an excessive process of exclusion. Another specific problem-solving skill is getting the balance of treatment right, in particular not relying too heavily on just pharmacological approaches, and also knowing when to refer a fibromyalgia patient.

The differential diagnosis of fibromyalgia includes hypothyroidism, lupus, inflammatory myopathy, hyperparathyroidism, osteomalacia, polymyalgia rheumatica, sleep apnoea, as well as the other functional somatic disorders listed in the text.

It is often better to do all the baseline investigations in one batch early on, rather than in a piecemeal fashion, to inspire confidence in the patient. A suggested list is laid out in Box 10.2.

---

Box 10.2 ○ *Suggested list of investigations for fibromyalgia (and allied conditions)*

▶ Full blood count (FBC).

▶ Erythrocyte sedimentation rate (ESR).

▶ Antinuclear antibody (ANA)/rheumatoid factor.

▶ Thyroid-stimulating hormone (TSH).

▶ C-reactive protein (CRP).

▶ Creatine kinase (CK)

▶ Calcium.

▶ Alkaline phosphatase.

▶ Blood glucose.

▶ Urinalysis for protein, blood and glucose.

---

This list includes additional tests recommended in the National Institute for Health and Clinical Excellence (NICE) guidelines for chronic fatigue syndrome (CFS)/myalgic encephalomyelitis (ME) as there is a large overlap in symptom clusters between fibromyalgia and CFS/ME.[11] Caution needs to be exercised with borderline positive results such as TSH and ANA. False-positive ANAs are common, whereas lupus is rare as a new presentation in primary care. Part of the specific problem-solving skills required by the GP includes the ability to relate specific decision-making processes to the prevalence and incidence of illness in the community.

## Biopsychosocial assessment

Although this is part of normal good general practice, it can be crucially important in helping to confirm the diagnosis and more specifically to inform the individualised management plan for a particular patient. Often this information is already known to the GP but it may be hidden in the database and sometimes a systematic enquiry may produce significant revelations.

It may be useful to produce a biopsychosocial formulation that attempts to deconstruct the patient's presentation into understandable components, namely biological, psychological and social, and then further into predisposing, precipitating and perpetuating categories. A small amount of extra time spent at this stage may save unnecessary and expensive referrals, and prove to be in the interests of both the patient and clinician. The reader is referred to the work of Simon Wessely for a more detailed account of the biopsychosocial formulation.[12]

## Treatment

The recent European League Against Rheumatism (EULAR) guideline provides a useful summary of evidence-based management. The development of this guideline involved a multidisciplinary taskforce from 11 different countries.[13] They identified about 150 suitable studies using the ACR criteria and produced a table that lists both the level and strength of evidence (see Table 10.1).

At the time of writing some of these drugs are unavailable in the UK (milnacipran and pirlindole) and others such as tropisetron are prohibitively expensive for routine use. The reader is advised to consult the individual data sheets and/or *British National Formulary* (BNF) for changing licensed indications.

In practical terms, low-dose amitriptyline (25 mg at night) seems the most logical choice as GPs are familiar with its use, it is cost-effective and current trials seem to suggest that it may produce consistent improvements in pain, sleep and fatigue. There does not seem to be any benefit in increasing the dose and any improvements seem to be short term (8–12 weeks). It may be a useful early adjunct to treatment while formulating and arranging more comprehensive and holistic management. There is good evidence that duloxetine in doses of 60–120 mg can produce improvement in pain in some fibromyalgia patients with a number needed to treat (NNT) of 6–7 to produce 50% pain relief.[14]

Although the evidence base is very variable for different treatment modalities, current opinion favours the tailoring of treatment to individual patients. GPs are in the key position to offer a patient-centred approach using the

Table 10.1  ○  *Evidence-based recommendations for the management of fibromyalgia*

| Recommendation | Level of evidence* | Strength of evidence† |
|---|---|---|
| **General** | | |
| Full understanding of fibromyalgia requires comprehensive assessment of pain, function and psychosocial context | IV | D |
| Optimal treatment requires a multidisciplinary approach with a combination of non-pharmacological and pharmacological treatment modalities tailored according to pain intensity, function and associated features (such as depression, fatigue and sleep disturbance) in discussion with the patient | IV | D |
| **Non-pharmacological management** | | |
| Heated-pool treatment, with or without exercise (balneotherapy) | IIa | B |
| Individually tailored exercise programmes, including aerobic exercise and strength training | IIb | C |
| Cognitive behavioural therapy (CBT) | IV | D |
| Other therapies such as relaxation, rehabilitation, physiotherapy, psychological support | IIb | C |
| **Pharmacological management** | | |
| Tramadol for pain management | Ib | A |
| Simple analgesics such as paracetamol and weak opioids may be considered | IV | D |
| Antidepressants: amitriptyline (tricyclic antidepressant, TCAD), fluoxetine (selective serotonin reuptake inhibitors, SSRI), duloxetine (serotonin-norepinephrine reuptake inhibitors, SNRI), milnacipran (SNRI), moclobemide (reversible inhibitors of monoamine oxidase type-A, RIMA), pirlindole (RIMA) reduce pain and often improve function | Ib | A |
| Tropisetron, pramipexole and pregabalin reduce pain | Ib | A |

*Notes*: * I = randomised controlled double-blind trials (RCT) | V = non-randomised open trials.

† 'A' is the strongest, based directly on category I evidence, i.e. meta-analysis of RCT. 'D' is the weakest, i.e. based on category IV evidence or extrapolated from category I, II or III evidence.

*Source*: adapted from EULAR.[13]

criteria laid out in the consultation observation tool (COT) of the MRCGP. This includes exploring the patient's health understanding, explaining the condition to the patient in appropriate language, involving the patient in significant management decisions, and making effective use of resources. At local level, contextual factors such as long waiting lists for CBT and local practice-based commissioning (PBC) initiatives will tend to influence referrals. CBT, for example, is probably best reserved for those patients with high levels of psychological distress. An important skill is knowing when to refer the minority of patients with fibromyalgia. Indications would include diagnostic uncertainty, significantly uncontrolled symptoms, management uncertainties and patient request for specialist opinion.

---

### A comprehensive and holistic approach to the fibromyalgia patient

A comprehensive approach to the fibromyalgia patient is also inevitably going to involve some degree of assessment of disability – many fibromyalgia patients will not be working. The fibromyalgia impact questionnaire may be useful to assess function (www.myalgia.com/FIQ/FIQ_questionnaire.pdf). Doctors vary widely in their assessment of disability in fibromyalgia as it is conceptually difficult to evaluate patients' perceptions of their functional ability. Changing national strategies such as those laid out in *Working for a Healthier Tomorrow* (including a 'fit for work' service and a more holistic approach integrating occupational health with mainstream health care) will alter the way fibromyalgia is handled.[15, 16] In particular, early intervention and an emphasis on the therapeutic aspects of work will challenge GPs and fibromyalgia patients alike.

As part of a holistic approach to the treatment of fibromyalgia patients the GP may need to facilitate self-help. In particular this involves getting the patient to share responsibility and ownership of the tailored management programme. The GP may be called upon to give advice about access to complementary and alternative medicines (CAM) and to comment on self-help websites and societies. Use of educational material is undoubtedly important, and giving the patient a selection of resources is useful – some of these are included at the end of this chapter. Education of carers and family is often equally crucial, although any discussion about the patient must of course always observe rules of confidentiality and preferably be joint consultations with the patient. Although a comprehensive approach to the management of fibromyalgia patients is inevitably going to involve other members of the team, studies suggest treating fibromyalgia in a specialised setting offers no clear advantages over primary care management.[17]

## Medically unexplained symptoms and chronic pain in rheumatology

The common prevalence of fibromyalgia in primary care has been discussed above. Even more common is the collective group of so-called MUPS, of which fibromyalgia is a subgroup. Some of the other conditions, such as IBS, CFS/ME, headache, non-cardiac chest pain, and atypical facial pain, have already been mentioned. Qualitative studies have shown that GPs feel pressurised to resort to somatic interventions, such as symptomatic prescribing, or investigation when patients actually seek to engage the GP by conveying the reality of their suffering, and do not necessarily want referrals or prescriptions.[18] In practice, missed organic pathology is rare whereas psychiatric morbidity is common and frequently missed.

It is estimated that 25% of GP patients in England have MUPS; pain is usually a significant component of these presentations. Studies from Scotland suggest that about 18% of the population have chronic pain.[19] In Western Europe as a whole studies again suggest that about 1 in 5 adults reports chronic pain. For the UK the average age of sufferers was 49, with back pain and arthritis being the commonest causes.[20] Unlike acute pain, which is often well defined with a clear-cut biomedical explanation, chronic pain tends to be different; it is not just acute pain that has gone on for a longer period. The International Association for the Study of Pain (IASP) defines chronic pain as 'pain without apparent biological value that has persisted beyond normal tissue healing time'. In practice this is set as three months. Once pain becomes chronic it often becomes more complex in nature, with associated psychological components that include poor-quality sleep, fatigue, low mood and cognitive difficulties such as poor concentration (note the overlap with fibromyalgia).

Chronic pain tends to be most prevalent in middle-aged people, especially women, and is one of the most common reasons for primary care consultations. It is clearly a major public health problem and at an individual level often causes severe personal distress. It also tends to be poorly managed as well as being a major cause of disability and reduced quality of life. When assessing pain it is important to ascertain what type or quality of pain the patient is experiencing as this can help in diagnosis and management. The patient's pain narrative is also crucially important. Histories should be 'received' rather than taken. The GP should actively listen to the exact words that the patient uses as well as their context and be acutely aware of cues and body language.

Nociceptive pain, classically caused by tissue damage, is often well localised (although it may be more diffuse if visceral rather than somatic), sharp, stabbing or gripping in nature, with typical examples being arthritis pain and trauma. Neuropathic pain, caused by neural dysfunction, can be central, peripheral or autonomic and is often described as persistent, burning, paroxysmal or like 'electric shocks'. Other features of neuropathic pain include allodynia (a painful response to stimuli that would not normally cause pain), hyperalgesia (an exaggerated response to a pain stimulus) and dysaesthesia (unpleasant, abnormal pain sensations). Complex regional pain syndromes are examples of musculoskeletal neuropathic pain.

A significant proportion of chronic pain is musculoskeletal in nature. The commonest subgroups of chronic pain are back pain, arthritis and pain following injury. In terms of the commonest anatomical sites of pain these are, in order, back pain, headache, joint pain, arm or leg pain, chest pain and abdominal pain. About 40% of patients with chronic pain will report pain at three or more sites. The traditional biomedical approach to chronic pain tends to view it as a symptom of an identifiable disease. The IASP lists over 600 clinical syndromes related to chronic pain. With increasing specialisation in secondary care, GPs, as generalists, are in the best position to use their all-round diagnostic skills to screen for red-flag symptoms. In terms of causes for diffuse musculoskeletal pain it is important to consider the following causes (see Box 10.3).

---

**Box 10.3 ○ *Causes of diffuse or widespread musculoskeletal pain***

▶ Inflammatory arthritis (including rheumatoid arthritis and spondyloarthropathies).

▶ Polymyalgia rheumatica.

▶ Polymyositis/dermatomyositis.

▶ Vasculitides.

▶ Hypo/hyperthyroidism.

▶ Multiple sclerosis.

▶ Neuropathies.

▶ Osteomalacia.

▶ Fibromyalgia.

▶ CFS/ME.

▶ Complex regional pain syndromes.

---

## Community orientation and holistic approach to patients with chronic musculoskeletal pain

Having assessed the patient with chronic musculoskeletal pain and excluded any red-flag conditions or specific diseases that could be treated or reversed, there will be a significant group of patients, as previously discussed, with ongoing chronic and distressing pain (which could be collectively labelled as 'chronic pain syndromes'). Endless searching for a nonexistent diagnosis should be avoided. How are these to be managed in primary care? Some of the management has already been discussed under the topic of fibromyalgia. However, consideration will now be given to a 'generic toolkit' that should prove helpful and practical in the management of any chronic musculoskeletal pain. Box 10.4 lists a ten-point toolkit for the generic management of patients with chronic musculoskeletal pain.

---

**Box 10.4** ○ *Ten-point toolkit for the generic management of chronic musculoskeletal pain.*

1 ▶ Carry out *individual assessment* (be person centred and holistic) including health beliefs (remembering that patients may have inner experiences that are subjective, mystical or religious that influence their health beliefs) – consider *COT* or *ICE tools* (see pp. 253–4).

2 ▶ Treat cause if possible (consider notes review).

3 ▶ Assess for anxiety and/or depression (which will be commonly present).

4 ▶ Assess need for analgesia/adjuvant therapy (and sleep management) (see p. 247).

5 ▶ Modify aggravating factors (e.g. physical, social environment).

6 ▶ Consider physical therapies (which engage the patient).

7 ▶ Consider psychological therapies such as CBT and look at coping strategies.

8 ▶ Think family. (Who are the patients' allies?)

9 ▶ Co-ordinate multidisciplinary care but avoid over-medicalisation.

10 ▶ Consider rehabilitation. (Look at return to work early.)

---

One of the early difficulties encountered by GPs in managing chronic musculoskeletal pain is how to explain the condition to patients in an acceptable manner. One study suggests that patients are most satisfied by explanations that make sense to the patient, remove blame, and suggest ideas for management. Explanations should certainly attempt to integrate psychological and biological factors rather than imply purely psychological causation. The GP also needs to be able to identify mistaken beliefs and fears as well as iatrogenic distress and anger. Excellent empathic listening skills are also vitally important at this point, especially when looking for cues and transference.

In tailoring the management of an individual patient it is important to understand not only the quality and severity of the pain but also how it is affecting the following domains:

▷ physical effects/manifestations
▷ functional effects
▷ interference with activities of daily living (including sexual difficulties)
▷ psychosocial functioning
▷ spiritual aspects (from the patient's perspective – 'Why am I experiencing such pain?' – which may or may not include a religious component).

As with fibromyalgia and other functional somatic disorders (FSDs), psychosocial factors often predict persistence of chronic musculoskeletal pain. For example, with chronic back pain psychosocial factors appear to be more predictive of chronicity than anatomical pathology. Such factors include poor job satisfaction, low pay, inadequate coping skills, somatisation, ongoing litigation, low education level, anxiety, low mood, and emotional distress. Although much of the research on musculoskeletal pain has focused on anatomical sites, such as low-back pain, a recent systematic review has identified that similar prognostic factors may prevail for poor outcome irrespective of the site of pain. Examining prospective observational cohort studies based in primary care, Mallen *et al.* identified 11 'generic' prognostic factors related to poor outcome. These were as follows: higher pain severity at baseline, longer pain duration, multiple pain site, previous pain episodes, anxiety and/or depression, higher somatic perceptions, adverse coping strategies, low social support, older age, higher baseline disability, and greater movement restriction.[21] Some of these factors may be difficult to quantify in the context of a busy general practice surgery. Nevertheless, they do raise the possibility of being able to target patients at higher risk of developing chronic pain and perhaps enabling earlier intervention.

The 'flag' system is well known to GPs, especially the concept of the 'red flag'. Main and Burton have expanded the flag concept to include red, yellow, blue, orange and black flags.[22] It provides a useful way of looking at chronic back pain from a holistic and biopsychosocial perspective (see Table 10.2).

Table 10.2 ○ *Flag system as applied to chronic back pain*

| Flag type | Parameter | Biopsychosocial category |
|---|---|---|
| Red flags | Organic pathology | Biomedical factors |
| | Concurrent medical problems | |
| Yellow flags | Iatrogenic factors | Psychological or behavioural factors |
| | Health beliefs | |
| | Coping strategies | |
| | Distress | |
| | Illness behaviour | |
| | Willingness to change | |
| | Family factors | |
| Orange flags | Psychiatric equivalent of red flags, i.e. significant mental illness | Psychiatric factors |
| Blue flags | Work status | Social and economic factors, and perceptions of workplace |
| | Litigation | |
| | Job satisfaction | |
| Black flags | Working conditions | Organisational aspects of occupation |
| | Social policy | |

Although the flag system has been devised for use with back pain it may be a useful *aide-mémoire* for assessing most types of chronic pain and FSD. The assessment of red flags has been dealt with elsewhere under specific disease headings.

In terms of yellow flags, the GP should be in a key position to take a good psychosocial history. Indeed, much of the information may already be recorded or known. It is, however, difficult to take a full history from scratch in a 10-minute consultation. Using the COT template of the MRCGP may prove useful. The experienced GP, in particular, may find the early identification of cues useful in identifying a predominantly psychosocial presentation without an excessively long consultation. Table 10.3 (overleaf) shows a one-page summary of the COT as used in the author's own practice. Other useful tools include the acronym ICE, namely asking the patient about his or her 'ideas, concerns and expectations'.

Table 10.3 ○ *One-page summary of the COT performance criteria (MRCGP)*

| | | | Performance criteria (PC) | Present |
|---|---|---|---|---|
| **Competences** | Discover the reasons for the patient's attendance | **a** | PC1 ▶ the doctor is seen to encourage the patient's contribution at appropriate points in the consultation | |
| | | | PC2 ▶ the doctor is seen to respond to signals (cues) that lead to a deeper understanding of the problem | |
| | | **b** | PC3 ▶ the doctor uses appropriate psychological and social information to place the complaint(s) in context | |
| | | **c** | PC4 ▶ the doctor explores the patient's health understanding | |
| | Define the clinical problem(s) | **a** | PC5 ▶ the doctor obtains sufficient information to include or exclude likely relevant significant conditions | |
| | | **b** | PC6 ▶ the physical/mental examination chosen is likely to confirm or disprove hypotheses that could reasonably have been formed OR is likely to address a patient's concern | |
| | | **c** | PC7 ▶ the doctor appears to make a clinically appropriate working diagnosis | |
| | Explain problem(s) to patient | **a** | PC8 ▶ the doctor explains the problem or diagnosis in appropriate language | |
| | | **b** | PC9 ▶ the doctor specifically seeks to confirm the patient's understanding of the diagnosis | |
| | Address patient's problem(s) | **a** | PC10 ▶ the management plan (including any prescription) is appropriate for the working diagnosis, reflecting a good understanding of modern accepted medical practice | |
| | | **b** | PC11 ▶ the patient is given the opportunity to be involved in significant management decisions | |
| | Make effective use of the consultation | **a** | PC12 ▶ makes effective use of resources | |
| | | | PC13 ▶ the doctor specifies the conditions and interval for follow-up or review | |

*Source*: Browning Street Surgery Marking Template, 2009.

In terms of predicting which patients with FSD or chronic pain have psychiatric co-morbidity (orange flags) Box 10.5 lists some useful predictors (especially depression, anxiety or somatisation) in patients who have physical symptoms.

---

Box 10.5 ○ ***Predictors of psychiatric co-morbidity in patients who have physical symptoms***

▶ Unexplained symptoms after the clinician's initial assessment.

▶ Multiple symptoms.

▶ Chronic or recurrent symptoms.

▶ Frequent healthcare use.

▶ Polypharmacy.

▶ Failure to respond to multiple medication trials for the same symptom.

▶ Intolerance of multiple medications ('nocebo' effect).

▶ Difficult encounter ('heartsink' – as perceived by the clinician).

▶ Number of **S4** predictors:

  **1 S**tress in past week

  **2 S**ymptom count high (on PHQ-15 symptom checklist)

  **3 S**elf-rated health is low

  **4 S**everity of symptoms is high (>5 on 10-point scale, where 0 is none and 10 is unbearable).

*Source*: adapted from Kroenke and Rosmalen.[23]

---

Pharmacological treatment of chronic musculoskeletal pain is clearly a specific management skill, but not to the exclusion of other approaches. Space does not permit a detailed discussion of this area and the reader is referred to the BNF and individual data sheets for up-to-date information about dosages and licensed indications. As a general principle the WHO analgesic ladder is a useful starting point:

**Level 1** ▶ non-opioid +/- adjuvant
**Level 2** ▶ opioid for mild to moderate pain +/- non-opioid +/- adjuvant
**Level 3** ▶ opioid for moderate to severe pain +/- non-opioid +/- adjuvant.

Non-opioids include paracetamol, non-steroidal anti-inflammatory drugs (NSAIDs) and COX-2 inhibitors. Opioids used in primary care are mainly various strengths of codeine moving up to dihydrocodeine, morphine, fentanyl and others. For a more detailed discussion of opioid prescribing in chronic pain the reader is referred to the British Pain Society guidelines

(2005).[24] Adjuvants or unconventional analgesics include low-dose tricyclic antidepressants such as amitriptyline, anticonvulsants such as gabapentin and pregabalin, and the analgesic tramadol. Although tramadol has opioid activity it has a complex mode of action involving serotonin and noradrenaline reuptake inhibition, which may explain its efficacy in treating 'difficult' pain such as neuropathic pain. It should be remembered that 70% of chronic pain patients will also suffer from significant sleep disturbance. Poor sleep can contribute to the patient's perception of pain intensity. Sleep disturbance needs to be addressed holistically including using appropriate analgesic regimes (including adjuvants such as amitriptyline), treating underlying depression, and accessing interventions targeting insomnia ('sleep hygiene'). Other pharmacological interventions include myofascial trigger point injections of local anaesthetic and/or steroid injection (risks of infection and fat necrosis) – these are best reserved for true trigger points rather than just tender spots. TENS and acupuncture may also be used, although there is no strong evidence for their use.

One of the major challenges for patients, GPs and society in general is the question of chronic pain and work. Patients with chronic musculoskeletal pain are at significantly increased risk of not working. The current sickness certification process focuses on what people cannot do and GPs often feel poorly equipped to offer patients work-related advice. Recent documents such as *Working for a Healthier Tomorrow* and the NICE guideline on long-term sickness absence and incapacity for work place a strong emphasis on early intervention with return to work plans and the use of CBT, coping strategies, exercise programmes, counselling, workplace modifications and solution-focused group sessions for patients with chronic musculoskeletal pain and disability.

Although much chronic pain can be managed in primary care the GP will sometimes need to co-ordinate a multidisciplinary approach. Most patients will not need the care of a full multidisciplinary team and a tailored approach is appropriate as previously discussed. Box 10.4 lists, in no particular order, some of the possible resources and referral options the GP can utilise in the management of these patients.

Some patients may require referral to specific pain management programmes with a comprehensive multidisciplinary input. Such programmes should focus on function rather than disease, management rather than cure, emphasise active rather than passive methods, and self-care rather than simply receiving treatment. Self-management/support groups may also be helpful at local level. To conclude, however, it is clear that the majority of patients with fibromyalgia, or other diffuse musculoskeletal pain, may be best served by the dedicated efforts of the truly generalist, well-informed, clinically con-

---

**Table 10.4** ○ *Multidisciplinary team – potential resources*

▶ GP.

▶ General Practitioner with a Special Interest (GPwSI) (in pain management).

▶ Pain consultant.

▶ Specialist nurse.

▶ Physiotherapist.

▶ Pharmacist.

▶ Psychologist.

▶ Social worker.

▶ Occupational therapist.

▶ Osteopath.

▶ Chiropractor.

▶ Complementary and alternative practitioners.

▶ Rehabilitation.

▶ Psychiatrist.

▶ Psychosexual counsellor.

fident GP practising, in the words of the RCGP motto, *'cum scientia caritas'* (science with compassion). The challenge to the GP is to transcend the formulaic world of guidelines, the Quality and Outcomes Framework (QoF) and evidence-based medicine, and, in the words of Sir William Osler, see 'the poetry of the commonplace, of the ordinary man, of the plain, toil-worn woman, with their loves and their joys, their sorrows and their griefs'.[25] Only then can the doctor fully appreciate that 'every patient you see is a lesson in much more than the malady from which he suffers'.[25]

---

## Self-assessment questions

Which is the **single most** accurate statement about the prevalence of fibromyalgia in the general adult population? Select **one** option only.

1 ▷ The overall prevalence is about 0.5%
2 ▷ The overall prevalence is about 2.5%
3 ▷ The overall prevalence is about 5.0%
4 ▷ The peak age of onset is between 20 and 25
5 ▷ It is more common in men than women

*Correct answer* ▷ **3**

Which of the following is *not* one of the generally recognised tender points in fibromyalgia? Select **one** option only.

1 ▷ Occiput, at the suboccipital muscle insertion
2 ▷ Trapezius, at the midpoint of the upper border
3 ▷ Second rib, at the second costochondral junction
4 ▷ Biceps, at the midpoint of the medial border
5 ▷ Greater trochanter, posterior to the trochanteric prominence

*Correct answer* ▷ **4**

Which of the following features is *not* consistent with a diagnosis of fibromy-algia? Select **one** option only.

1 ▷ History of widespread pain
2 ▷ Morning stiffness
3 ▷ Cold intolerance
4 ▷ Raised ESR
5 ▷ Cognitive impairment

*Correct answer* ▷ **4**

A 50-year-old woman with a previous diagnosis of fibromyalgia joins your practice list. Which of the following statements is *most* likely to be correct? Select **one** option only.

1 ▷ She would be unlikely to be depressed
2 ▷ It would be unusual for her to have irritable bowel-type symptoms
3 ▷ Her fibromyalgia is likely to have resolved
4 ▷ Her sleep pattern is likely to be normal
5 ▷ There would be a significant chance of her having suffered sexual abuse in childhood

*Correct answer* ▷ **5**

A 60-year-old woman with established fibromyalgia consults with you to discuss the best option for treatment. Her main symptoms are widespread pain, fatigue and cognitive impairment. She is armed with multiple print-outs from the web. Which **one** of the following modalities would you be *least* likely to recommend?

1 ▷ An antidepressant
2 ▷ Heated-pool treatment
3 ▷ Tramadol for her pain
4 ▷ Acupuncture
5 ▷ CBT

*Correct answer* ▷ **4**

**References**

1 • Fauci AS (ed.). *Harrison's Rheumatology* (16th edn) New York: McGraw Hill, 2006.

2 • Wolfe F, Smyth HA, Yunus MB, *et al.* The American College of Rheumatology 1990 Criteria for the Classification of Fibromyalgia *Arthritis and Rheumatism* 1990; **33(2)**: 160–72.

3 • Wolfe F, Clauw DJ, Fitzcharles MA, *et al.* The American College of Rheumatology Preliminary Diagnostic Criteria for Fibromyalgia and Measurement of Symptom Severity *Arthritis Care and Research* 2010; **62(5)**; 600–10.

4 • Clauw DJ. Fibromyalgia: update on mechanisms and management *Journal of Clinical Rheumatology* 2007; **13(2)**: 102–9.

5 • Boisset-Pioro MH, Esdaile JM, Fitzcharles MA. Sexual and physical abuse in women with fibromyalgia syndrome *Arthritis and Rheumatism* 1995; **38(2)**: 235–41.

6 • Castro I, Barrantes F, Tuna M, *et al.* Prevalence of abuse in fibromyalgia and other rheumatic disorders at a specialized clinic in rheumatic diseases in Guatemala City *Journal of Clinical Rheumatology* 2005; **11(3)**: 140–5.

7 • Hamilton WT, Gallagher AM, Thomas JM, *et al.* The prognosis of different fatigue diagnostic labels: a longitudinal survey *Family Practice* 2005; **22(4)**: 383–8.

8 • Stone J, Wojcik W, Durrance D, *et al.* What should we say to patients with symptoms unexplained by disease? The 'number needed to offend' *British Medical Journal* 2002; **325(7378)**: 1449–50.

9 • Hatcher S, Arroll B. Assessment and management of medically unexplained symptoms *British Medical Journal* 2008; **336(7653)**: 1124–8.

10 • Smith R. In search of 'non-disease' *British Medical Journal* 2002; **324(7342)**: 883–5.

11 • Baker R, Shaw EJ. Diagnosis and management of chronic fatigue syndrome or myalgic encephalomyelitis (or encephalopathy): summary of NICE guidance *British Medical Journal* 2007; **335**: 446–8.

12 • Wessely S, Hotopf M, Sharpe M. *Chronic Fatigue and its Syndromes* Oxford: Oxford University Press, 1998.

13 • Carville S F, Arendt-Nielsen S, Bliddal H, *et al*. EULAR evidence-based recommendations for the management of fibromyalgia syndrome *Annals of the Rheumatic Diseases* 2008; **67(4)**: 536–41.

14 • Uceyler N, Hauser W, Sommer C. A systematic review on the effectiveness of treatment with antidepressants in fibromyalgia syndrome *Arthritis and Rheumatism* 2008; **59(9)**: 1279–98.

15 • Black C. *Working for a Healthier Tomorrow* London: The Stationery Office, 2008, www.dwp.gov.uk/health-work-and-well-being/resources/ [accessed October 2011].

16 • National Institute for Health and Clinical Excellence. *Managing Long-Term Sickness Absence and Incapacity for Work* [NICE Public Health Guidance 19] London: NICE, 2009.

17 • Garcia-Campayo J, Magdalena J, Magallón R, *et al*. A meta-analysis of the efficacy of fibromyalgia treatment according to level of care *Arthritis Research & Therapy*, 2008, www.arthritis-research.com/content/10/4/R81 [accessed October 2011]

18 • Ring A, Dowrick C, Humphris G, *et al*. Do patients with unexplained physical symptoms pressurise general practitioners for somatic treatment? A qualitative study *British Medical Journal* 2004; **328(7447)**: 1057–61.

19 • NHS Quality Improvement Scotland. *Management of Chronic Pain in Adults* Edinburgh: NHS Quality Improvement Scotland, 2006.

20 • Dickman A, Simpson K H. *Chronic Pain* (Oxford Pain Management Library) Oxford: Oxford University Press, 2008.

21 • Mallen C D, Peat G, Thomas E, *et al*. Prognostic factors for musculoskeletal pain in primary care: a systematic review *British Journal of General Practice* 2007; **57(541)**: 655–61.

22 • Main C J, Sullivan M J L, Watson P J. *Pain Management: practical applications of the biopsychosocial perspective in clinical and occupational settings* (second edn) Edinburgh: Churchill Livingstone, 2008.

23 • Kroenke K, Rosmalen JGM. Symptoms, syndromes, and the value of psychiatric diagnostics in patients who have functional somatic disorders *Medical Clinics of North America* 2006; **90(4)**: 603–26.

24 • British Pain Society. *Opioids for Persistent Pain: good practice* London: British Pain Society, 2005, www.britishpainsociety.org/book_opioid_main.pdf [accessed October 2011].

25 • Osler W. The student life. In: *Aequanimitas* Philadelphia: P Blakiston, 1906, pp. 404–5.

## Appendix: criteria for fibromyalgia and measurement of symptom severity

| Widespread pain index (WPI) | Score (one for each tick) | Symptom severity (SS) (circle one for each option A–D) | 0 | 1 | 2 | 3 | Total SS (0–12) |
|---|---|---|---|---|---|---|---|
| Shoulder girdle, left | | A – fatigue | No Problem | Mild | Moderate | Severe | |
| Shoulder girdle, right | | | | | | | |
| Upper arm, left | | | | | | | |
| Upper arm, right | | | | | | | |
| Lower arm, left | | | | | | | |
| Lower arm, right | | B – waking unrefreshed | No Problem | Mild | Moderate | Severe | |
| Hip (buttock, trochanter), left | | | | | | | |
| Hip (buttock, trochanter), right | | | | | | | |
| Upper leg, left | | | | | | | |
| Upper leg, right | | C – cognitive symptoms | No Problem | Mild | Moderate | Severe | |
| Lower leg, left | | | | | | | |
| Lower leg, right | | | | | | | |
| Jaw, left | | | | | | | |
| Jaw, right | | D – number of somatic symptoms | No Symptoms | Few Symptoms | Moderate Symptoms | Many Symptoms | |
| Chest | | | | | | | |
| Abdomen | | | | | | | |
| Upper back | | | | | | | |
| Lower back | | | | | | | |
| Neck | | Total SS (0–12) | | | | | |
| Total WPI (0–19) | | | | | | | |

Notes: Criteria 1, 2 and 3 needed for diagnosis of fibromyalgia syndrome.
1) Diagnose fibromyalgia syndrome if WPI ≥7 and SS ≥5 or WPI 3–6 AND SS ≥9.
2) Symptoms present for at least three months.
3) No alternative explanation for the pain.

Source: Wolfe F, Clauw DJ, Fitzcharles MA, et al. The American College of Rheumatology Preliminary Diagnostic Criteria for Fibromyalgia and Measurement of Symptom Severity.[3]

# Acute arthropathies

*Elspeth Wise*

## Introduction

The term 'acute arthropathies' covers a number of conditions that can potentially be seen in primary care. Some of these are quite common, for example
gout, whereas others are quite rare. Included in this chapter are a number
of diagnoses that it is essential not to miss, as early diagnosis can prevent
irreversible joint damage.

Some possible causes of an acute arthropathy are as follows:

▷ sepsis
▷ gout
▷ inflammatory arthritis including rheumatoid arthritis and the
  seronegative spondyloarthropathies
▷ osteoarthritis
▷ trauma
▷ and others.

The management of these different conditions has changed dramatically
over recent years, in particular the management of the inflammatory arthri-
tidies. In the case of rheumatoid arthritis, there is very good evidence to
show that early referral to secondary care enables appropriate treatment to be
started.[1] Studies have also shown that, even this early on in the disease process, joint damage is occurring. Aggressive treatment can arrest this process
and can allow the joint to repair before irreversible damage occurs.

At the end of this chapter you will be:

▷ able to describe the differential diagnoses of an acute monoarthritis and
  an acute polyarthritis
▷ aware of red-flag symptoms and signs
▷ able to recognise potential emergencies and when they should be
  referred to secondary care.

## Initial management in primary care

In order to cover the differential diagnoses this chapter will look at the features of possible clinical presentations. In case study 1, Mr Smith is a 52-year-old teacher who rarely attends your surgery. He comes to see you in a morning surgery with a single painful, swollen joint.

And, in case study 2, Mrs Jones is a 42-year-old housewife and mother of three children. She presents with multiple painful joints.

---

**Box 11.1 ○ *Case study 1***

---

As already mentioned, Mr Smith is a 52-year-old teacher who very rarely attends the surgery. He has no past medical history of note and takes no prescribed medications. Mr Smith noted some slight pain in the affected joint yesterday evening. Overnight the pain has become more intense and Mr Smith indicates that the joint is now swollen and red. On examination the affected joint is inflamed, warm and swollen. The joint is tender to the touch and the swelling feels boggy and not bony. Both passive and active movements are painful.

In summary, Mr Smith has an acutely inflamed single joint, i.e. a monoarthropathy.

---

**Box 11.2 ○ *The classic signs of acute inflammation***

---

▶ *Calor* (heat).

▶ *Dolor* (pain).

▶ *Rubor* (erythema or redness).

▶ *Tumor* (swelling).

These are accompanied by loss of function.

---

The differential diagnosis of an acute monoarthropathy includes:

▷ gout
▷ septic arthritis
▷ inflammatory arthritis – reactive arthritis and the other seronegative spondyloarthropathies, and occasionally rheumatoid arthritis
▷ trauma, e.g. a ruptured anterior cruciate
▷ acute exacerbation of osteoarthritis
▷ haemophilia with bleeding into the joint capsule.

What further questions could help decide the diagnosis?

▷ Which joint is affected?

▷ Are there any aggravating/relieving factors?
▷ Is there a diurnal variation?
▷ Is there morning stiffness?
▷ Is there history of trauma?
▷ Has Mr Smith been unwell recently in any other way?
  ☐ In particular, check for gastrointestinal (GI) upset, urinary
    disturbance or rash.
▷ Has there been any history of trauma?
▷ Are there any risk factors for infection, e.g. diabetes mellitus, an
  immunodeficiency state or an underlying joint disease, e.g. RA/
  prosthesis?
▷ Check for evidence of multisystem disease, e.g. rash, problems with eyes,
  GI symptoms, pulmonary symptoms.

---

## Investigations

None may be required. However, you may wish to consider checking the full
blood count (FBC), C-reactive protein (CRP)/erythrocyte sedimentation rate
(ESR), glucose, uric acid, clotting and auto-antibodies. You may also want to
check for possible sources of infection with, for example, cervical or throat
swabs.

If you have the skills, you may wish to aspirate the joint fluid to send for
microscopy, culture and sensitivities.

---

## Possible diagnoses

Looking at each of the possible diagnoses in turn:

### *Sepsis*

Joint sepsis is uncommon but it is a diagnosis that it is essential not to miss as
there is an associated high fatality (about 11%) and evidence of bone destruction can be seen within seven days.[2]

If Mr Smith were to have a septic arthritis he would be expected to feel
generally unwell. He may or may not have a temperature and the affected
joint will be painful at rest. The pain will be exacerbated by both active and
passive movements. There would be no diurnal variation and no history of
morning stiffness as the symptoms will be persistent throughout the day. He
may have a history of trauma to the joint although spread can be haema-

togenous from an infection elsewhere. Any joint could be affected with no particular predilection for any area.

---

**Box 11.3 ○ *History red flags***

---

▸ Constant, progressive, non-mechanical pain.

▸ Systemic steroid usage.

▸ Systemically unwell – fever, sweats, malaise, temperature, weight loss.

▸ Trauma.

---

On examination Mr Smith may or may not have a fever. The joint would be hot, swollen and tender with reduced passive movements. Prosthetic joints and joints already damaged by chronic arthritis are at increased risk.

No investigations would need to be performed in primary care. If there is any suspicion of possible joint sepsis Mr Smith should be urgently referred to secondary care for joint aspiration. DO NOT wait for blood tests. DO NOT aspirate – refer and allow secondary care to investigate. If the affected joint was prosthetic Mr Smith should be referred to orthopaedics. If not, referral to either rheumatology or orthopaedics may be appropriate and may vary from region to region.

Septic arthritis may easily be confused with gouty arthritis as patients with gout can have a fever. It is also important to remember that an infected bursitis at the elbow and knee may also be confused with joint sepsis. If there is any doubt the patient should be referred.

*If, when planning to inject a joint, a cloudy looking aspirate is obtained, the patient and the aspirate should be sent to hospital and the joint not injected.*[2]

### Gout

Gout is a common cause of an acute hot joint in primary care and is exquisitely painful. It is the most common cause of an inflammatory arthritis in men aged over 40.

Gout typically presents as a severely painful, swollen, inflamed and erythematous joint with symptoms developing quite quickly over a few hours. It classically affects the 1st metatarsophalangeal (MTP) joint, where it is known as podagra. About 90% of cases of gout affect the 1st MTP joint and it is the first joint affected in 70% of patients. In a patient with no prior history of gout and an affected joint, other than the 1st MTP joint, sepsis must first be ruled out as a possible cause.

If Mr Smith were to present with gout, it is likely that the 1st MTP joint would be affected. The pain in the joint would be constant and exacerbated by any pressure. Patients may often attend the surgery wearing footwear that puts no pressure on the joint, e.g. slippers or flip-flops. Both active and passive movements of the joint are painful, and the pain does not vary throughout the day. Mr Smith may or may not have an associated temperature.

---

Box 11.4 ○ **Other important factors to consider**

▸ **Sex** ▷ gout is commoner in males and is unusual in pre-menopausal females.

▸ **PMH** ▷ is more likely in patients with renal impairment, hypertension, obesity, increased cell turnover (e.g. psoriasis), chemotherapy, haemopoetic malignancies.

▸ **DH** ▷ diuretics, i.e. the thiazide diuretics and furosemide (losartan and fenofibrate are uricosuric and so can reduce the risk of gout).

▸ **SH** ▷ diet, alcohol intake.

▸ **FH** ▷ gout, psoriasis.

---

If the history is classical of podagra then it is possible to diagnose gout confidently without any further investigations. If other joints are involved then it may be essential to rule out septic arthritis. The presence of gouty tophi would make the diagnosis of gout more likely, but a high level of suspicion for septic arthritis should remain. In order for septic arthritis to be ruled out, joint aspiration should be performed with the aspirate being examined under the microscope to check for organisms/crystals. Uric acid crystals are negatively birefringent when examined under polarised light. Serum urate may or may not be raised during an acute attack and should not be used to rule in/rule out a diagnosis.

Gout is associated with the metabolic syndrome (a term used to describe patients with glucose intolerance, hypertension, central obesity and dyslipidaemia) and so opportunistic checking of cardiovascular risk factors including body mass index, hypertension, smoking status, glucose and lipid levels is worthwhile.

### INITIAL MANAGEMENT OF GOUT

If you believe that Mr Smith has gout, it is worth educating him with regards to possible causes, e.g. meat, shellfish, beer and spirits, all of which are high in purines, precursors of uric acid. Advising Mr Smith to ice the affected joint can help ease his pain. There are then three options for managing the acute attack:

▷ **colchicine** ▶ this drug is very effective in treating acute gout[3]

▷ **non-steroidal anti-inflammatory drugs (NSAIDs)** ▶ traditionally indometacin has been used but other NSAIDs are equally as effective

▷ **steroids** ▶ can be used orally, intramuscularly or intra-articularly, but should only be prescribed if there is certainty that sepsis is not present. Intra-articular injections are probably used most commonly, but in patients used to taking oral steroids or already on a low dose this may be a useful option.

Initiation of allopurinol is contraindicated during an acute attack. If Mr Smith were known to have gout and were already taking allopurinol regularly, he should continue on his current treatment.

### Inflammatory arthritis

Inflammatory joint disease is an important cause of a monoarthropathy.

---

Box 11.5 ○ *Characteristics of inflammatory arthritis*

---

▶ Morning stiffness (significant if >one hour) and stiffness after rest.

▶ Pain and stiffness better with activity.

▶ Symptoms worse in the morning and improve during the day (diurnal variation).

▶ Joint symptoms improve with anti-inflammatory drugs.

▶ Constitutional symptoms: fatigue, malaise, loss of appetite, low-grade fever.

---

It would be worth enquiring as to whether or not Mr Smith has had any previous similar episodes. Has he had a recent infection? And is there any relevant family history of inflammatory joint disease of any type? Examples include psoriasis and ulcerative colitis/Crohn's disease.

On examination, the affected joint is swollen and warm. The overlying skin should not be significantly inflamed unlike a joint affected by sepsis or gout.

As Mr Smith has presented with a monoarthropathy, if he has inflammatory joint disease the most likely cause is one of the spondyloarthritides. Rheumatoid arthritis would be a possible diagnosis although it more commonly affects multiple joints in a symmetrical pattern. It will be covered later in the chapter.

### The spondyloarthritides

This is a group of inflammatory arthritides that share a number of features:

▷ there is no association with any known auto-antibodies, in particular rheumatoid factor. There is an association with the HLA-B27 genotype
▷ they can all cause a monoarthritis
▷ there is a tendency to affect the sacro-iliac joint
▷ anterior uveitis can commonly occur.

Included in this group of conditions are: psoriatic arthritis, reactive arthritis (including Reiter's syndrome) and enteropathic arthritis. These conditions affect 1–2% of the population, which is roughly the same as those affected by rheumatoid arthritis.

#### REACTIVE ARTHRITIS

Reactive arthritis is an inflammatory arthritis triggered by a distant infection. It commonly affects a single joint although, rarely, multiple joints can be affected. Other symptoms may occur concurrently and these include: conjunctivitis, uveitis, keratoderma blenorrhagica (a pustular psoriasis affecting the palms of the hands and the soles of the feet) and balanitis circinata. Reiter's syndrome was a term used to describe the triad of arthritis, conjunctivitis and non-specific urethritis, although its diagnostic title (Reiter's syndrome) is falling out of current usage.

The joint symptoms typically occur between one to three weeks after the precipitating infection. The infection, though, may be relatively asymptomatic and so be forgotten by the patient. Common associated infections include diarrhoea, urethritis, prostatitis or cervicitis and the organisms involved include *Campylobacter, Clostridium, Salmonella, Shigella, Yersinia* or *Chlamydia*. The onset of the joint symptoms may be acute and there is often an associated fever and weight loss.

Investigations should be performed in order to establish the source of the infection, i.e. stool and urine cultures, urethral and vaginal swabs. The joint may be aspirated with the aspirate sent for microscopy, culture and sensitivity, although this is not essential. Blood tests including ESR and CRP may be performed. Checking to see if the patient is HLA-B27 positive is not of any benefit.

Symptoms in the majority of patients will resolve. Anti-inflammatories, especially non-steroidal anti-inflammatory agents, are the main treatment of choice. Analgesics may also be used to help treat the symptoms. It is also worthwhile treating any remaining infection if found. If patients have an associated uveitis they should be referred to an ophthalmologist. Occasionally, some patients develop recurrent episodes and these may go on to develop a chronic inflammatory joint disease. Any patients with recurring symptoms should be referred to a rheumatology service as disease-modifying antirheumatic drugs (DMARDs) may be used.

### The other spondyloarthropathies

These include psoriatic arthritis, ankylosing spondylitis and enteropathic arthritis. Each of these conditions can cause a monoarthritis or oligoarthritis.

Ankylosing spondylitis more commonly presents as inflammatory back pain but a peripheral arthritis may also occur with the lower limbs particularly being affected. Treatment of ankylosing spondylitis is generally with NSAIDs but, when peripheral joints are also affected, DMARDs may be added (see Chapter 13). It would be unusual for a patient with ankylosing spondylitis to present with a monoarthropathy but it is worth remembering that it can be easily missed as a cause of back pain.

Psoriatic arthritis occurs in 5–10% of patients with psoriasis. It is therefore worth checking both the skin and, in particular, the nails (nail changes are usually present in 85–90%) in patients presenting with inflammatory joint symptoms. Psoriatic arthritis commonly affects multiple joints and in particular the small joints of the hands, but it can be the cause of a single hot, swollen joint. Initial treatment in mild cases is NSAIDs but all suspected cases should be referred.

Enteropathic arthritis occurs in patients with ulcerative colitis and Crohn's disease. It usually affects the knees and ankles as a monoarthritis, and its presence reflects disease activity in the bowel. Patients should be treated with NSAIDs or steroids and should be referred to a rheumatologist.

Investigations may be performed in primary care when these conditions are suspected, but referral should not be delayed until the results are available. Blood tests including FBC, U&Es, LFTs, ESR and CRP may be requested, along with an X-ray of the affected joint(s). In many areas, rheumatology services have developed 'Early Arthritis Clinics' where patients are seen and assessed quickly, and these investigations can also be performed there.

For more information on the spondyloarthritides, see Chapter 13.

### Osteoarthritis

An acute exacerbation of osteoarthritis may present with an acute arthropathy. This may be caused by calcium pyrophosphate disease, which is also known as pseudogout. If Mr Smith were to present with an acute exacerbation, it would be expected that he would give a history of having had mechanical pain due to joint degeneration in the affected joint prior to this episode.

---

Box 11.6 ○ *Characteristics of mechanical joint pain*

▶ Pain on exertion that is relieved by rest (rest pain occurs late in the disease).

▶ Pain worst in the evenings.

▶ Morning stiffness and stiffness after sitting lasting <30 minutes.

▶ Systemically well.

▶ Disability depending on the joint affected.

---

During an acute exacerbation patients may develop a history characteristic of inflammatory joint pain, particularly if the affected joint has an effusion.

Risk factors for osteoarthritis include obesity, a history of significant trauma to the affected joint, occupation/sport and a positive family history. These should be enquired about in the history.

Common joints involved are:

▷ distal interphalangeal (DIP) joints (Heberden's nodes)
▷ proximal interphalangeal (PIP) joints (Bouchard's nodes)
▷ base of the thumb (1st carpometacarpal joint)
▷ hips
▷ knees
▷ lumbar/cervical spine.

On examination the affected joint may be warm and swollen with evidence of an effusion. The overlying skin should not be significantly inflamed. Crepitus may be felt on movement.

### INVESTIGATIONS

No investigations are usually required for an acute exacerbation of osteoarthritis. If there is significant diagnostic uncertainty over the cause, blood tests, including ESR and CRP, may be performed and referral to a rheumatologist considered. X-rays are generally only required if red flags are present, or if consideration is being made to referring the patient to secondary care.

### MANAGEMENT

Non-steroidal anti-inflammatory agents may be of benefit during an acute attack. Caution should be exercised if considering using them long term as they are known to affect both cardiac and renal function. They may also affect a patient's blood pressure and cause occult GI blood loss. If they are used on a regular basis the patient's blood pressure, renal function and FBC should be checked annually.

Intra-articular steroid injections may also be of benefit during an acute exacerbation of osteoarthritis.

For chronic management of osteoarthritis, see Chapter 8.

## TRAUMA

Trauma may cause an acutely inflamed joint. There is usually a good history of an injury and the swelling developing shortly afterwards. Examples include joint sprains and cruciate ligament or meniscal injuries of the knee. For a further discussion regarding the management of musculoskeletal trauma, see Chapter 18.

## HAEMOPHILIA

This is an uncommon inherited coagulation disorder causing spontaneous bleeding. Haemarthroses may occur and may present as an acute monoarthropathy. In someone Mr Smith's age a diagnosis of haemophilia should have already been made and a plan in place for how he should be treated.

---

Box 11.7 ○ *Case study 2*

As already mentioned, Mrs Jones is a 42-year-old housewife and mother of three children. She does not have any significant past medical history and has only really attended the surgery for contraception, antenatal care and cervical screening. Mrs Jones presents with multiple painful joints of recent onset, i.e. she has an acute polyarthropathy. Her hands are particularly affected.

---

Possible causes of a polyarthropathy are:

▷ rheumatoid arthritis
▷ osteoarthritis
▷ hypermobility
▷ psoriatic arthritis and the other spondyloarthritides
▷ connective tissue diseases
▷ vitamin D deficiency
▷ viral polyarthritis
▷ rarely gout.

Other more unusual causes include: iatrogenic, malignancy and sarcoidosis.

What further questions could help decide the diagnosis? Which joints are affected?

▷ Are there aggravating/relieving factors?
▷ Is there diurnal variation?
▷ Is there morning stiffness?
▷ Is there a history of trauma?
▷ Has Mrs Jones been unwell recently in any other way?
▷ Does she have any other symptoms suggestive of a multisystem disease, e.g. rash or pulmonary symptoms?

### Rheumatoid arthritis

Rheumatoid arthritis is a disease that should not be missed in this situation as delay in referral, and delay in appropriate treatment, can lead to joint damage.[1] Prior to the use of MRI and ultrasound in assessing these patients, it was believed that only around 20% of patients had joint damage at the time of their initial rheumatology appointment. With more sophisticated techniques it has been found that 80% of patients who have normal radiographs on presentation can have MRI evidence of joint damage.[1]

What features could help make the diagnosis of rheumatoid arthritis in Mrs Jones?

The pattern of joints affected can assist in making a diagnosis. Rheumatoid arthritis commonly causes a symmetrical polyarthropathy that tends to affect the small joints of the hands and feet. The metacarpophalangeal, proximal interphalangeal and wrist joints, in particular, tend to be involved (see Figure 11.1 overleaf).

The history should have the features of inflammatory pain, as shown in Box 11.8.

---

Box 11.8 ○ *Characteristics of inflammatory arthritis*

---

▶ Morning stiffness (significant if >one hour) and stiffness after rest.

▶ Pain and stiffness better with activity.

▶ Symptoms worse in the morning and improve during the day (diurnal variation).

▶ Joint symptoms improve with anti-inflammatory drugs.

▶ Constitutional symptoms: fatigue, malaise, loss of appetite, low-grade fever.

Figure 11.1 ○ *Joints affected in rheumatoid arthritis*

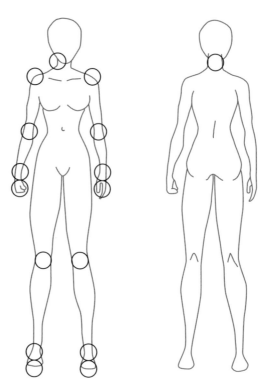

The constitutional symptoms are often forgotten when taking a history, but they are incredibly important and, if present, can help make the diagnosis. Patients with rheumatoid arthritis feel unwell when their joint disease is active. They may describe that they feel as if they have influenza. These patients, when asked, will also often describe problems with loss of function due to the joint problems. For example, they may struggle with simple things like taking lids off jars, chopping vegetables, doing up buttons, etc.

It is also worthwhile enquiring about any relevant family history. Rheumatoid arthritis is an autoimmune condition and what triggers its development is unknown. There is a known association with other autoimmune diseases, so it may be helpful to ask about any family history of hypothyroidism, Type 1 diabetes mellitus and pernicious anaemia.

Examination should reveal swollen, warm and tender joints with evidence of synovitis (a boggy feeling to the swelling). As there can be variation in the symptoms throughout the day, there can also be variation in the signs. Sometimes the signs may have settled significantly by the late afternoon, so it can be worth bringing the patient back to an early appointment in the morning where synovitis may be more obvious.

Recently the National Institute for Health and Clinical Excellence (NICE) published a guideline on the early management of rheumatoid arthritis in adults.[4] It highlights the impact that rheumatoid arthritis has on an individual and how early referral is important.

---

**Box 11.9 ○ *NICE guidance on rheumatoid arthritis in adults*[4]**

Refer for specialist opinion any person with suspected persistent synovitis of undetermined cause. Refer urgently if any of the following apply:

▶ The small joints of the hands or feet are affected

▶ More than one joint is affected

▶ There has been a delay of three months or longer between onset of symptoms and seeking medical advice.

Do not avoid referring urgently any person with suspected persistent synovitis of undetermined cause whose blood tests show a normal acute-phase response or negative rheumatoid factor.

---

As already discussed in the section on spondyloarthritides, it is not necessary to perform any investigations in primary care and referral should not be delayed until the results of investigations are available. Blood tests may be performed whilst awaiting review, including FBC, U&Es, LFTs, ESR, CRP and rheumatoid factor. A negative rheumatoid factor does not rule out a diagnosis of rheumatoid arthritis. More recently, anti-CCP antibodies have been discovered. These are more sensitive and specific than rheumatoid factor and, *if present, can signify the presence of more erosive disease. At present these are generally being performed in secondary care but in the future they may start to be used in primary care so X-rays of the affected joints may also be requested.*

As mentioned before, many areas have Early Arthritis Clinics, where patients with suspected inflammatory arthritis are seen as quickly as possible to enable early treatment with disease-modifying agents. Whilst awaiting review, the joint pain and synovitis may be treated with NSAIDs or steroids. Generally, non-steroidals are used first line but, at times, it may be appropriate to use either oral or intramuscular steroids.

### Osteoarthritis

Osteoarthritis may cause a monoarticular or a polyarticular arthropathy. When many joints are affected, the pattern of joint involvement is different from that of rheumatoid arthritis, with larger joints such as the hips and knees likely to be involved. In the hands the distal interphalangeal joints and the carpometacarpal joints of the thumb tend to be affected. Although, in some patients, the metacarpophalangeal joints can be inflamed, making it difficult to differentiate from rheumatoid arthritis. If there is uncertainty the patients should be referred for a specialist opinion.

Mrs Jones is rather young to be presenting with osteoarthritis of the hands but, if it were to be the cause of her joint problems, she would be expected to have a history of mechanical joint pain.

---

**Box 11.10 ○ *Characteristics of mechanical joint pain***

▶ Pain on exertion that is relieved by rest (rest pain occurs late in the disease).

▶ Pain worst in the evenings.

▶ Morning stiffness and stiffness after sitting lasting <30 minutes.

▶ Systemically well.

▶ Disability depending on the joint affected.

---

Women can often present with a polyarthropathy during the perimenopause, which may be related to underlying osteoarthritis. This responds well to hormone replacement therapy, although other treatments should be considered first.

No investigations are required if the diagnosis is not in doubt. If there are any concerns, X-rays of the affected joints may be arranged.

Management of a polyarthropathy due to osteoarthritis involves using analgesics, supports and braces, and appropriate footwear. For further discussion regarding the management of osteoarthritis, see Chapter 8.

### Hypermobility

Hypermobility is an excessive range of movement of a joint or joints, which may be due to variations in the joint surface or lax ligaments (see Chapter 15). Patients may present with pain in a single joint but patients with the hypermobility syndrome can present with polyarthralgia. Hypermobility is commonly overlooked as a diagnosis and these patients appear to be at increased risk of developing fibromyalgia.[5] It is therefore important that, as GPs, we recognise this condition and treat it appropriately to prevent complications from occurring.

If Mrs Jones's joint pains were due to hypermobility it would be expected that any joint could be affected. There should be no significant history of stiffness and in particular morning stiffness, and Mrs Jones should feel well in herself. Hypermobility-associated joint pain can vary throughout the menstrual cycle and with changes in weather. A history of being supple when a teenager, having knee problems as a child, having growing pains and being clumsy as a child can help establish a diagnosis.

A screening tool for hypermobility is the nine-point Beighton Score, which can easily be performed in primary care.[5] It is important to appreciate that this may overlook some affected joints and it gives no indication as to the degree of hypermobility.

Table 11.1 ○ *Brighton revised diagnostic criteria for benign joint hypermobility syndrome, 1998*

| The ability to: | Right | Left |
| --- | --- | --- |
| **1** Passively dorsiflex the fifth metacarpophalangeal joint to >90° | 1 | 1 |
| **2** Passively appose the thumb to the volar aspect of the forearm | 1 | 1 |
| **3** Passively hyperextend the elbow to >10° | 1 | 1 |
| **4** Passively hyperextend the knee to >10° | 1 | 1 |
| **5** Actively place hands flat on the floor without bending the knees | 1 | |
| | | |
| Total | 9 | |
| | | |

*Source*: Grahame R, Bird HA, Child A. The revised (Brighton 1998) criteria for the diagnosis of benign joint hypermobility syndrome (BJHS).[11]

The hypermobility syndrome is diagnosed using the Brighton criteria, which includes having a Beighton score of 4/9 or greater.[5] No investigations are required.

## TREATMENT

Simple analgesics such as paracetamol with or without codeine can be helpful. Amitriptyline at a low dose (5–10 mg nocte) can be beneficial in cases of chronic pain. For further management, see Chapter 15.

### Connective tissue disorders

These are very rare in primary care but most GPs will have a couple of patients affected and will probably see one or two new presentations during their career. The connective tissue disorders are an overlapping group of diseases, each of which affects more than one organ, although the musculoskeletal system is most commonly involved. They include systemic lupus erythematosus, systemic sclerosis, the **CREST** syndrome (**C**alcinosis, **R**aynaud's, **Oe**sophageal dysmotility, **S**clerodactyly and **T**elangiectasia), Sjögren's syndrome, polymyositis and dermatomyositis. Joint pain is the presenting complaint in 50% of cases.

If Mrs Jones were presenting with a connective tissue disorder she would complain of stiffness, pain and swelling in the affected joints. The arthritis/arthralgia is typically symmetrical and may be flitting, intermittent or persistent. The metacarpophalangeal joints and proximal interphalangeal joints are commonly affected, although the wrists, knees, ankles, elbows and shoulders may also be involved. The symptoms are usually worse in the morning. Connective tissue disorders are multisystem diseases and so it is worth performing a systemic review when considering this diagnosis. In particular, it is worth enquiring about rashes, the presence of Raynaud's syndrome and general constitutional symptoms such as fatigue, weight loss and fever.

Examination of the joints may be relatively unrewarding, with little evidence of synovitis.

It is worth performing investigations in these patients. These should include an FBC, ESR, CRP (which is generally normal in patients with lupus, but if raised should trigger investigations to rule out an intercurrent infection), LFTs, U&Es and a urine dipstick. Other tests could include auto-antibody testing, in particular checking for: rheumatoid factor, antinuclear antibodies, extractable nuclear antigens, anti-DNA antibodies and complement levels.[6]

## MANAGEMENT

Once a diagnosis of a connective tissue disorder is considered, these patients should be referred for a definitive diagnosis to be made. Simple analgesics and non-steroidals can be used to ease the arthralgia/arthritis in the mean time. For further management, see Chapter 14.

### Fibromyalgia

Fibromyalgia is a difficult condition to both diagnose and treat. Any delay in diagnosis is very distressing for patients, and GPs have an important role in supporting them throughout this time.

Fibromyalgia is a chronic condition comprising symptoms of generalised pain, sleep and mood disturbances, significant fatigue, paraesthesia, poor concentration, headaches, abdominal pain and bowel and urinary symptoms. The prevalence of the condition is around 2% and there is an overlap with chronic fatigue syndrome and ME. Fibromyalgia may be precipitated by a traumatic event, including both physical and psychological trauma. It is more likely to occur in patients with inflammatory joint disease or hyper-mobility. Patients are often female and symptoms develop between the ages of 30 and 50.

Mrs Jones has presented with multiple painful joints but it is worth clarify-ing with her exactly where she feels the pain. If the pain is generalised and the muscles also affected then fibromyalgia is a possibility.

On examination there would be no obvious signs of joint disease. The classic tender points for fibromyalgia should be examined (see Chapter 10).

Fibromyalgia is often made as a diagnosis of exclusion. Other causes for the symptoms should be investigated, including: hypothyroidism, connective tissue disorders, hyperparathyroidism, vitamin D deficiency (osteomalacia), myeloma and polymyalgia rheumatica. The patient must have ≥11/18 classic tender points present.

It is possible to diagnose patients in primary care, although these patients are often referred and diagnosed in secondary care. They may have multiple investigations by different specialties prior to a formal diagnosis being made and this can be very distressing for the patient.

The initial management of fibromyalgia involves educating the patient about his or her diagnosis. The patient needs to be aware that this is a chronic condition and that it is often impossible to 'cure' his or her symptoms. Low-dose amitriptyline, i.e. 10 mg nocte, can be useful as a first line. For further management, see Chapter 10.

### Vitamin D deficiency

Vitamin D deficiency has traditionally been known as a cause of osteomala-cia in adults and rickets in children. The symptoms of osteomalacia are pain and proximal muscle weakness. More recently it is becoming increasingly clear that vitamin D deficiency is more widespread in the UK than was origi-nally thought and that the pain can be more diffuse.[7] Vitamin D deficiency is also felt to be related to cardiovascular disease, Type 2 diabetes mellitus and the development of some cancers.[7] Serum vitamin D levels can easily be checked and vitamin D supplements exist. For further details, see Chapter 9.

### Gout

Gout can affect multiple joints, with anywhere between 3–14% of attacks presenting as a polyarthritis. When this occurs, small joints, such as the dis-tal interphalangeal joints, tend to be affected. Patients are more likely to be female and taking diuretics.

### Analysis of case study 1 with respect to the six domains of Being a GP

#### DOMAIN 1: PRIMARY CARE MANAGEMENT

▷ To recognise the symptoms of the different causes of a monoarthropathy.
▷ To recognise potential emergencies so that patients can be referred appropriately.
▷ To recognise the symptoms and signs of inflammatory joint disease to enable early referral.

#### DOMAIN 2: PERSON-CENTRED CARE

▷ To understand the impact of the specific conditions on the patient and to treat the initial presentation appropriately for that person.

#### DOMAIN 3: SPECIFIC PROBLEM-SOLVING SKILLS

▷ To have the diagnostic skills necessary to enable a differential diagnosis to be made.

#### DOMAIN 4: A COMPREHENSIVE APPROACH

▷ To be aware of the red flags in presentations with joint disease.

#### DOMAIN 5: COMMUNITY ORIENTATION

▷ To recognise potential emergencies and how to access urgent treatment in your locality.
▷ To be aware of what services are available locally and what is the best pathway for referral.

#### DOMAIN 6: A HOLISTIC APPROACH

▷ To understand the impact that musculoskeletal disorders can have on the individual and his or her life. To educate the patient about his or her condition in order to facilitate the patient's management.

## Analysis of case study 2 with respect to the six domains of Being a GP

### DOMAIN 1: PRIMARY CARE MANAGEMENT

▷ To recognise the symptoms of the different causes of a polyarthropathy.
▷ To recognise the symptoms and signs of inflammatory joint disease, in particular rheumatoid arthritis, to enable early referral.

### DOMAIN 2: PERSON-CENTRED CARE

▷ To understand the impact of the specific conditions on the patient and to treat the initial presentation appropriately for that person.

### DOMAIN 3: SPECIFIC PROBLEM-SOLVING SKILLS

▷ To have the diagnostic skills necessary to enable a differential diagnosis to be made.

### DOMAIN 4: A COMPREHENSIVE APPROACH

▷ To be aware of the red flags in presentations with joint disease.

### DOMAIN 5: COMMUNITY ORIENTATION

▷ To recognise potential emergencies and how to access urgent treatment in your locality.
▷ To be aware of what services are available locally and what is the best pathway for referral.

### DOMAIN 6: A HOLISTIC APPROACH

▷ To understand the impact that musculoskeletal disorders can have on the individual and his or her life. To search for educational resources that will enhance your ability to act as the advocate of your patient's care.

**References**

1 • Emery P. Treatment of rheumatoid arthritis *British Medical Journal* 2006; **332(7534)**: 152–5.

2 • Coakley G, Mathews C, Field M, *et al.,* on behalf of the British Society for Rheumatology Standards, Guidelines and Audit Working Group. BSR & BHPR, BOA, RCGP and BSAC guidelines for the management of the hot swollen joint in adults *Rheumatology* 2006; **45(8)**: 1039–41.

3 • Zhang W, Doherty M, Bardin T, *et al.* EULAR evidence based recommendations for gout. Part II: Management. Report of a task force of the EULAR Standing Committee for International Clinical Studies Including Therapeutics (ESCISIT) *Annals of the Rheumatic Diseases* 2006; **65(10)**: 1312–24.

4 • National Institute for Health and Clinical Excellence. *Clinical Guideline 79, Rheumatoid Arthritis: national clinical guideline for management and treatment in adults* London: Royal College of Physicians, 2009, www.nice.org.uk/CG79 [accessed October 2011].

5 • Keer R, Grahame R. *Hypermobility Syndrome: recognition and management for physiotherapists* London: Butterworth-Heinemann, 2007.

6 • Lupus UK. *Lupus: a GP guide to diagnosis* Romford, Essex: Lupus UK, 2000.

7 • Pearce S H, Cheetham T D. Diagnosis and management of vitamin D deficiency *British Medical Journal* 2010: **340**; b5664.

# Rheumatoid arthritis

## Ongoing management

# 12

*Peter Lanyon*

### Introduction

The management of rheumatoid arthritis (RA) has recently undergone a period of unprecedented transition. In the past, the diagnosis was often delayed, and treatment was empirical and frequently ineffective at preventing the development and progression of disability. The magnitude of the disabling effects is highlighted by the employment outcomes in a recent study of affected individuals, 40% of whom will have health-related work loss within three to five years of diagnosis.[1] In addition to pain and disability, people with RA can have overwhelming fatigue as a result of systemic inflammation, altered physical functioning and low mood.

We now have a much greater understanding of risk factors for this disease, better ways to assess disease activity, and, for the first time, targeted biological therapies that have a real prospect of inducing disease remission. This knowledge has also advanced our awareness of the co-morbidities associated with rheumatoid disease, particularly cardiovascular and infection risks, and the impact of the illness on individuals and their families.

It can be difficult for people in the early stages of a chronic disease to negotiate the health care that they need and to make informed choices about their healthcare provider. Many are unaware of the services and treatment that they are entitled to receive. This can leave them vulnerable to poorly controlled symptoms that significantly reduce quality of life and threaten their employment status. Although there is National Institute for Health and Clinical Excellence (NICE) guidance for RA management[2] and Arthritis and Musculoskeletal Alliance (ARMA) Standards of Care,[3] these are not yet universally implemented, and recent studies have highlighted that access to 'best care' for people with RA is extremely variable.[4]

This places the management of RA not only as a prime model for inflammatory disease, but also for the general management of chronic disease in primary care. The new potential of earlier detection and intervention, enhanced management, improved patient self-efficacy, and earlier management of co-morbidities and disease flares, places the GP in a key position to influence the outcome.

## Aims

At the end of this chapter you will be able to:

1 ▷ Recognise the clinical expression of RA, when to refer, and the key components of assessing disease activity
2 ▷ Understand the principles of pharmacological management and monitoring, and as a Directed Enhanced Service (DES) for disease-modifying antirheumatic drugs (DMARDs) in general practice
3 ▷ Appreciate the role of the multidisciplinary team (MDT) – and also accessing secondary care and the nurse specialist
4 ▷ Detect the co-morbidities associated with RA and manage them in primary care
5 ▷ Be vigilant to the potential for ongoing joint damage and disability, even when the disease is apparently quiescent
6 ▷ Recognise potential emergencies and when to refer back urgently to secondary care
7 ▷ Find educational resources that will enhance your ability to act as the advocate of your patient's care.

## Initial management in primary care

### Risk factors for disease

RA is an autoimmune disease affecting 450,000 people in the UK, and 12,000 new cases are diagnosed annually. It affects all ages, with a peak incidence between ages 50–70, and the impact on an individual will vary according to his or her age and stage in life.

The autoimmunity is characterised by the presence of antibodies to IgG ('rheumatoid factor') and to citrullinated peptides. Citrullination is a process of post-translational modification of arginine residues, and occurs in normal health but is enhanced in the synovial cells in RA. Antibodies to citrullinated proteins are highly specific. They are detected in 60% of RA patients, but only in 1–2% of healthy people. They can be detected five to ten years before the onset of disease.

For an individual, the risk of developing RA is determined by the interaction of several genes with environmental factors and 'chance' effects. The largest genetic risk is amongst individuals who carry HLA-DR1 alleles that share in common an amino-acid motif within the antigen-binding site of the HLA groove, termed the 'shared epitope'.[5] This epitope is thought to present potential 'arthritogenic peptides' to the immune system, leading to stimulation and proliferation of T cells within the joint. These cells subsequently induce activation of macrophages, B cells, fibroblasts and osteoclasts, which leads to the clinical presentation of joint inflammation, swelling and bone erosion. A second susceptibility gene termed PTPN22, which has a role in T and B cell signalling, has recently been identified.[6]

*Cigarette smoking* is the largest environmental risk factor, and leads to increased citrullination of proteins in the lung.[7] Smokers also have a more severe disease course and an increased risk of lung and cardiovascular co-morbidities.

The GP therefore has a crucial role to support smoking cessation in newly diagnosed patients, and in their first-degree relatives, as smoking significantly interacts to increase the risk in genetically susceptible individuals.

*Hyperlipidaemia* is also a risk factor. Compared with healthy people, those who develop RA are more likely to have had an atherogenic lipid profile at least ten years prior to diagnosis. Statin therapy appears to ameliorate some of this risk, compared with hyperlipidaemia patients who did not receive a statin.[8]

**285**

### Clinical expression

The key to early identification is the detection of inflamed synovium (synovitis). This causes an increase in size and number of synovial cells, and increased production of synovial fluid. There are three cardinal features that confirm the presence of synovitis at any joint:

1 ▷ Capsular pattern of swelling (in other words, distending the capsule of the joint and recognisable from the shape this produces)
2 ▷ Joint line tenderness
3 ▷ 'Stress pain' at end-of-range movement due to increased pressure within the joint.

When the disease starts suddenly, with involvement of the hands, feet or large joints, the diagnosis is usually made rapidly. However, many people have insidious symptoms that wax and wane before becoming permanent. This is a diagnostic challenge, as laboratory tests can be normal in early disease, particularly if there is small-joint synovitis of insufficient 'bulk' to drive elevation of C-reactive protein (CRP) or erythrocyte sedimentation rate (ESR). In these situations a GP should pay much more attention to the subjective reporting of symptoms. Sometimes there is a flitting migratory episode of pain and mild erythema that lasts 24–48 hours at each joint site, termed 'palindromic' disease. This particular subgroup is strongly associated with anti-cyclic citrullinated peptide (CCP) antibodies.

### Initial primary care management

When managing a patient with suspected early RA, the GP will use his or her communication skills to take a comprehensive history. This will cover pain, fatigue and difficulties with activities of daily living (ADL), psychological aspects (e.g. altered body image) and social aspects, particularly employment (discussed in more detail later). The GP will have also undertaken a notes review to see if there have been any previous episodes.

Skills in problem solving will then help the GP to come to an accurate diagnosis and to explain the findings to the patient. A further course of action will then be discussed with the patient. This, and the GP's knowledge of local referral networks, will enable an appropriate referral to be made. At this point the doctor should offer the patient some educational material and contact details for support groups.

RA is a lifelong condition, and the GP will need to work in partnership with the patient, treating him or her with empathy and compassion, while respecting the patient's autonomy at all times. In primary care the doctor will have an essential role in providing continuity of care and acting as the patient's advocate in his or her relationship with all members of the MDT.

The first goal of treatment is symptom control, with *pain management* being the most important priority, and this may require non-steroidal anti-inflammatory drugs (NSAIDs) either alone or in combination with analgesics. The choice of NSAID will depend on the patient's other co-morbidities such as cardiovascular risk and gastrointestinal disease. All NSAIDs should be given for the shortest time possible and with a proton-pump inhibitor to protect the stomach.

Current treatment strategies are based on three key principles:

▷ **Early Intervention** ▶ early RA is both quantitatively and qualitatively different from established disease, and is more amenable to intervention at this early stage. This 'window of opportunity' is within the first three months[2]
▷ **Treat to Target** ▶ this means achieving a low disease activity state, with remission being a realistic goal of treatment
▷ **Tight Control** ▶ therapy should be escalated and modified until inflammation is controlled; this initially requires assessment and adjustment at least every month.

### Secondary care referral

Any person whom the doctor suspects has RA should be referred to a specialist rheumatology provider. Delay in referral or receiving definitive diagnosis and treatment can result in significant costs to the individual, particularly those who are employed.

The GP should discuss this course of action and, where local choice of provider exists, have knowledge of local services in order to recommend providers that demonstrate compliance with both NICE guidance and ARMA Standards of Care.

If the patient has had symptoms affecting the small joints of the hands and feet, affecting more than one joint, and there has been a delay of more than three months between onset of symptoms and seeking medical advice, this referral should be made urgently.[9]

The GP should explore the patient's concerns and beliefs about his or her condition. This is because all treatment must take into account the patient's needs, and preferences must be individually tailored to the stage of disease and degree of disease activity. At an early stage the GP should explain to the patient how to access available resources, and encourage him or her to do so. Examples of resources include the Arthritis Research Campaign (ARC), ARMA, the National Rheumatoid Arthritis Society (NRAS) and Arthritis Care.

The reason for referral is to enable access to a full MDT comprising a rheumatologist, a named clinical nurse specialist, a physiotherapist and an occupational therapist. There should also be access to podiatry, orthotics and dietetics, and to other medical teams who specialise in managing aspects of RA, such as orthopaedic surgeons.

The nurse specialist will usually co-ordinate the patient's secondary care, provide advice on drug therapies and other treatments, and monitor these treatments for efficacy and toxicity. An integral role of all MDT members is to provide education, as this is the cornerstone for promoting patient self-management and leads to improved concordance and risk management. This education should be ongoing and based on individual needs, and include telephone advice line support.

### Assessing your patient's disease activity and response to treatment

Patient-centred care can only be achieved by accurate and reproducible assessments of disease activity. The DAS (disease activity score) 28 comprises four domains assessed by examination of 28 peripheral joints:[10]

1 ▷ A physician count of the number of swollen joints
2 ▷ A physician count of the number of tender joints
3 ▷ A patient-determined general health status on a 0–100 visual analogue score (VAS)
4 ▷ A laboratory measure of inflammation, either CRP or ESR.

Using an algorithm (www.das-score.nl) disease activity can be defined as either remission (DAS <2.6), low activity (DAS <3.2) or high activity (DAS >5.1).

The VAS and the tender-joint count are subjective and patient focused, and each tender joint contributes twice as much 'weight' to the DAS as each swollen joint. So if there is concomitant fibromyalgia, a common accompaniment to RA, the DAS will tend to be higher due to a higher VAS and more widespread tenderness. However, the DAS can appear artificially low if there is predominately foot and ankle disease, as these sites are not included in the 28 joint count, or if there is isolated small-joint synovitis that does not cause elevation of CRP or ESR. However, despite these caveats it is a rapid and reproducible tool that is used to tailor the treatment for an individual patient.

The DAS score can also be used to demonstrate and assign a numerical value to clinical improvement for each patient, and can also therefore indicate how well each rheumatology unit is adhering to NICE guidance.

### Predicting the long-term outcome for your patient

Because RA is a lifelong disease, caution and vigilance in assessing response to treatment is needed in all patients. Individual outcome is difficult to predict, but these features at disease onset associate with a poorer prognosis:

1 ▷ Antibody positivity – either rheumatoid factor or anti-CCP antibodies, with the presence of both associated with the worst prognosis
2 ▷ The number of swollen joints – the more joints affected at baseline the worse the prognosis
3 ▷ The degree of baseline functional disability
4 ▷ Older age
5 ▷ Lower educational status
6 ▷ Female gender – women have a worse prognosis than men.

Although there is no current evidence that poor-prognosis patients should be treated differently, these are the patients who require the greatest vigilance.

The long-term prognosis is paralleled by a decline in radiographic status with the development of new erosions.

However, the degree of joint inflammation that is detected by clinicians has historically been described as 'waxing and waning', with a decline in inflammation in the later stages of disease. We now know that this is incorrect; recent studies demonstrate that, even within joints that clinicians consider to be 'inactive', there can be ultrasound or magnetic resonance imaging (MRI) evidence of ongoing synovial proliferation and erosion.

## Management at the primary/secondary care interface

### *Communication*

In an ideal world, there should be seamless communication between the primary and secondary care teams. This can be facilitated by:

▷ empowering patients as an integral part of the team by promoting self-care and management, and helping them to become knowledgeable about their condition and treatment
▷ rapid written correspondence, copied to patients, following consultations
▷ encouraging patients to carry copy letters and monitoring booklets (patient-held documentation)
▷ clear shared-care protocols for transfer of prescribing between secondary and primary care
▷ ensuring rapid access to urgent GP appointments
▷ provision of GP and patient access to a Secondary Care Helpline with rapid access to specialist nurse or consultant when required
▷ joint community/hospital education programmes to educate, promote networking and aid service planning and provision
▷ provision of clear guidance as to what to do in the event of problems.

### *Disease-modifying drugs and steroids*

After pain control, the most important strategy is to start DMARDs as soon as possible; any delay will affect symptom control, quality of life, and functional ability up to five years after diagnosis. This 'window of opportunity', i.e. the time from symptom onset to initiation of a DMARD, should be less than three months.[2] Early initiation is also associated with fewer drug side effects and drug withdrawals.

Initiating two DMARDs simultaneously is superior to sequential monotherapy, both in terms of initial symptom control and ability to achieve remission, without an increase in toxicity.[7] It takes 4–12 weeks to obtain a DMARD response, and glucocorticoids are often used as an additional short-term 'bridge' to gain more rapid symptom control.

▷ All patients who start steroids should be considered for osteoporosis prophylaxis according to current guidelines (see Royal College of Physicians website for most recent guidance: www.rcplondon.ac.uk).
▷ All patients should also be given a steroid card.

Whichever DMARD is started, it is important to closely monitor the response; a DAS 28 should initially be recorded in secondary care at least monthly, and treatment optimised if the patient is not responding to his or her management plan. When a stable and effective dose of DMARD is reached, many secondary care services will seek to devolve prescribing and monitoring to primary care, termed 'shared care' (see p. 294).

The most frequently used DMARDs are described in more detail below. While other agents have been used in the past (e.g. gold, D-penicillamine, azathioprine, cyclosporin), these are rarely used in routine care due to greater toxicity and less efficacy.

All DMARDs should be used with caution or are contraindicated if there is hepatic or renal impairment. Both methotrexate and leflunomide are teratogenic and should be avoided in men and women who wish to conceive. These drugs are also 'immunosuppressive' and live vaccines should be avoided; influenza and pneumococcal vaccinations are safe and recommended.

### Methotrexate

Methotrexate is the preferred initial drug, and is the cornerstone of all treatment regimes, either as monotherapy or as part of combination therapy.[11] Compared with other DMARDs, it has greater efficacy, quicker onset of action, and fewer treatment withdrawals. Up to 80% of people who start methotrexate are still taking it five years later, which compares favourably with the retention rates for other drugs used in long-term conditions.

All patients should receive the NPSA (National Patient Safety Agency) methotrexate booklet, which contains detailed information, highlights the importance of only taking the drug *once a week*, and records the current dose and monitoring results.

*Although 2.5 mg and 10 mg tablets are available, GPs should only prescribe 2.5 mg tablets, as this results in fewer administration errors than mixed-strength tablets.*

The usual starting dose is 10–15 mg once weekly, with escalation to 25–30 mg weekly depending on clinical response and toxicity.[11] Folic acid 5 mg is co-prescribed at least weekly to reduce the risk of marrow depression and mucosal toxicity (resulting in mouth ulcers). Elderly patients may require lower doses, particularly if there is any renal impairment, and methotrexate must not be prescribed if the GFR is below 30. If maximum oral dose is not effective or causes side effects, weekly subcutaneous administration is an effective alternative. If there is no therapeutic response to methotrexate, it is much less likely that there will be response to another DMARD. The dose of methotrexate can be increased if the patient develops mouth ulcers after advice is taken from secondary care.

FBC, U&E and LFT should be monitored every two weeks until the dose and results are stable for six weeks, then monthly until the dose and disease is stable for one year. This is often done as part of a DES or Local Enhanced Service (LES) within primary care.

Thereafter the monitoring can be reduced to 2–3 monthly, unless there is renal impairment.

Liver function abnormalities can occur, usually only with long-term use, and alcohol intake should be restricted to recommended limits.

The most *serious early side effect* is pneumonitis, which causes fever, dry cough and breathlessness. Although this is a rare complication, the doctor or nurse should suspect this if the above symptoms occur, particularly when there is no other cause such as an upper respiratory tract infection (URTI). Methotrexate should be *immediately stopped* in conjunction with secondary care advice, and if your patient is unwell or breathless should be admitted directly to hospital. The treatment is high-dose steroids, but the condition can be fatal, particularly if not detected early.

Which is the **single least appropriate** management option of a patient with RA taking methotrexate who develops mouth ulcers?

1 ▷ Discussion with relatives
2 ▷ Discussion with the rheumatology consultant
3 ▷ Increasing the dose of folic acid
4 ▷ Stop the methotrexate
5 ▷ Advise the patient to use a mouthwash

*Correct answer* ▷ **3**

### Sulfasalazine

The use of this drug as first-line monotherapy is declining, as it has greater toxicity and slower onset than methotrexate. It does have the advantage that it can be used in women who wish to conceive; in this situation folic acid should be added. It may cause reversible oligozoospermia in men. The usual dose is 500 mg once daily, increased by 500 increments each week up to 2 g per day. It is contraindicated where there is a history of allergy to sulphonamides or aspirin. Monitoring FBC, renal and liver function is required monthly for the first three months, and then three-monthly until two years, after which routine monitoring is not required.

### Leflunomide

This newer immunomodulatory drug has similar efficacy to methotrexate but a higher incidence of side effects, and so is usually used after methotrexate or sulfasalazine. The usual dose is 10–20 mg daily. The commonest side effects are marrow toxicity, GI intolerance, rash, abnormal LFTs and hypertension, and there is a *significant drug interaction with warfarin*.

The half-life of the drug is long (two to four weeks) and therefore if side effects occur the drug may need to be washed out with cholestyramine (seek specialist advice). Rare cases of severe liver injury have been reported, and the manufacturers have recently recommended and increased monitoring frequency of FBC and LFT very two weeks for six months, then, if stable, reduced to two-monthly unless co-prescribed with another immunosuppressant or potentially hepatotoxic agent.

*Blood pressure* and *weight* should be checked at each monitoring visit. Women planning to have children should either discontinue the drug two years prior to conception or have a rapid removal of its active metabolite by following the washout procedure. Men should continue to use effective contraception for three months after stopping leflunomide.

### Hydroxychloroquine

This has a lower efficacy than other DMARDs and is usually used in combination therapy, particularly with methotrexate, rather than as monotherapy. It has an extremely good safety profile, does not require routine blood monitoring and also has a mild beneficial effect on lipid profiles. Potential side effects include skin rashes/allergy, mild gastrointestinal (GI) disturbance and ocular toxicity. The latter is extremely rare and no routine ophthalmologic monitoring is required unless therapy continues for at least five years. If patients develop any changes in visual acuity or develop blurred vision, treatment should be stopped pending ophthalmology review.

### Biological therapies

A major breakthrough in understanding the pathogenesis of RA was the identification of the pivotal role in inflammation of tumour necrosis factor-alpha (TNF). This is the key cytokine responsible for the articular consequences of RA (joint pain, cartilage loss, bone erosion). TNF also mediates release of inflammatory markers by the liver and the systemic disease manifestations of fatigue, weight loss and mood disturbance. These pivotal effects were confirmed when clinical trials of anti-TNF agents resulted in a rapid, profound and sustained clinical improvement and halted bone erosion. Five agents are currently approved for clinical use:

▷ etanercept (a soluble TNF receptor)
▷ adalimumab (a humanised anti-TNF antibody)
▷ infliximab (a chimeric anti-TNF antibody)
▷ certolizumab (a humanised anti-TNF antibody)
▷ golimumab (a human anti-TNF antibody).

In a recent trial in early RA, at the end of one year 50% of patients receiving a combination of etanercept and methotrexate achieved clinical remission, compared with 28% of patients receiving methotrexate alone. A significant difference between the two treatments appeared by the second week.[12] The probability of stopping work was also significantly lower amongst those taking etanercept and methotrexate (8.6%) compared with methotrexate alone (24%).

However, anti-TNF therapy costs £9000 per year, and in a healthcare system with finite resources there has to be a balance between the needs of an individual patient and the needs of the community as a whole. NICE has issued guidance on the use of these agents, and they are currently approved for use only when the disease remains highly active (DAS > 5.1) despite an adequate trial for at least six months of at least two DMARDs, one of which should have been methotrexate. Despite NICE approval, there is still wide geographical variation in the ability of patients to access anti-TNF therapy, and it is during this period of continued active disease whilst awaiting treatment that the risk of job loss is greatest. If no response to anti-TNF therapy occurs within six months (indicated by a failure to improve the DAS by at least 1.2), treatment is discontinued and either another anti-TNF or rituximab initiated.

Neutralisation of TNF has potential disadvantages to the immune system, and the long-term outcome of therapy (> 10 years) is unknown. To address safety concerns, there is a national registry of those who have received treatment. It is not yet known whether there is a significantly increased long-term risk of malignancy, over and above the known lymphoma risks that occur with longstanding rheumatoid disease.

Anti-TNF therapy will accelerate current tuberculosis (TB), and reactivate latent TB and viral hepatitis, and all patients should have been screened for these conditions prior to treatment.

*There is a small but significant risk of serious infections (requiring IV antibiotics or hospitalisation), particularly in the first six months of treatment. Specialist advice should be sought when any patient taking anti-TNF therapy develops an unusual or severe infection, and you should consider prompt use of antibiotics, particularly in out-of-hours situations and stopping treatment until the infection has cleared.*

Because the drug is prescribed in secondary care, there may be no record in the primary care prescribing notes, as there are no Read codes for DMARD or anti-TNF therapy. Until this coding issue has been resolved, each GP practice will need to decide how to code this important information.

The risk of cardiovascular disease is also reduced amongst patients who respond to anti-TNF therapy.

### Other biological drugs

The success of anti-TNF has led to the development of other drugs that target different aspects of the immune response. Rituximab is an intravenous monoclonal antibody that binds to the surface of B lymphocytes, resulting in their depletion from the peripheral circulation for at least six months. It has similar efficacy to anti-TNF therapy, and is currently approved by NICE for use in combination with methotrexate when anti-TNF therapy fails.

Tocilizumab is an interleukin-6 receptor antibody, which has similar efficacy and has NICE approval for use when rituximab has failed.

---

### Ongoing management in primary care

### Shared care

The doctor who has clinical responsibility for a patient should undertake prescribing. Aligning the clinical and prescribing responsibilities enhances patient safety, as the prescriber is also responsible for ensuring that any necessary monitoring has been undertaken and that the results have been checked. There must be proper written handover procedures from hospital specialists to GPs, with an agreement to jointly manage a patient under a shared-care guideline; patients should never be uncertain about where to obtain supplies of their medication. Once shared care has occurred, the GP will be responsible for ensuring the continued monitoring and prescribing of the recommended drugs. Each party in the shared-care agreement has his or her own responsibilities.

### Primary care responsibilities

▷ Having sufficient knowledge of the therapeutic issues to prescribe for your patient, and in accordance with the local shared-care guideline.
▷ Ensuring dose reduction/avoidance if patients develop renal impairment.
▷ Vigilance regarding co-prescribing; in particular avoiding other antifolate drugs (e.g. trimethoprim/sulfamethoxazole with methotrexate).

▷ Ensuring adequate contraception for men and women of child-bearing age taking methotrexate or leflunomide.
▷ Ensuring those at risk receive pneumovax and annual influenza immunisation.
▷ Maintaining the patient-held record with the results of investigations and changes in dose.
▷ Stopping DMARD treatment can cause a relapse of symptoms, and you should report any adverse drug events to the secondary care team, particularly if this causes cessation of treatment.
▷ If your patient does not attend for monitoring, ensuring that you do not continue to prescribe.

### Secondary care responsibilities

Initiating DMARD and continuing prescribing until the dose and monitoring interval are stable.

▷ Ensuring that the patient is educated and provided with written information about his or her treatment (e.g. NPSA guidance and copies of clinic letters), contact telephone number and the importance of attending monitoring.
▷ Issuing to primary care GP the locally approved shared-care guidelines detailing monitoring arrangements.
▷ If dose changes in previously stable patients are made in secondary care this should be clearly communicated to the GP and patient in writing.
▷ Regular review in the out-patient clinic to assess disease activity and recommending any adjustments to treatment.
▷ Telephone support to the GP by a member of the medical team if serious adverse events occur.
▷ Additional support for patients, via the rheumatology telephone helpline.

The GP will be responsible for reviewing the results of monitoring tests and taking appropriate action on abnormal results. Usually this happens as part of a DES or LES as mentioned above.

Further information is available with the British Society for Rheumatology (BSR) guidelines for DMARD monitoring (www.rheumatology.org.uk), but the following are considered threshold levels for withholding the DMARD until discussed with the secondary care team:

▷ WBC $< 3.5 \times 109/l$
▷ neutrophils $< 2.0 \times 109/l$
▷ platelets $< 150 \times 109/l$

▷ AST, ALT > twice upper limit of reference range

▷ mild to moderate renal impairment

▷ MCV > 105 fL – check serum B12, folate and TFT, and discuss with specialist team if necessary

▷ oral ulceration, nausea and vomiting, diarrhoea

▷ unexplained acute widespread rash (refer urgently to dermatology)

▷ new or increasing dyspnoea or dry cough (discuss urgently with specialist team)

▷ severe sore throat, abnormal bruising – immediate FBC and withhold until the result of FBC is available.

### Recognising the impact of disease

A diagnosis of chronic illness can precipitate distressing emotion due to the inevitable impact on quality of life and the loss that accompanies living with disease and treatment, e.g. concerns regarding drugs and conception, being no longer able to enjoy a favourite hobby, being no longer able to work, etc. Fear, loneliness, depression, anger and anxiety are common and, if unacknowledged, can be overwhelming and disabling. All members of the MDT should be alert to the emotional consequences of RA. Tackling distress is multifaceted:

▷ good symptom control (pain relief) is essential

▷ simple strategies of listening, acknowledging the normality of distressing emotion, helping patients to recognise and develop simple coping strategies, e.g. pacing, distraction, relaxation, gentle exercise

▷ provision of practical help, e.g. helping to get financial support, child care, disabled badges for parking, devices to aid ADL, help with employment

▷ in some instances patients may require more specialist skilled help from trained counsellors or psychologists.

### Occupational issues

Work ability is significantly curtailed by RA. In a recent survey by the NRAS, two thirds of those respondents not currently employed had prematurely stopped work as a result of their disease. For those in employment, there may be a need to change occupation, reduce hours or work part time. The most significant barriers to work are pain, physical limitations (particularly commuting to work), fatigue and having to take time off work due to ill health or sudden exacerbations of disease (flares).[13] These can be compounded by a lack of understanding or support from the employer, including a reluctance to make 'reasonable adjustments', and a lack of understanding from colleagues. Patients should be encouraged to discuss their illness with their employers, in order to facilitate flexible working arrangements such as increased work from home, or later start times to accommodate morning stiffness. Other factors that facilitate people to remain in work are rapid access to primary and secondary care for management of flares, and better awareness of their rights at work. The NRAS produces very useful guides for people with RA and their employers, which cover aspects of fatigue, benefits and driving (DVLA) advice. The 'Access to Work' programme can also be accessed to provide practical support for adjustments needed to help support a return to work.

### Management of co-morbidities

The improved treatment of RA is already changing the spectrum of disease complications, with extra-articular manifestations (nodules, cervical spine instability and vasculitis) becoming much less common. However, there remains an excess mortality, particularly from *ischaemic heart disease* (IHD), much of which is silent. This is not solely attributable to heightened traditional cardiovascular risk factors, with RA itself being a separate, independent factor due to the cumulative effect of inflammation.

The greatest priority is to address *smoking*, as this is a risk factor for a more severe disease course. It is also important to control blood pressure (which may also be raised because of NSAIDs) and to check fasting lipids annually. When assessing if your patient meets the threshold for intervention, the estimated ten-year risk should be increased by 1.5–2-fold due to the presence of rheumatoid disease. All patients should be encouraged to exercise and control weight. In addition to the consequences of excess weight on joints, truncal adipose tissue produces pro-inflammatory cytokines that contribute to disease activity and can directly cause elevation of CRP.

All patients receiving immunosuppressive drugs (steroids, methotrexate, leflunomide or biological agents) should receive influenza and pneumococcal vaccination. For those not immune to varicella zoster, if there is significant chickenpox exposure, you should seek specialist advice from your local microbiology department regarding passive immunisation with varicella zoster immune globulin (VZIG).

There is also an increased risk of lymphoma in RA, which is mainly related to long-term disease activity rather than immunosuppression, but when this does arise it is likely that B cell-directed therapy (rituximab) would be effective treatment for both diseases.

### Emergency situations – when to refer back urgently

#### FLARES

Many patients with stable disease will be reviewed annually in secondary care, and if the disease is genuinely in remission a flare is a rare occurrence. The usual symptoms are a sudden increase in generalised pain and stiffness; if the flare symptoms are confined to a single joint you should carefully assess this to ensure there are no features to suggest joint sepsis.

Flares can sometimes be precipitated by viral infection, physical trauma, stressful life events or steroid dose reduction. In many situations the patient will have access to advice from the rheumatology department advice line or nurse specialist. If the patient consults the GP initially, the options to treat flares include either:

▷ the addition of NSAIDs
▷ escalation of DMARD dose or
▷ a short course of oral steroids; you should liaise directly with
   secondary care so that an agreed management plan and earlier
   follow-up can be agreed.

#### SUSPECTED SEPSIS

Patients with arthritis are also more prone to develop joint sepsis. If any of the affected joints are red or the patient is systemically unwell, sepsis should be considered, particularly for the latter or if the patient is taking either steroids, immunosuppressive or biological drugs. Remember that elderly patients with sepsis may not always be pyrexial, particularly if this is masked by steroids or NSAIDs. If sepsis is suspected, this is a medical emergency, and the patient should be admitted immediately. In addition to the risk of joint sepsis, *anti-TNF therapy increases the risk of skin and soft-tissue infections*; if significant infection occurs this should be managed in conjunction with rheumatology advice, which will usually include temporary cessation of treatment.

#### NEW-ONSET NEUROLOGICAL SYMPTOMS

Rheumatoid disease of the cervical spine can result in vertebral body subluxation, either at the level of the atlantoaxial joint, or at lower levels in the cervical spine. This is more likely to occur in the setting of poorly controlled longstanding disease, and is usually heralded by subtle loss of hand and upper-limb function, often associated with sensory disturbance and increasing neck pain. Eliciting the signs of cervical cord compression, i.e. long tract signs, can be difficult, as the assessment of both power grip and reflexes can be difficult in the presence of marked rheumatoid deformities. If this complication is suspected, direct urgent referral to a neurosurgeon is advised.

Entrapment neuropathies – usually either at wrist, elbow or tarsal tunnel – can occur due to direct compression from synovitis. If these develop then management is by injection of steroid (particularly if synovitis present) or surgery depending on degree of compromise and local access to hand surgery.

## PERSISTENT UNEXPLAINED DYSPNOEA

If there is severe, persistent or unexplained dyspnoea, vigilance is needed for the possibilities of either methotrexate-induced pneumonitis or rheumatoid lung disease or silent IHD, and arrange further investigation.

---

Box 12.1 ○ *Case study 1 – early disease*

**Mrs Green consults you with a three-month history of generalised arthralgia associated with poor sleep, fatigue, low mood and morning stiffness. She is peri-menopausal and also under stress at work.**

Your assessment of Mrs Green will initially involve primary care management; the initial history will explore her symptoms and problems with ADL. Using communication skills, you will explore her beliefs about her health and her concerns for the future. A review of her notes may reveal entries from colleagues documenting similar symptoms and previous investigations. A full examination at this point did not reveal synovitis, but using your problem-solving skills you were sufficiently concerned about the degree of physical impairment to refer her to secondary care.

**At this appointment there was no detectable synovitis in her hands, and blood tests and X-rays were normal. She was reassured that she did not have RA and in view of her other symptoms a diagnosis of fibromyalgia was made. She is discharged from secondary care but returns to see you two months later as she is still struggling. She does not understand what fibromyalgia is.**

You discuss her concerns and expectations. She is struggling with her job as a secretary. You elicit the symptoms of depression using your listening and consultation skills. She cannot meet her workload demands and her line manager is losing patience with her. You explore the possibility of issuing a sick note. Holistically, her health and her life are now suffering, and she is developing psychological symptoms. You re-examine her and it is now clear that she has developed synovitis. You both come to the decision that she needs urgent reassessment and you use your knowledge of local networks to phone the local rheumatology team.

## Analysis of case study 1 with respect to the six domains of Being a GP

### DOMAIN 1: PRIMARY CARE MANAGEMENT

▷ To recognise the clinical expression of RA, when to refer, and the key components of assessing disease activity.

### DOMAIN 2: PERSON-CENTRED CARE

▷ To understand the impact of rheumatoid disease on the individual and his or her concerns.

### DOMAIN 3: SPECIFIC PROBLEM-SOLVING SKILLS

▷ To understand the principles of pharmacological management and monitoring, and as a DMARD Directed Enhanced Service in general practice.

### DOMAIN 4: A COMPREHENSIVE APPROACH

▷ To detect the co-morbidities associated with RA and manage them in primary care.
▷ To be vigilant to the potential for ongoing joint damage and disability, even when the disease is apparently quiescent.

### DOMAIN 5: COMMUNITY ORIENTATION

▷ To appreciate the role of the MDT – also accessing secondary care and the nurse specialist.
▷ To recognise potential emergencies and when to refer back urgently to secondary care.

### DOMAIN 6: A HOLISTIC APPROACH

To understand the impact that disorders of rheumatoid disease can have on individuals and their lives. To search for educational resources that will enhance your ability to act as the advocate of your patient's care.

*At this appointment two weeks later, the rheumatologist agrees that she does now have RA, which unfortunately is very active, aggravated by the diagnostic delay. Her ESR is 85 and CRP 72, and although her rheumatoid factor is negative her CCP anti-*

*bodies, which were not tested initially, were strongly positive. She is commenced on methotrexate and a reducing course of oral steroids.*

The clinic letter is faxed through to your surgery but is not filed in the notes, so that when she returns you cannot find the letter. (You make a note to review information management in the practice.) It would be far more efficient to have electronic transfer of letters. Eventually it is located. Mrs Green is angry and upset that, in her opinion, she has been mismanaged. You discuss her concerns and give her time to talk. She is worried about the future and her job. She is also worried about any medication that she might have to take. You arrange to see Mrs Green next week at a longer consultation to give you both more time to discuss matters more holistically. In the mean time you decide to update your knowledge of current methods of managing RA and look on the NICE website for the recently released guideline.

*When Mrs Green returns, she discusses her worries about having another baby; she has a 2-year-old and she and her husband were planning an addition to the family. She has been advised at the hospital to avoid conception while taking methotrexate. She also discusses work and whether she should take time off until her disease comes under control.*

You update her records with the methotrexate prescription and the advice about contraception. You also add her to the register for influenza vaccination and pneumovax recall. This problem of newly diagnosed RA has to be managed holistically.

Unfortunately, over the next 12 months, despite steroids and combination DMARDs, her disease remained active. She was unable to return to her secretarial job and after nine months, with no prospect of further recovery, she lost her job. Because her disease had remained active despite treatment, she became eligible for anti-TNF therapy. Within one month of starting this she no longer required any analgesia and achieved complete remission within three months. She subsequently returned to full-time secretarial work for a new employer.

---

### Learning points

This case highlights the importance of early, accurate diagnosis, which can be difficult if the symptoms have been insidious, when synovitis can be difficult to detect. If there is ongoing clinical suspicion, the newer diagnostic tools of anti-CCP antibodies and ultrasound should be used, particularly as the long-term prognosis is much worse if diagnosis is delayed beyond three months. Probably as a result of this delay, conventional DMARD therapy was not effective in this patient, as the 'window of opportunity' to gain early control of the disease had been missed. The occupational implications are that permanent ill-health retirement should not be considered as inevitable unless anti-TNF therapy has been accessed.

---

Box 12.2 ○ *Case study 2 – established disease*

---

**Ms Blue is 32 years' old and developed RA ten years ago. The first time that you see her in surgery is when she comes to report that her arthritis is 'terrible'. She tells you that her rheumatologist doesn't seem to understand the amount of pain that she is in. Her hand function is poor.**

Using specific problem-solving skills you elicit a history of ongoing pain and difficulty in coping with ADL, which does not tally with the letters from the hospital clinic. You wonder if Ms Blue's distress may be caused by other co-morbidities apart from active RA. Using communication skills you explore the possibility of depression and decide to use the PHQ-9, but this yields a low score, making depression unlikely. You do not elicit any other possible causes for her distress. You are concerned about her poor hand function and the fact that she is young and needs to retain employment, and you note that she has been assessed at each clinic visit by a different junior doctor. You refresh your memory on management of RA by searching useful websites such as GP Notebook and NHS Evidence. Here you find the recently published guideline on RA and realise that her care has probably been suboptimal. You work out a DAS very roughly using the web-calculator supplied and her score is above 5.1, indicating active disease. You discuss this with a GP colleague who has worked in the local rheumatology clinic and he agrees that her care is suboptimal, but that a referral for a second opinion may have to be handled tactfully in case Ms Blue ever wishes to return to that hospital for care in the future.

**You ask Ms Blue to return to surgery by telephoning her; you are careful to allay her anxieties when she realises that it is her doctor phoning and record the conversation in her records. You discuss your concerns about her ongoing disease activity when she calls in later in the week. She is very worried herself because of her ongoing fatigue and difficulties at work, and is happy to accept your advice that a second opinion is necessary.**

You use your knowledge of the local health network to contact a neighbouring rheumatologist to ask if he will see Ms Blue. You are mindful that referring her to another unit will incur a higher charge because this will be a new appointment and is more expensive than a follow-up. You also feel that the current provider is not making good use of your practice money at the moment. You decide to discuss this failure in care with colleagues at a practice meeting so that the practice can review the management of other rheumatology patients at this unit. You may decide to refer them to another provider, particularly if the current provider is not meeting the standards of care for people with inflammatory arthritis (NICE and ARMA guidelines).

At the neighbouring Trust she is noted as having a large number of tender joints, a high pain VAS, and a DAS of 5.8, indicating highly active disease. Ultrasound confirms that despite the low CRP she still has ongoing synovitis in many small joints. This explains the discrepancy between her previous clinical assessments and her symptoms. She receives anti-TNF therapy but despite six months of treatment her disease remains active. She is subsequently treated with rituximab, to which she responds, and has a significant improvement in her hand function.

## *Analysis of case study 2 with respect to the six domains of* Being a GP

### DOMAIN 1: PRIMARY CARE MANAGEMENT

▷ To recognise the features of uncontrolled RA and how this manifests in the patient.

### DOMAIN 2: PERSON-CENTRED CARE

▷ To understand the impact of poorly controlled rheumatoid disease on the individual and his or her concerns. To understand that other co-morbidities such as depression may also be affecting the outcome.

### DOMAIN 3: SPECIFIC PROBLEM-SOLVING SKILLS

▷ To use the DAS 28 to assess disease activity and applying this to the patient. Also to know where to find resources such as NICE guidance and apply these to the case mentioned.

### DOMAIN 4: A COMPREHENSIVE APPROACH

▷ To detect the co-morbidities associated with RA and manage them in primary care.
▷ To be vigilant to the potential for ongoing joint damage and disability even when the disease is apparently quiescent.

### DOMAIN 5: COMMUNITY ORIENTATION

▷ To appreciate the role of the MDT and understand when a patient may be receiving less than adequate care. Look at community resources that may help this patient stay in work (a local job centre, for example).

### DOMAIN 6: A HOLISTIC APPROACH

▷ To understand the impact that disorders of rheumatoid disease can have on the individual and his or her life. To search for educational resources that will enhance your ability to act as a key clinician in your patient's care.

## Learning points

All patients with RA should undergo a composite DAS at regular intervals, in order to confirm an adequate response to their management plan, and this should be indicated in the written communications from secondary care and copied to patients. If a patient does not achieve a low disease activity state, there should be an indication of planned further treatment strategies. Commissioners should ensure that the service they are purchasing for your patients is compliant with the 2009 NICE RA guidance.

### *Useful websites*

▷ Arthritis Care, **www.arthritiscare.org.uk**.
▷ Arthritis and Musculoskeletal Alliance (ARMA), **www.arma.uk.net**.
▷ Arthritis Research Campaign (ARC), **www.arc.org.uk**.
▷ British Society for Rheumatology (BSR), **www.rheumatology.org.uk**.
▷ National Rheumatoid Arthritis Society (NRAS), **www.nras.org.uk**.
▷ National Patient Safety Agency (NPSA), **www.npsa.nhs.uk**.

### *Further reading*

▷ Chakravarty K, McDonald H, Pullar T, *et al*. BSR/BHPR guideline for disease-modifying anti-rheumatic drug (DMARD) therapy *Rheumatology* (Oxford) 2008; **47(6)**: 924–5.

### References

1 • Han C, Smolen J, Kavanaugh A, *et al*. Comparison of employability outcomes among patients with early or long-standing rheumatoid arthritis *Arthritis and Rheumatism* 2008; **59(4)**: 510–14.

2 • Deighton C, O'Mahony R, Tosh J, *et al*. on behalf of the Guideline Development Group. Management of rheumatoid arthritis: summary of NICE guidance *British Medical Journal* 2009; **338**: b702.

3 • Arthritis and Musculoskeletal Alliance. *Standards of Care for People with Inflammatory Arthritis* London: ARMA, 2004.

4 • King's Fund. *Perceptions of Patients and Professionals on Rheumatoid Arthritis Care* London: King's Fund, 2009.

5 • du Montcel ST, Michou L, Petit-Teixeira E, *et al*. New classification of HLA-DRB1 alleles supports the shared epitope hypothesis of rheumatoid arthritis susceptibility *Arthritis and Rheumatism* 2005; **52(4)**: 1063–8.

6 • Rieck M, Arechiga A, Onengut-Gumuscu S, *et al*. Genetic variation in PTPN22 corresponds to altered function of T and B lymphocytes *Journal of Immunology* 2007; **179(7)**: 4704–10.

7 • Klareskog L, Padyukov L, Alfredsson L. Smoking as a trigger for inflammatory rheumatic diseases *Current Opinion in Rheumatology* 2007; **19(1)**: 49–54.

8 • Nurmohamed MT, Dijkmans B A. Dyslipidaemia, statins and rheumatoid arthritis *Annals of the Rheumatic Diseases* 2009; **68(4)**: 453–5.

9 • National Institute for Health and Clinical Excellence. *Clinical Guideline 79, Rheumatoid Arthritis: national clinical guideline for management and treatment in adults* London: Royal College of Physicians, 2009, www.nice.org.uk/CG79 [accessed October 2011].

10 • Fransen J, van Riel P L. The Disease Activity Score and the EULAR response criteria *Clinical and Experimental Rheumatology* 2005; **23(5 Suppl 39)**: S93–9.

11 • Visser K, Katchamart W, Loza E, *et al.* Multinational evidence-based recommendations for the use of methotrexate in rheumatic disorders with a focus on rheumatoid arthritis *Annals of the Rheumatic Diseases* 2009; **68(7)**: 1086–93.

12 • Brown A K, Conaghan P G, Karim Z, *et al.* An explanation for the apparent dissociation between clinical remission and continued structural deterioration in rheumatoid arthritis *Arthritis and Rheumatism* 2008; **58(10)**: 2958–67.

13 • National Rheumatoid Arthritis Society. *I Want to Work. Employment and rheumatoid arthritis: a national picture. National Rheumatoid Arthritis Society survey* Maidenhead: NRAS, 2007.

# Spondyloarthropathy

# 13

*Philip S. Helliwell and Laura C. Coates*

## Aims of this chapter

This chapter will introduce the (seronegative) spondyloarthropathies: ankylosing spondylitis, psoriatic arthritis, reactive arthritis and the arthritis related to inflammatory bowel disease. Together they constitute a group linked by genes, notably HLA-B27, and shared clinical features. Historically, they were first characterised clinically by Verna Wright and his team in Leeds – the genetic evidence followed. The aims of the chapter are as follows:

▶ to describe the shared clinical features
▶ to discuss in more detail the individual diseases:
  ▪ ankylosing spondylitis
  ▪ psoriatic arthritis
  ▪ reactive arthritis
  ▪ arthritis related to inflammatory bowel disease
▶ to discuss treatment options in the context of primary and secondary care, and the role of the multidisciplinary team.

The key learning points are to:

▶ recognise clinical features of these disorders and their significance
▶ recognise the role of treatment in both primary and secondary care
▶ acknowledge the genetic background to these disorders
▶ explain the aetiology and natural history of spondyloarthropathies
▶ understand the roles of the primary and secondary healthcare team including allied health professionals
▶ understand the indications for referral within a suitable timeframe to the most appropriate healthcare practitioner.

## Introduction

The spondyloarthropathies emerged as a clinical concept in the early 1970s as a result of work by Verna Wright, Professor of Rheumatology at Leeds.

Wright recognised that a number of arthropathies shared common clinical features:

▷ absence of rheumatoid factor (seronegative)
▷ a predilection for lower-limb oligoarthritis (fewer than five joints clinically involved)
▷ absence of rheumatoid nodules
▷ spinal involvement with sacroiliitis
▷ eye inflammation and skin disorders resembling psoriasis
▷ enthesitis
▷ familial aggregation.

The research group led by Wright set about describing the clinical associations of ankylosing spondylitis,[1] inflammatory bowel disease,[2] reactive arthritis,[3] Behcet's disease (then believed to be a member of this group)[4] and psoriatic arthritis.[5] This group also recognised the familial clustering of these diseases and a number of impressive family pedigrees were collected.[1,6,7] The culmination of this work, frenetically carried out in a period in the late 1960s and early 1970s, was the book *Seronegative Polyarthritis*, setting out and reviewing the evidence for this distinct group of disorders.[8] Although much of the work on familial clustering had been done before the discovery of HLA-B27, the association with this genetic marker confirmed the innate susceptibility of people who develop these disorders.[9] Since that time new molecular techniques have led to greater enlightenment about pathogenesis and susceptibility, and recent developments in therapeutics means that we now have powerful drugs with which to treat these disorders. However, much of the pioneering clinical work remains valid.

**Ankylosing spondylitis**

*Introduction*

Ankylosing spondylitis primarily affects the spine, but in a significant proportion of people the peripheral joints and entheses are involved. The latter is especially true for juvenile-onset ankylosing spondylitis, which may present as a painful hip or knee many years before the spinal symptoms appear.

*What causes ankylosing spondylitis?*

A major breakthrough in understanding this disease came in the early 1970s with the discovery of the association with the HLA antigen B27, present in over 90% of cases. This association has been confirmed many times since but more recent association with the IL12/23 gene has moved things along a little more. How does the presence of HLA-B27 influence the onset of the disease? Unfortunately, the precise pathogenesis has yet to be elucidated but several facts are known:

▷ only certain isotypes of B27 are associated with ankylosing spondylitis
▷ B27 helps present foreign (bacterial) antigens to the immune system, but it may do this in a faulty way, thus leading to abnormal recognition signals
▷ some parts of the B27/bacterial antigen complex may be antigenically similar to self-antigens in the musculoskeletal system, thus initiating an immunological reaction to self
▷ it is also possible that B27 causes increased reactivity to bacterial antigens that themselves 'cross-react' with self-antigens in the musculoskeletal system.

Why are bacterial antigens thought to be so important in this disorder? First, there is an animal model of this disease, the B27 transgenic mouse, which develops many of the clinical features of ankylosing spondylitis. Interestingly, rearing these animals in a germ-free environment prevents development of the disorder. Second, gut inflammation is common in ankylosing spondylitis – much of this may be subclinical and situated in the terminal ileum. Sometimes the inflammation is clinically apparent and may manifest as the association between inflammatory bowel disease and this disorder. Persistent inflammatory change in the gut wall leads to a breakdown of the natural barrier between gut bacterial commensals and the blood.

### How common is ankylosing spondylitis?

Exact figures are unknown and current prevalence and incidence are probably underestimates. The disease is probably slightly more common in men than women, although a common belief that women do not get ankylosing spondylitis has led to under-diagnosis in the past. The prevalence has been reported as 0.1% of the population but this may be low for reasons discussed below.

### Clinical features

Although primarily a disease of the spine, peripheral symptoms may be the first to appear, particularly in children. It is not uncommon for a child of eight to ten years to present with a swollen knee or painful hip, which may persist for some years prior to the appearance of spinal symptoms. Adults may occasionally present with a swollen lower-limb joint or with enthesitis, experienced as heel pain (either plantar fasciitis or at the Achilles insertion) or musculoskeletal pain around the chest wall. Rarely, rheumatologists are referred patients who have presented with iritis (uveitis) to the ophthalmology department. In a few cases advanced ankylosis is found by chance following an accident or an abdominal X-ray for another reason. Associated disease of the aortic valve is becoming less common, as is renal involvement due to amyloidosis.

In adults the pain often starts in the lumbar spine but may be felt anywhere in the spine, even at onset of symptoms. The characteristics of inflammatory back pain are given in Box 13.1. It is worth asking about associated diseases, both in the person presenting and in the family. Patients may have also already tried over-the-counter non-steroidal anti-inflammatory drugs (NSAIDs) and a good clinical response to these is a pointer to inflammatory back pain.

---

**Box 13.1 ○ *Inflammatory back pain history***

- Insidious onset.
- Night pain, especially causing the patient to awaken in the latter half of the night.
- Severe, prolonged, early-morning and inactivity stiffness.
- Buttock pain, often alternating (due to sacroiliitis).
- Worsened (stiffness and pain) by rest or prolonged sitting and relieved by exercise.

---

## What is the natural history and prognosis?

There is no doubt that ankylosing spondylitis is a heterogeneous disease. People with this disorder progress at different rates but several longitudinal surveys have shown that most patients do demonstrate progression of spinal changes. In our clinic we still have a few patients with total ankylosis but these people have had their disease for 20 or 30 years. Successive clinic evaluations show that the majority of non-ankylosed patients deteriorate only very slowly. However, as mobility is progressively lost (a situation which we try to avoid by regular follow-up and monitoring with targeted treatment) other problems emerge. There is an increased risk of cardiac conduction abnormalities and aortic valve disease, although these are uncommon. Renal amyloidosis is infrequently seen, but a slowly rising serum creatinine, possibly associated with NSAID treatment, requires surveillance.

With progressive loss of movement in the thoracic spine and rib cage, chest infections become more of a problem because the patient is unable to generate enough forced expiration to cough. This is when cigarette smokers are particularly at risk. Finally, and most importantly, people with an ankylosed spine are vulnerable to devastating injury, sometimes overlooked initially (see Box 13.2). A rigid, fused spine behaves like a long bone in response to injury, and may break catastrophically. When occurring in the cervical spine this may be immediately obvious, but fractures through the spine at lower levels may be diagnosed late.

---

Box 13.2 ○ *Case study 1 – ankylosing spondylitis*

A 60-year-old man with a 27-year history of ankylosing spondylitis slips and falls on ice, landing on his back. He later reported going down with a 'right crack' but he picked himself up and carried on. Over the next few days he noticed a sharp pain in the lower thoracic spine. He also noticed that when he coughed or sneezed he had a shooting pain down both legs. His legs also felt a 'bit funny' and he had difficulty opening his bowels. He visited his GP who gave him analgesia and recommended rest, observing that he may have 'slipped a disc'. Four months later he attended his usual clinic appointment whereupon he was admitted and his magnetic resonance imaging (MRI) scan showed a complete, unstable fracture at T10/11 with compromise of his spinal cord at that level. He was referred for surgical stabilisation.

---

### How is the diagnosis made?

For classification purposes the following should be present:

▷ inflammatory back pain
▷ restriction of spinal movement
▷ radiological abnormalities in the sacroiliac joints.

However, the radiological changes take an average of eight years to develop, so these criteria are of limited use for early classification, and indeed diagnosis. Most rheumatologists would diagnose ankylosing spondylitis with a history of inflammatory back pain responding well to NSAIDs. Many would also require an abnormal MRI scan of the sacroiliac joints or spine (the early features are quite typical).

The role of testing for HLA-B27 remains controversial. In the UK the prevalence of this antigen in the 'normal' population is about 7%, which impairs the usefulness of the test in diagnosis. Some German authors would argue that the test, although reasonably expensive, is a 'one off' (you only need testing once) and that a positive test combined with a history of inflammatory back pain (see Box 13.1) makes the chance of having ankylosing spondylitis very high. However, during many years of practice we have seen the consequences of indiscriminate testing for B27 in our clinics as people with mechanical back pain (very common – lifetime prevalence over 60%) and a positive HLA-B27 test have visited the world wide web and are already convinced of their diagnosis before consultation has started. Nor does MRI help to solve the conundrum in these cases as changes may not be present consistently and MRI inflammation may be influenced by use of NSAIDs. There is no question of the powerful utility of new diagnostic tests but the art of clinical diagnosis remains the most valuable tool in assessment.

### When should a referral be made?

There is no doubt that the end result of ankylosing spondylitis, with total ankylosis of the spine and a stooped posture, is devastating, so early referral is recommended. This is especially true nowadays as powerful biologic drugs are now available for this condition (see pp. 318–19). However, many patients are quite diffident about their symptoms, and many deny a history despite obvious and marked spinal radiographic changes. It may therefore be difficult to both identify and persuade these people that hospital treatment is required. Another problem, less so nowadays, is that there is a perception that women do not get this disease, and so appropriate diagnosis and referral is delayed.

### Treatment for ankylosing spondylitis

The first-line treatments, and indeed the only treatments for many years, were NSAIDs and physiotherapy. The response to NSAIDs is remarkable for most patients with ankylosing spondylitis, so much so that some classification criteria include a good response to NSAIDs as a criterion. The only limitations to NSAIDs in these disorders are adverse effects, mostly dyspepsia. The dose of NSAIDs required for symptom relief may be higher than usual: typical doses are 1 to 1.5 g of naproxen, 90 to 120 mg etoricoxib and up to 2.4 g of ibuprofen. Long-term uninterrupted use of such doses, or indeed any dose of NSAIDs, is now discouraged not only because of gastrointestinal side effects but also because of adverse effects on the cardiovascular system. However, these patients are truly dependent on NSAIDs and they will report deterioration within one half-life of discontinuing these drugs.

Traditional disease-modifying antirheumatic drugs (DMARDs) are generally ineffective in ankylosing spondylitis so the option of achieving disease control with these drugs, including steroids, is not available in ankylosing spondylitis. NSAID therapy should be coupled with education and physical therapy as daily stretching has been shown to retard disease progression and to help in symptom relief. People will find many excuses to justify their avoidance of these exercises – no time, no space, or being too painful are common reasons. To help people maintain the exercises the main patient organisation in the UK, the National Ankylosing Spondylitis Society (www. nass.co.uk), often co-organises weekly exercise and hydrotherapy sessions in collaboration with a local physiotherapy department. The physiotherapists involved in this scheme often do this on a voluntary basis and the group ethos invoked in these sessions is an integral part of their success.

The anti-TNF (tumour necrosis factor) drugs are particularly effective in ankylosing spondylitis – probably more so than in any other rheumatic disease. According to the National Institute for Health and Clinical Excellence (NICE) guideline the criteria for accessing these drugs are simply:

▷ failure of at least two NSAIDs, either due to inefficacy or adverse effects
▷ a certain level of disease activity as measured by the Bath Ankylosing Spondylitis Disease Activity Index (BASDAI) – a self-completed questionnaire containing a series of questions about pain and stiffness (see Box 13.3), where patients must exceed a score of 4 to be eligible
▷ no contraindications to treatment
▷ once started, demonstration that the drugs are effective (also measured by the BASDAI).

---

Box 13.3 ○ *Questions used in the BASDAI*

**Responses are made on 10 cm visual analogue scales.**
**The total score range is 0–10.**

1 ▶ How would you describe the overall level of fatigue/tiredness you have experienced?

2 ▶ How would you describe the overall level of ankylosing spondylitis neck, back or hip pain you have had?

3 ▶ How would you describe the overall level of pain and swelling in joints other than the neck, back or hips you have had?

4 ▶ How would you describe the overall level of discomfort you have had from any areas tender to touch or pressure?

5 ▶ How would you describe the overall level of discomfort you have had from the time you wake up?

6 ▶ How long does your morning stiffness last from the time you wake up?

There is no doubt that these drugs have transformed the lives of many patients with this disease. Moreover it is not just the people with early disease who benefit. People with advanced longstanding disease may benefit dramatically from a symptom point of view, although existing ankylosis will of course remain unchanged. A question mark still exists about the ability of anti-TNF drugs to inhibit radiological progression but this is probably just a matter of designing the right studies, with the correct follow-up. This is something that may not be ethically sound given the efficacy of these drugs on symptoms. The only downside of their use is the potential for adverse effects, although most people take them without any obvious problem. The main adverse effects are the risk of serious infection (both mycobacterial and others) and the potential to induce tumours. However, the latter may only appear after many years of use, and use is – relatively speaking – still in its infancy.

Treatment guidelines have been produced by the Assessment of Spondyloarthropathies Group (ASAS).[10] NICE guidelines on the use of anti-TNF drugs are available online at www.nice.org.uk/guidance/TA143.[11]

### Patient education, work and non-pharmacological treatments

A comprehensive patient education leaflet is available to download from the Arthritis Research UK website at www.arthritisresearchuk.org/. This booklet explains the clinical features and treatment options available and emphasises the need for regular exercises/stretching and for monitoring. Physiotherapists are ideally placed to fulfil this role and to advise on work, driving and other problems with participation.

### Conclusions

People with ankylosing spondylitis seem to be a bit more stoic than most. This may explain why diagnosis is made so late: in some cases complete ankylosis can occur before presentation. Mechanical back pain is common and symptoms can overlap with those of ankylosing spondylitis. However, it is fairly straightforward to be aware of the red-flag aspects of low-back pain and to be able to recognise inflammatory back pain. Although ankylosing spondylitis often presents in early adulthood it is as well to remember that late presentations can occur both *de novo* and in those with established disease.

### Further reading

▷ Khan M A. *Ankylosing Spondylitis: the facts* Oxford: Oxford University Press, 2002 [an easy-to-read guide by an international expert; the writer suffers from the disease].

▷ Dougados M, van der Heijde D. *Fast Facts: ankylosing spondylitis* Oxford: Health Press, 2004.

---

## Psoriatic arthritis

### Introduction

Psoriatic arthritis is a multifaceted articular disorder usually, although not exclusively, associated with psoriasis. It is important to recognise psoriatic arthritis because, untreated, it can cause long-term joint damage and disability with impact on quality of life. As there are shared genetics, pathophysiology and co-morbidities, psoriasis and psoriatic arthritis have been collectively termed 'psoriatic disease'.

315

### How common is psoriatic arthritis?

The prevalence of psoriasis in the UK is about 2%. The prevalence of psoriatic arthritis within this population is about 15%. This figure may be an underestimate as psoriasis can go unrecognised, especially if it is in 'hidden' areas such as behind the ears, the hair-line and the natal cleft (see Figure 13.1 on p. 476). In addition, in about 15% of people the arthritis starts before the psoriasis and may for that period of time be mislabelled. Finally, using ultrasound examination of tendons (see p. 330) many people with psoriasis also have (asymptomatic) abnormalities usually seen in psoriatic arthritis.

### Clinical features

A number of characteristic clinical features are seen in this disorder.

▷ The arthritis on the whole involves fewer joints than in rheumatoid arthritis, although the same joints may be involved (see Figure 13.2 on p. 476). However, it is not uncommon to see just one or two joints involved in this condition (see Figure 13.3 on p. 476).

▷ Enthesitis is inflammation at the attachment of tendons and ligaments to bone. The major enthesis of the body is at the Achilles insertion, and this is commonly involved in psoriatic arthritis (note this is at the insertion and not the tendon itself – see Figure 13.4 on p. 476). There are hundreds of entheses in the body, however, and this may explain why some people present with widespread pain unrelated to joints (around the chest wall and spine for example).

▷ Dactylitis is defined as uniform swelling of a digit and is also described as a 'sausage' finger or toe (see Figure 13.5 on p. 477). This may occur in isolation or along with inflammation in other areas. It is an adverse prognostic sign in this disease.

▷ Spondylitis may resemble ankylosing spondylitis. Patients present with inflammatory back pain (insidious onset, nocturnal pain, early-morning stiffness, improved with exercise and worsened by rest) and buttock pain (due to sacroiliitis). Spondylitis may be asymptomatic in as many as 30% of patients with psoriatic arthritis.

▷ Inflammation of distal interphalangeal joints is characteristic, especially in the presence of nail disease (see Figure 13.6 on p. 477). This may be indistinguishable from osteoarthritis except it may occur in young men and in the absence of signs of osteoarthritis elsewhere.

### How to diagnose psoriatic arthritis – what are the key features?

Articular complaints are increasingly common in the general population, as age advances. People with psoriasis are no exception but the possibility of psoriatic arthritis should be kept in mind if patients present with musculoskeletal complaints. As a guide, a screening questionnaire has been developed, which includes only 5 questions, and a manikin (see Figure 13.7, overleaf). This instrument has a sensitivity of 92% and a specificity of 75% in people with psoriasis. People presenting with dactylitis and enthesitis at major sites are easier to spot, as are those presenting with generalised articular complaints. Inflammatory back pain may be present and the presence of distal interphalangeal joint inflammation/enlargement in a young person is suggestive. A raised acute-phase reactant – erythrocyte sedimentation rate (ESR), plasma viscosity (PV) or C-reactive protein (CRP) – is suggestive of inflammatory arthritis, but normal inflammatory markers do not exclude joint inflammation. Rheumatoid factor is usually negative.

If characteristic clinical features are present but no psoriasis evident (remember the 'hidden' areas have to be examined to be sure disease is not present; most patients find this either amusing or invasive or both), it is worth seeking a previous personal or family history of psoriasis, as these conditions are highly genetic.

Figure 13.7 ○ **The PEST screening questionnaire for psoriatic arthritis**

In the drawing below, please tick the joints that have caused you discomfort (i.e. stiff, swollen or painful joints).

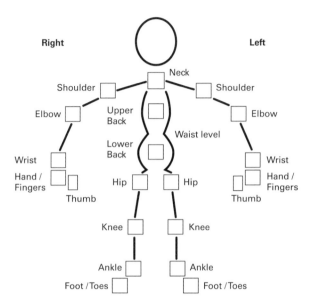

Score 1 point for each question answered in the affirmative.

A total score of 3 or more is indicative of psoriatic arthritis (sensitivity 0.92, specificity 0.78, positive predictive value 0.61, negative predictive value 0.95).

▶ Have you ever had a swollen joint (or joints)?

▶ Has a doctor ever told you that you have arthritis?

▶ Do your fingernails or toenails have holes or pits?

▶ Have you had pain in your heel?

▶ Have you had a finger or toe that was completely swollen and painful for no apparent reason?

*Source*: Ibrahim G, Buch M, Lawson C, *et al.* Evaluation of an existing screening tool for psoriatic arthritis in people with psoriasis and development of a new instrument: the PEST questionnaire.[12] Copyright© *Clinical and Experimental Rheumatology.* Used with permission.

It is worth noting that a recent community survey of people with psoriasis found undiagnosed psoriatic arthritis in about 14%. The average disease duration was ten years; it was not all recent-onset arthritis. People have to consult to be diagnosed, of course, but it is worth keeping a high index of suspicion in people with psoriasis presenting with musculoskeletal complaints.

### Natural history and prognosis

About a third of patients with psoriatic arthritis have oligoarticular (fewer than five joints involved), non-progressive disease and can be treated symptomatically or with intermittent intra-articular injections of steroids. However, it is identifying this group at an early stage that is the crux. Adverse prognostic signs at presentation include polyarticular disease, previous steroid use (for any reason), male sex and a raised inflammatory marker such as the ESR or CRP. In this larger progressive group, joint destruction will occur with time such that, after ten years, significant impact on disability and quality of life will occur. In about 5% of people a rapidly advancing and destructive form of arthritis occurs with the end result being arthritis mutilans (see Figure 13.8 on p. 477). Mortality is increased in psoriatic disease with an increased prevalence of the metabolic syndrome and cardiovascular disease. For this reason identification and treatment of the usual risk factors for cardiovascular disease (obesity, smoking, hypertension, cholesterol) is important. People with psoriatic disease are also more likely to have liver abnormalities independent of alcohol use – this makes treatment with traditional agents such as methotrexate problematic, although not impossible.

### When to refer and who to refer to

If any of the above clinical features are present then a referral to a rheumatologist is indicated. Any swollen joint in the presence of psoriasis is an indication for referral. Sometimes generalised pain or recurrent enthesitis (bilateral tennis elbow, for example) may be the presenting feature. The foot is an important source of pathology in this disease, so podiatrists should be familiar with dactylitis and enthesis or combinations of the two. Since joint destruction is a function of time it is best, as with other inflammatory rheumatic diseases, to refer patients early. No specific radiology or blood tests are necessary prior to referral, although if the acute-phase response (ESR, PV or CRP) is elevated it indicates a worse prognosis. If your local hospital runs combined rheumatology/dermatology clinics then it would be appropriate to refer to this service, particularly in the presence of skin disease.

### Treatment

It is fair to say that psoriatic arthritis has lagged behind other rheumatic diseases in terms of good clinical trial evidence, but the situation is changing rapidly. There has been an explosion in the number of publications on this condition in the last ten years, and these have been fuelled by the new biologic therapies. Greater interest in these disorders has resulted both in laboratory and clinical science. However, there is still a lot to be done. It is unknown which patients to target for early intensive treatment and good evidence is lacking for many of the treatments in use, including methotrexate. A number of publications have appeared in the last few years and it is now possible to find international treatment recommendations for psoriatic arthritis.[13] There are also NICE criteria for the use of biologic drugs such as anti-TNF (www.nice.org.uk/Guidance/TA104).[14]

The ideal treatment for a patient with this disease will help both the skin and the joints. It will be a convenient, and preferably infrequent, regime. This sounds far fetched, but the new biologic drugs can fill this role. It is not hard to see why patients are keen to start them; on the whole, patients hate covering themselves with greasy, sometimes smelly, unguents such as tar and dithranol every day. A pill or injection that does the same job is much more attractive. Of the traditional disease-modifying drugs, methotrexate is the one that can work for both aspects of the disease, although ciclosporin and azathioprine have been used in the past for the joints and are still used for the skin, particularly ciclosporin. Combination therapy with ciclosporin and methotrexate is sometimes used for added effectiveness. It is also worth making the point that, although 100% of the skin may be affected by psoriasis, once treatment is successful that person will have virtually normal-looking skin again. There is very little scarring or lasting damage. Conversely, joint inflammation can cause lasting damage to the cartilage and bone – the former does not have the regenerative capacity of skin. This may explain why dermatologists are more likely to give 'pulses' of therapy and rheumatologists continuous therapy for this disease.

A simple algorithm was developed by an international group involved in investigating and treating psoriatic disease (see Figure 13.9). For each feature of the disease a hierarchy of treatment is followed, working downwards. As can be seen from the figure, sometimes the same drug can be used for different features of the disease. A third of patients can be managed successfully by symptomatic treatment alone.

For example, a patient with a knee affected by oligoarticular disease can be managed successfully by intermittent intra-articular steroid injections. Specialist advice is recommended to be certain that the correct treatment is given to the patient.

Figure 13.9 ○ *Treatment algorithm for psoriatic arthritis*

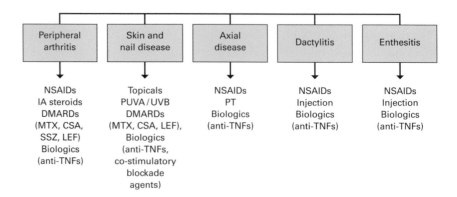

*Note*: injection for dactylitis and enthesitis indicates injection of corticosteroid. For dactylitis the injection is placed into the tendon sheath, joint or both. For enthesitis the injection is placed at the enthesitis, such as would be given for lateral epicondylitis.

*Key*: DMARDs = disease-modifying anti-rheumatic drugs | IA = intra-articular | LEF = leflunomide | MTX = methotrexate | NSAIDs = non-steroidal anti-inflammatory drugs | PUVA = psoralen plus ultraviolet light A | SSZ = sulfasalazine | TNF = tumour necrosis factor | UVB = ultraviolet light B.

*Source*: adapted from Kavanaugh A F, Ritchlin C T; GRAPPA Treatment Guideline Committee. Systematic review of treatments for psoriatic arthritis: an evidence based approach and basis for treatment guidelines.[15]

Clearly, the biologic drugs (mainly anti-TNF) are drugs of 'last resort' after all else has failed and thus are usually given in the most severe cases. However, it is worth noting that this disease can remain oligoarticular and the NICE guideline for use of anti-TNF in psoriatic arthritis requires only three tender and swollen joints (they can be the same joint) and failure of at least two conventional DMARDs. This is a fair reflection of the disease's impact because oligoarticular disease can be particularly disabling – persistent dactylitis in the index finger of the dominant hand can interfere with most daily and work activities, while enthesis at the Achilles insertion can make normal walking impossible.

It should also be remembered that this is a multifaceted disease that crosses specialist boundaries. The ideal specialist scenario for treating this condition is in combined dermatology/rheumatology clinics so that assessment and appropriate targeted therapy can be discussed. This also stops patients making duplicate appointments for what is essentially the same disease – important when so many patients are young and still working.

### How to monitor the progress of the disease

The aims of treatment are to prevent joint damage and associated disability. Damage can occur insidiously and most rheumatologists will be on the alert for this by carrying out both physical examination and imaging, usually plain radiography. However, X-ray change occurs slowly so radiographs would not usually be repeated more frequently than annually. As an elevated acute-phase response may predict those who progress radiologically, a measure of this will also be checked regularly. It may also be necessary to monitor the effects (and side effects) of DMARDs such as methotrexate, sulfasalazine, ciclosporin and leflunomide. Shared-care guidelines are available nationally, although many localities adapt these for their own.[16] Some secondary care clinics will also monitor the impact of the disease by administering questionnaires to assess function and quality of life. In psoriatic disease these can be affected by both the skin and the joint disease. Indeed, one study showed that people with psoriatic arthritis had equivalent reduction in function and quality of life despite less joint damage in the psoriatic arthritis group.[17]

All DMARDs should be used with caution in women of child-bearing age. Methotrexate and leflunomide in particular should be discontinued well before conception. People on DMARDs and biologic drugs should have annual influenza vaccination. Pneumococcal vaccine is also recommended for this group.

### Conclusion

Psoriatic arthritis is a complex, heterogeneous disease that is often unrecognised. Two thirds of people will develop joint destruction and disability with reduced quality of life. Early recognition and treatment may prevent these complications.

### Further reading

▷ Mease P, Helliwell P (eds). *Atlas of Psoriatic Arthritis* London: Springer, 2007.

---

## Reactive arthritis

### Introduction

Reactive arthritis, formerly referred to as Reiter's disease (this eponym is now discredited due to activities during the Second World War),[18] covers a wide spectrum of disorders from the classical triad of arthritis, urethritis and conjunctivitis in response to gut or sexually acquired infections, to rheumatic fever. A simple classification, based on the carriage of HLA-B27, is given in Table 13.1.

Table 13.1 ○ *Classification of reactive arthritis*

| HLA-B27 associated | Non-HLA-B27 associated |
|---|---|
| Sexually acquired reactive arthritis (SARA) – triggers such as *Chlamydia* spp. | Post-viral arthritis – triggers such as rubella and parvovirus |
| Enterocolic reactive arthritis – triggers such as *Shigella*, *Salmonella*, *Yersinia* and *Campylobacter* | Post-streptococcal group A (rheumatic fever) |
| Similar clinical features to above conditions but no antecedent infection found | Others (e.g. Lyme disease) |

*Source*: adapted from Keat A. Reiter's syndrome and reactive arthritis in perspective.[19]

### How common is reactive arthritis?

The commonest form of reactive arthritis is probably post-viral reactive arthritis, but the incident infection is rarely identified. Parvovirus, the cause of erythema infectiosum, also called 'fifth disease' or 'slapped-cheek syndrome', is the classic cause but few cases of early arthritis have evidence of *recent* parvovirus infection. The prevalence of classic reactive arthritis to some extent depends on the prevalence of HLA-B27; past epidemiological surveys have shown that the chance of getting reactive arthritis following infection with, for example, *Shigella* is about 20% if you also carry the B27 antigen and about 1% if you do not. However, recent figures disagree, suggesting that the association with HLA-B27 may be with persistence of the arthritis rather than incidence.[20]

### Clinical features

In B27-associated reactive arthritis the classical triad of arthritis, urethritis and conjunctivitis may not always be seen. In our experience the commonest presentation is a young person, usually a male with preceding opportunistic sexual contact, presenting to A&E with a swollen knee or ankle. Post-dysenteric reactive arthritis may occur in minor epidemic form if many people are affected. Back and buttock pain due to inflammation in the spine and sacroiliac joints may be present. In addition the following features may be present:

▷ enthesitis at major entheses such as the Achilles tendon insertion and the plantar fascia; entheses around the patella may contribute to knee pain

▷ dactylitis of a finger, or more likely a toe

▷ sacroiliitis and spondylitis, which may become more persistent and ultimately resemble ankylosing spondylitis.

▷ a pustular skin rash on the soles and palms. This is rather grandly called keratoderma blennorrhagica, the intriguing feature being the resemblance to pustular psoriasis (see Figure 13.10 on p. 477). At the same time nail dystrophy, similar to that seen in psoriasis, may occur. Not infrequently a rash appears on the glans penis, called circinate balanitis because of the way in encircles the glans (see Figure 13.11 on p. 478).

Rheumatic fever will not be discussed in this chapter. As previously mentioned, unrecognised viral infection may precede reactive arthritis. However, as well as parvovirus, Hepatitis B and C, and rubella (as well as rubella vaccination) may precede the non-HLA-B27-associated reactive arthritis. This may resemble early rheumatoid arthritis with involvement (synovitis, stiffness and pain) of the small joints of the hands and feet. Other forms of reactive arthritis include the arthritis that follows infection with the tick-borne virus of Lyme disease and a reactive arthritis associated with tuberculosis (also known as Poncet's disease), neither of which are necessarily linked to the carriage of HLA-B27.

### How to diagnose reactive arthritis – what are the key features?

It is always good to recognise reactive arthritis since, on the whole, the prognosis is better than with other arthritides. A definite preceding infection is not always present, but if it is it makes life a lot simpler. Generally the arthritis follows the infection by a minimum of 12 days and a maximum of 21 days. B27-associated reactive arthritis tends to have such a distinctive clinical pattern that, when seen, a trigger is actively sought. Typically the young person with a hugely swollen lower-limb joint, and perhaps some entheseal tenderness, has had some preceding infection, usually sexually acquired. Although urethritis in males may be clinically very obvious to patient and doctor, in females this may not be as prominent and cervicitis may go unnoticed – this probably explains the apparent male predominance of this disorder.

A raised acute-phase reactant (ESR, PV or CRP) is suggestive of inflammatory arthritis and the CRP may be in the 100s in an acute case. Rheumatoid factor is usually negative. Ultimately, in the absence of a clear trigger, the diagnosis is presumptive but a good outcome would be part of this process. In the absence of a trigger, but with typical clinical features, chronic cases may well just be classified as undifferentiated spondyloarthropathy. In cases of early arthritis where a trigger is suspected it is always worth enquiring about contact with children, aged four to eight, and any recent illness.

---

Box 13.4 ○ *Case study 2 – post-dysenteric reactive arthritis*

---

A 30-year-old man went out with his team-mates after a game of cricket. They visited a local restaurant and had different dishes. Two days later he developed colicky abdominal pain and profuse diarrhoea, which lasted several days. His GP visited and a stool sample grew *Campylobacter* species. No specific treatment was given other than oral rehydration. Twelve days later he developed a painful, swollen left knee, and had aches in his right ankle. He went to A&E with his swollen knee, which was X-rayed. This confirmed that his knee was swollen. An orthopaedic referral was made and he was admitted for aspiration, in theatre, under aseptic conditions. The aspirated fluid showed many inflammatory cells but was (eventually) culture negative, and no crystals were seen. He was nevertheless treated with intravenous antibiotics on the assumption that he had an infected joint. By this time his ankle had become very swollen, prompting a referral to a rheumatologist, who diagnosed post-dysenteric reactive arthritis. Full doses of NSAIDs were given, with some symptom relief, but persistent pain and swelling in his ankle and knee prompted the rheumatologist to give him intra-articular injections of steroids. A few days later he was up and about and discharged. He was given a two-week review appointment for the rheumatologist but did not attend; nor did he ring to say why he was not attending. It was assumed that his arthritis had fully resolved.

---

## Analysis of case study 2 with respect to the six domains of Being a GP

### DOMAIN 1: PRIMARY CARE MANAGEMENT

▷ Recognition of the presentation, signs and symptoms of acute infective diarrhoea and acute inflammatory arthritis.
▷ Understanding the likely sequelae of such a problem for the patient and his social and economic wellbeing.

### DOMAIN 2: PERSON-CENTRED CARE

▷ Understanding the impact of the diarrhoea on this patient. He had asked for a home visit from his GP, so obviously felt very unwell. Then he developed swollen, painful joints and went to the A&E department. It is possible that he has a chaotic lifestyle and does not cope well with illness.

**DOMAIN 3: SPECIFIC PROBLEM-SOLVING SKILLS**

▷ Making a diagnosis of acute infective diarrhoea and, subsequently, inflammatory arthritis.
▷ Understanding the differential diagnoses of septic arthritis and how to diagnose this.

**DOMAIN 4: A COMPREHENSIVE APPROACH**

▷ Understanding why this patient presented to A&E rather than making a routine GP appointment.
▷ Assessing whether there are enough urgent GP appointments to see patients when required.
▷ Making note of the fact that he did not attend review with the rheumatologist and flagging this up. This is so that, when he next presents to primary care, he can be questioned about his arthritis.

**DOMAIN 5: COMMUNITY ORIENTATION**

▷ Where possible, diagnosing and treating the patient in primary care. This patient chose to use hospital emergency services.

**DOMAIN 6: A HOLISTIC APPROACH**

▷ Understanding that this illness will affect the patient socially and economically. Look at the reasons for his chaotic approach to his health care (presenting to A&E and not attending follow-up appointments). Perhaps he has other co-morbidities such as alcohol abuse?

### Natural history and prognosis

Most cases of reactive arthritis in which a recognised trigger is found settle spontaneously within a few weeks. People who are HLA-B27 positive are more likely to have persistent disease. In epidemics of gastrointestinal infection most cases settle within three to six months but some may grumble on for up to 12 months. A small minority, about 15%, become chronic. With time the disorder comes to resemble another member of the spondyloarthropathy group, ankylosing spondylitis or psoriatic arthritis, particularly if the skin and nail changes become more prominent.

325

## When to refer and who to refer to

Many of the cases of acute reactive arthritis are self-referring to the hospital A&E department. Young men arriving in casualty on a weekend with a hot, swollen knee are almost always cases of reactive arthritis. The differential diagnosis of a hot, swollen joint includes infection and gout, so aspiration is necessary to rule out these other important and treatable conditions. A sample of synovial fluid should be sent for microscopy and culture. Many of these cases will settle quickly with just treatment with NSAIDs, but if symptoms persist over a couple of weeks they should be referred for urgent rheumatology review.

## Treatment

Given the benign nature of many cases of this condition, all that is required is symptomatic treatment. NSAIDs are particularly effective but people tend to require, and tolerate, larger than usual doses, such as indomethacin 225 mg or naproxen 1500 mg. Since only short-term use is necessary, these doses can be justified. In case of intolerance or contraindication an intramuscular dose of a depot steroid preparation should suffice. If only one or two joints are involved intra-articular injections are usually very effective.

In cases that become chronic, i.e. those lasting more than three months, disease-modifying drugs may be necessary. This may particularly be necessary in cases in which no triggering infection is found but presenting with the classical clinical features of reactive arthritis. Traditionally sulfasalazine has been the first DMARD to be used in this condition but clinical trial evidence of efficacy is sparse. Of the other traditional disease-modifying drugs methotrexate is the next most likely drug to be used, although azathioprine has been used in the past. As for psoriatic arthritis, the biologic drugs (mainly anti-TNF) are drugs of 'last resort' after all else has failed and thus are usually given to the most severe cases.

A number of trials have examined the efficacy of treating the primary infection as a way of aborting or curtailing reactive arthritis, but results, apart from certain notable exceptions, have been disappointing. The exceptions are *Chlamydia* urogenital infection, Lyme disease and rheumatic fever. Longer-term studies with antibiotics have also been disappointing, although one study did report improved outcomes. The rationale for these studies was the identification of bacterial cell wall products in the joints of affected individuals.

### How to monitor the progress of the disease

As with the other conditions the aims of treatment are to prevent joint damage and the associated disability. Fortunately, many cases are self-limiting but may recur, particularly if the inciting agent is again encountered, such as someone reacquiring a venereal disease. Damage can occur in both peripheral joints and spine, and most rheumatologists will attempt to watch for this by both physical examination and imaging, usually plain radiography. The acute-phase response may be markedly elevated at presentation and is a good marker of disease resolution. It may also be necessary to monitor the effects (and side effects) of DMARDs such as sulfasalazine and methotrexate. All DMARDs should be used with caution in men and women of child-bearing age. Methotrexate and leflunomide in particular should be discontinued well before conception. People on DMARDs and biologic drugs should have annual influenza vaccination, and pneumococcal vaccine is also recommended for this group.

### Conclusion

Reactive arthritis is a fascinating disease that is probably becoming less prevalent. In cases where an infective trigger can be found, resolution usually occurs in a few months, although some cases become chronic. Other cases who appear clinically and radiologically to have reactive arthritis, but in whom no trigger can be found, are more likely to develop chronic arthritis.

### Further reading

▷ Hannu T, Inman R A, Granfors K, *et al*. Reactive arthritis or postinfectious arthritis? *Best Practice and Research Clinical Rheumatology* 2006; **20(3)**: 419–33.
▷ Leirisalo-Repo M. Reactive arthritis *Scandinavian Journal of Rheumatology* 2005; **34(4)**: 251–9.

---

### The arthritis of inflammatory bowel disease

### Introduction

The association of inflammatory bowel disease (IBD) with arthritis and spondylitis was studied extensively, as with the other spondyloarthropathies, in Leeds in the late 1960s and early 1970s under the guidance of Verna Wright. The prevalence of peripheral arthritis and spondylitis is probably greater in ulcerative colitis (UC) than Crohn's disease (regional enteritis): in Leeds 11.5% and 20% of subjects with UC having peripheral arthritis and spondylitis respectively.[1,21] Numerous other studies have reported the association and, on average, the prevalence of musculoskeletal involvement is probably less than the original figures from Leeds (less than 10% for both peripheral and axial arthritis). The prevalence may be changing (see section on 'Natural history and prognosis', pp. 330–1).

The peripheral arthritis particularly involves the large lower-limb joints (hip, knee and ankle) and the severity of the arthritis often parallels that of the colitis. In fact, in UC, following total colectomy, the peripheral arthritis – but sadly not the axial disease – may resolve completely. Peripheral manifestations, such as iritis, also seem to be associated with the peripheral arthritis.

### Clinical features

There are two aspects to this association. The clinical features of the spondylitis are the same as for ankylosing spondylitis, with the exception that a number of people with IBD (up to 40% in some series) have subclinical sacroiliitis. The clinical features of the peripheral arthritis have been hinted at in the 'Introduction' (pp. 309–310). Classically the arthritis is in a large lower-limb joint, it is non-erosive and often parallels the activity of the bowel disease. However, more recently the Oxford group has described a more chronic symmetrical peripheral arthritis that progresses independently of the bowel disease.[21] In addition to these two features it is worth seeking for signs of enthesitis, particularly at the major entheses (see section on 'Psoriatic arthritis', pp. 315–21).

The history should also focus on extra-articular features such as iritis and skin disease, as these may be more common in people who also develop musculoskeletal manifestations of the disease.

Sometimes the articular disease precedes the inflammatory bowel disease, rather like the arthritis of psoriatic arthritis preceding the skin disease. In the latter case the frequency of this presentation is 15% but there are no reliable figures for inflammatory bowel disease. A typical case is given in Box 13.5.

---

Box 13.5 ○ *Case study 3 – arthritis of inflammatory bowel disease*

A 35-year-old woman attended the rheumatology clinic for many years with a seronegative, non-erosive arthritis. The arthritis affected mainly the small joints of the hands and feet but on occasions an effusion was found in the knee. She smoked and drank alcohol moderately. Treatment was with NSAIDs and hydroxychloroquine. She never really achieved symptom control and frequently visited her GP. She was struggling to keep a job as a supermarket cashier.

Her GP referred her back to the rheumatology clinic and her treatment was changed to methotrexate. This unfortunately had limited effect. At every clinic visit she complained of abdominal pain and this was thought to be related to use of NSAIDs and smoking. An upper gastrointestinal endoscopy was normal. After one particularly prolonged period of diarrhoea her GP referred her for a gastroenterology opinion and ultimately Crohn's disease was diagnosed, at age 42. Treatment with mesalazine and steroids improved both gut and joint symptoms. She is currently well controlled on anti-TNF drugs.

---

## Analysis of case study 3 with respect to the six domains of Being a GP

### DOMAIN 1: PRIMARY CARE MANAGEMENT

▷ This patient really had a 'shared care' arrangement between specialist and primary care.

▷ The monitoring of her DMARDs was undertaken within general practice and a 'shared-care agreement' had been prepared by specialist care and a copy filed in the primary care notes. This outlined the responsibility of all parties in the agreement: the specialist, the GP and the patient.

▷ When the patient was unwell, the GP had referred her back into specialist care, which is appropriate.

### DOMAIN 2: PERSON-CENTRED CARE

▷ Fortunately, this patient's GP was aware of her difficulties at work and was doing his best to improve the control of her arthritis.

### DOMAIN 3: SPECIFIC PROBLEM-SOLVING SKILLS

▷ The GP had to be aware of the symptoms of uncontrolled inflammatory arthritis (pain, swelling, fatigue, morning stiffness and raised ESR and CRP) to be able to refer this patient back into specialist care.

### DOMAIN 4: A COMPREHENSIVE APPROACH

▷ When looking after this patient, the GP was aware of other co-morbidities with her arthritis. He felt that she had low-grade depression and also an increased risk of cardiovascular disease.
▷ He outlined her risks and helped her to stop smoking by referral to Help-to-Quit.

### DOMAIN 5: COMMUNITY ORIENTATION

▷ The GP decided to perform an audit on all his patients with inflammatory arthritis and look at their cardiovascular risk factors. He would therefore improve the health of his practice population and comply with recommendations for revalidation.

### DOMAIN 6: A HOLISTIC APPROACH

▷ The GP was also aware of the effect of this illness on the patient's husband and children, and the financial strain of possibly losing her job at the supermarket.

## How to diagnose the musculoskeletal manifestations of inflammatory bowel disease

There are no agreed classification or diagnostic criteria. If the patient fulfils the criteria for ankylosing spondylitis, that is sufficient for the axial disease. For the peripheral disease the presence of at least one swollen joint for a minimum of six weeks would seem a reasonable minimum definition. There is also the added consideration of enthesopathy. The same considerations apply here to those for psoriatic arthritis – the major enthesis is the Achilles insertion but other common sites are the plantar fascia, around the patella, around the pelvis and around the shoulder. Pain and tenderness at these sites, and particularly if there is swelling at the Achilles insertion may indicate inflammatory enthesopathy (inflammation at the site of tendon insertions). The difficulty is distinguishing inflammatory from degenerative enthesopathy, and ultrasound and/or MRI may be helpful in this respect.

## Natural history and prognosis

The number of referrals with this tentative diagnosis seem to be falling. There are a number of possible explanations for this. First, the disease may genuinely be less common. Second, there may be less awareness of the condition. Third, other physicians may be more willing to treat the arthritis than previously. I think there is probably some truth in each of these hypotheses but it is also worth noting that IBD is now treated more aggressively than previously and with drugs that have the potential to suppress arthritis as well as enteritis (many of the pathological processes are common to these disorders), so that the articular manifestations are suppressed by the treatment aimed primarily at the bowel disease.

### When to refer

Any musculoskeletal manifestation in people with known IBD should be referred for assessment by a rheumatologist. Interestingly, like psoriatic arthritis sine psoriasis (or psoriatic arthritis preceding the development of psoriasis) the clinical manifestations of the arthritis of IBD may precede the bowel manifestations. In fact, it is likely the bowel manifestations are present but pre-clinical or ignored (by both patient and doctor) until they become more severe. Such a case is illustrated in Box 13.5.

### Treatment

Since the activity of the peripheral arthritis often mirrors the activity of the bowel disease, treatment aimed at intestinal inflammation often improves the arthropathy. It has been found that the opposite is true also when the bowel disease was less of a consideration for the patient. The use of NSAIDs in IBD is problematic. Many gastroenterologists will argue that NSAIDs can cause an exacerbation of IBD and will ban their use. Often a more pragmatic approach can be taken, particularly if the NSAIDs are effective, as they often are in ankylosing spondylitis. There is an impression that the COX-2 inhibitors are better than traditional NSAIDs but adverse publicity in other areas such as the cardiovascular system have meant decreased prescribing of this class of drugs generally.

A number of drugs are beneficial for both the bowel and the joints: corticosteroids, of course, and sulfasalazine (now replaced by mesalazine by gastroenterologists). It is our practice to convert a patient with IBD on mesalazine to sulfasalazine, with the co-operation of the gastroenterologist. The patient gets the benefit of the drug for both gut and joints whereas with mesalazine there is no benefit for the joints. Other DMARDs used by both specialties include azathioprine and ciclosporin. However, the big breakthrough was with anti-TNF drugs, efficacious for bowel, joint and spine. Interestingly, the TNF receptor drug, etanercept, is ineffective for IBD so if an anti-TNF drug is required for both articular and bowel disease either infliximab or adalimumab (currently available) should be used.

### Conclusions

Peripheral arthritis and ankylosing spondylitis occur in association with IBD. The peripheral arthritis is usually non-erosive and may fluctuate in severity with that of the intestinal inflammation. Eradicating the intestinal disease often eliminates the peripheral arthritis but the axial disease seems to progress independently.

Traditional DMARD treatment is common for both bowel and joints. Anti-TNF monoclonal antibodies work for both, indicating the shared pathophysiology of these manifestations.

### Acknowledgement

This chapter draws, with permission, upon the following publication: Helliwell P. Psoriatic arthritis: its presentation and management in primary care. Reports on the Rheumatic Diseases (Series 6), *Hands On* 3. Arthritis Research UK; summer 2009.

### Further reading

▷ Irving P, Rampton D, Shanahan F (eds). *Clinical Dilemmas in Inflammatory Bowel Disease* Oxford: Blackwell, 2006.

---

### Possible self-assessment questions

Which is the **single most** likely place to search for hidden psoriatic plaques? Select **one** option only.

1 ▷ Under the arms
2 ▷ In the nostrils
3 ▷ In the mouth
4 ▷ Between the buttocks
5 ▷ On the shins

*Correct answer* ▷ **4**

Inflammatory back pain has several characteristics. Which is the **single most** appropriate characteristic? Select **one** option only

1 ▷ Radiation down the leg
2 ▷ Interference with bowels
3 ▷ Improved after a period of rest
4 ▷ Wakes the patient in latter half of night
5 ▷ Paraesthesia

*Correct answer* ▷ **4**

**References**

1 • Macrae I, Wright V. A family study of ulcerative colitis, with particular reference to ankylosing spondylitis and sacro-iliitis *Annals of the Rheumatic Diseases* 1973; **32**: 16–20.

2 • Haslock I, Wright V. The arthritis associated with intestinal disease *Bulletin on the Rheumatic Diseases* 1973; **24**: 740–54.

3 • Iveson J M L, Nanda B S, Hancock J A H, *et al*. Reiter's disease in three boys *Annals of the Rheumatic Diseases* 1975; **34**: 364.

4 • Wright V, Moll J M H. Behcet's syndrome. In: V Wright, J M H Moll (eds). *Seronegative Polyarthritis* Amsterdam: North Holland, 1976, pp. 353–70.

5 • Moll J M H, Wright V. Psoriatic arthritis *Seminars in Arthritis and Rheumatism* 1973; **3**: 51–78.

6 • Moll J M H, Wright V. Familial occurrence of psoriatic arthritis *Annals of the Rheumatic Diseases* 1973; **32**: 181.

7 • Eastmond C J, Rajah S M, Tovey D, *et al*. HLA typing in seronegative oligoarthritis *Annals of the Rheumatic Diseases* 1979; **38**: 564–5.

8 • Wright V, Moll J M H. *Seronegative Polyarthritis* Amsterdam: North Holland, 1976.

9 • Brewerton D A, Caffrey M, Hart F D, *et al*. Ankylosing spondylitis and HL-A27 *Lancet* 1973; **1**: 904–7.

10 • Zochling J, van der Heijde D, Burgos-Vargas R, *et al*. ASAS/EULAR recommendations for the management of ankylosing spondylitis *Annals of the Rheumatic Diseases* 2006; **65(4)**: 442–52.

11 • National Institute for Health and Clinical Guidance. *Adalimumab, Etanercept and Infliximab for Ankylosing Spondylitis* (NICE technology appraisal guidance 143) London: NICE, 2008, www.nice.org.uk/guidance/TA143 [accessed October 2011].

12 • Ibrahim G, Buch M, Lawson C, *et al*. Evaluation of an existing screening tool for psoriatic arthritis in people with psoriasis and development of a new instrument: the Psoriasis Epidemiology Screening Tool (PEST) questionnaire *Clinical and Experimental Rheumatology* 2009; **27(3)**: 469–74.

13 • Ritchlin C T, Kavanaugh A, Gladman D D, *et al*. Treatment recommendations for psoriatic arthritis *Annals of the Rheumatic Diseases* 2009; **68(9)**: 1387–94.

14 • National Institute for Health and Clinical Guidance. *Etanercept and Infliximab for the Treatment of Adults with Psoriatic Arthritis* (NICE technology appraisal guidance 104) London: NICE, 2006, www.nice.org.uk/Guidance/TA104 [accessed October 2011].

15 • Kavanaugh A F, Ritchlin C T; GRAPPA Treatment Guideline Committee. Systematic review of treatments for psoriatic arthritis: an evidence based approach and basis for treatment guidelines *Journal of Rheumatology* 2006; **33(7)**: 1417–21.

16 • Chakravarty K, McDonald H, Pullar T, *et al*. BSR/BHPR guideline for disease-modifying anti-rheumatic drug (DMARD) therapy in consultation with the British Association of Dermatologists *Rheumatology* 2008; **47(6)**: 924–5.

17 • Sokoll K B, Helliwell P S. Comparison of disability and quality of life in rheumatoid and psoriatic arthritis *Journal of Rheumatology* 2001; **28(8)**: 1842–6.

18 • Jeffcoate WJ. Should eponyms be actively detached from diseases? *Lancet* 2009; **367(9519)**: 1296–7.

19 • Keat A. Reiter's syndrome and reactive arthritis in perspective *New England Journal of Medicine* 1983; **309**: 1606–15.

20 • Leirisalo-Repo M. Reactive arthritis *Scandinavian Journal of Rheumatology* 2005; **34**: 251–9.

21 • Wright V, Watkinson G. The arthritis of ulcerative colitis *British Medical Journal* 1965; **2**: 670–5.

22 • Orchard T R, Wordsworth B P, Jewell D P. Peripheral arthropathies in inflammatory bowel disease: their articular distribution and natural history *Gut* 1998; **42**: 387–91.

# Connective tissue diseases

## 14

*Graham Davenport*

**Aims of this chapter**

▶ To describe how connective tissue disorders (CTDs) present in primary care and the main differences between them.
▶ To identify when to consider an underlying CTD in a patient, red-flag symptoms and indications for investigation and referral to specialist care.
▶ To clarify the GP and practice team's role in the monitoring of treatment for CTDs.
▶ To describe the options for managing CTD patients holistically in primary care.

CTDs are chronic inflammatory autoimmune disorders that can affect all connective tissues, i.e. joints, skin, muscles and blood vessels, and therefore have multiple effects on many different organs throughout the body.

The incidence of CTDs in the primary care population is relatively low apart from rheumatoid arthritis (RA) and polymyalgia rheumatica, which are covered in separate chapters.

Patients with CTDs are usually managed in secondary or tertiary care but, in view of the multisystem effects of CTDs, GPs and their teams will be involved in their care to varying degrees.

GPs cannot expect to be knowledgeable about all of the rare CTDs but they need to be aware of:

▶ common presentations
▶ differential diagnoses
▶ which investigations to carry out
▶ how to monitor the treatment prescribed in secondary care
▶ how to support these patients through a lifetime of chronic illness.

## The most common presentations of CTD

Patients with CTD commonly present with one or more of the following:

▷ Raynaud's phenomenon
▷ generalised arthralgia or arthritis
▷ non-specific syndromes.

Raynaud's phenomenon is due to intermittent vasospasm of the peripheral arteries, which causes temporary ischaemia.[1] It is categorised as primary or secondary.

Primary Raynaud's phenomenon:

▷ is usually benign
▷ has no underlying cause
▷ is commoner in young females
▷ is often seen in general practice.

Secondary Raynaud's phenomenon:

▷ occurs in CTD
▷ is often associated with other features that suggest individual organ involvement
▷ is commoner in males and the elderly
▷ may be caused by occlusive arterial disease, drugs (e.g. beta-blockers), polycythaemia and occupational hazard (e.g. vibrating tools).

Classically, the fingers go through a sequence of colour changes from initially being white, due to vasospasm, then, as reperfusion occurs, the fingers go blue and finally red, at which point there is often associated pain and burning (see Figure 14.1 on p. 478). Necrosis may occur with secondary Raynaud's.

**Practical tip** ▶ to aid diagnosis, ask the patient to photograph his or her hands, perhaps using a mobile phone, the next time it occurs.

---

Box 14.1 ○ *Case study 1*

---

**Mrs Carter, a 27-year-old housewife, attends your surgery complaining of cold, blue hands.**

Take a moment or two to consider the following questions:

▶ What *important points in the history* do you need to cover?
▶ What would you look for on *examination*?
▶ How would you *investigate* her?
▶ How would you *manage* her?

The important points in the history to cover are:

▷ distinctive colour changes from pallor through to cyanosis and erythema
▷ frequency of attacks
▷ symptoms brought on by exposure to cold
▷ occupational, smoking and drug history (beta-blockers, ergotamine and clonidine can precipitate symptoms)
▷ symptoms of possible underlying CTD, i.e. arthralgia, skin rashes, dry eyes and acid reflux.

Upon examination, the GP should:

▷ look for fingertip ulceration
▷ check blood pressure
▷ check peripheral pulses.

A GP should request the following investigations:

▷ full blood count (FBC)
▷ erythrocyte sedimentation rate (ESR)
▷ antinuclear antibodies (ANA)
▷ renal and liver function, immunoglobulins and electrophoresis
▷ dipstick urine for protein or blood.

She should be advised to:

▷ stop smoking, if appropriate
▷ keep hands and feet warm
▷ exercise regularly.

You should stop any drug that may be causing Raynaud's. If symptoms persist, nifedipine can be prescribed, initially at 20 mg a day. Other drug treatments used include prazosin. Referral to a rheumatologist should be considered.

**Warning** ▶ occasionally, an acute episode can be prolonged. Persistently pale fingers may warrant emergency admission for intravenous iloprost infusions to prevent irreversible ischaemia and tissue necrosis.

## Self-assessment questions

Which of the following statements are true of Raynaud's? Select **true** or **false** for each.

**A** ▷ Is usually associated with CTD
**B** ▷ Can be precipitated by calcium channel blockers
**C** ▷ Fingers change colour from white to blue to red
**D** ▷ Is always mild and reversible

Which of the following diseases are associated with Raynaud's? Select **one or more** of the following diseases:

▷ systemic sclerosis
▷ systemic lupus erythematosus
▷ dermatomyositis
▷ RA
▷ osteoarthritis

### ANSWERS

**A** ▷ *False* ▶ Only about 10% of Raynaud's is due to CTD
**B** ▷ *False* ▶ Calcium channel blockers, e.g. nifedipine, are used to treat Raynaud's
**C** ▷ *True*
**D** ▷ *False* ▶ Raynaud's may develop into a severe condition that requires urgent treatment in hospital

All of the diseases are associated with Raynaud's, except for osteoarthritis.

---

## Systemic lupus erythematosus

▷ Systemic lupus erythematosus (SLE) is a multisystem autoimmune disease.
▷ It is common in women and those from non-white ethnic backgrounds.
▷ Lupus nephritis can occur in up to 50% of patients.

SLE has widespread clinical manifestations as a result of the different symptoms and signs, and its effect on the various organs (see Figure 14.2 on p. 478). It is a multifactorial disease caused by a complex set of environmental and genetic factors. Some infections such as the Epstein–Barr virus and certain drugs, such as hydralazine, can trigger the disease.

Arthritis will occur in 70–90% of patients with SLE; alopecia is common as are mouth ulcers. Photosensitivity occurs in 10–60%. Skin rashes are particularly common, in particular the malar or 'butterfly' rash (see Figure 14.3 on p. 479).

**Practical tip** ▸ the classic 'butterfly' malar rash of SLE does not affect the nasolabial folds, which helps to distinguish it from acne rosacea and seborrhoeic dermatitis.

The other complications associated with SLE are as follows.

### Acute hot joint

An acute hot joint in a CTD, such as SLE, should not be considered a flare-up of disease activity until septic arthritis has been excluded. Sepsis is much commoner in the immunosuppressed and needs to be excluded by aspiration.

Sepsis cannot be treated by oral antibiotics in primary care but needs admission for assessment and intravenous antibiotics.

### Cerebral lupus

Cerebral lupus is a serious condition occurring in up to 1 in 6 of SLE patients and can cause prolonged headaches, seizures, strokes, acute psychotic episodes and severe depression.

Cerebral lupus is usually associated with a flare-up in disease activity elsewhere. GPs must exclude other causes such as corticosteroid psychosis, sepsis and malignant hypertension.

Non-steroidal anti-inflammatory drugs (NSAIDs) can cause cerebral symptoms of headache, confusion and giddiness, which may be mistaken for cerebral lupus.

**Practical tip** ▸ depression in SLE is common but only a small proportion will be due to cerebral lupus.[2]

### Premature coronary artery disease

Premature coronary artery disease due to accelerated atherosclerosis results in women with SLE having an increased risk of myocardial infarction.[3]

Regular annual screening of SLE patients for cardiovascular risk factors is recommended, with a low threshold for intervention, i.e. the target blood pressure in SLE is 130/80 and the target low-density lipoprotein (LDL) is

339

<2.6 mmol/l. Prophylactic low-dose aspirin should be used in all SLE patients.[4]

**Practical tip** ▶ statins have recently been shown to have a disease-modifying effect in SLE and, therefore, may have a dual benefit in these patients.[5]

### Diagnosis

Blood tests will often show anaemia. Leucopenia and thrombocytopenia are common. ANAs are usually positive. Extractable nuclear antigens (ENAs), which are antibodies to antigens extracted from DNA, may be positive. In particular, the following are associated with SLE:

▷ anti-Sm
▷ anti-RNP
▷ anti-Ro
▷ anti-La.

The particular pattern of positivity of these ENAs will define the clinical type of CTD.

Renal function should be monitored, including glomerular filtration rate. Urinalysis for blood, protein and casts should be carried out to monitor the development of lupus nephritis. CRP and ESR investigations should be implemented; usually the CRP is normal in SLE but the ESR is raised. Complement levels may be depleted.

Once a diagnosis is made, the patient should be referred to secondary care for assessment and treatment.

### Treatment

Although SLE is treated with drug therapies such as antimalarials, immunosuppressives and corticosteroids in secondary care, GPs have an important role in providing holistic care.

Primary care should provide prompt treatment for infections and also advise the patient on:

▷ avoiding exposure to the sun
▷ cardiovascular risk management, e.g. hypertension and hyperlipidaemia[6]
▷ osteoporosis prevention.

The GP should also screen for depression and provide pre-pregnancy coun-selling, the latter to ensure optimal disease control and drug therapy before pregnancy.

**Practical tip** ▶ asymptomatic proteinuria may be the only indication of autoimmune nephritis in SLE, and quantitative assessment, renal function investigations and renal biopsy will probably be required.

### Presentation with arthritis and arthralgia

SLE is one of the commonest CTDs to present with arthritis and arthralgia. Arthritis in SLE is often asymmetrical and usually non-erosive, but there is invariably considerable arthralgia, pain and early-morning stiffness, with a marginally raised ESR.

A proportion of patients with SLE develop Jaccoud's arthritis (see Figure 14.4 on p. 479) with ulnar deviation, swan-neck deformities and subluxa-tions. Absence of erosions and reversibility of the swan-neck deformities in early disease help to distinguish Jaccoud's arthritis from RA.

Severe arthralgias also occur in Sjögren's syndrome and systemic sclerosis (SS).

Apart from the association with arthritis and arthralgia, SLE can also commonly present with:

▷ Raynaud's phenomenon
▷ non-specific symptoms such as lethargy, malaise, fever, headaches and fibromyalgia
▷ mouth ulcers, skin rashes, lymphadenopathy and splenomegaly
▷ commonly, tenosynovitis of flexor finger tendons
▷ multiple allergies antiphospholipid syndrome (APS) (in about 20% of patients).

SLE may present in teenage life with growing pains, migraines and per-sistent 'glandular fever'.

**Note** ▶ Infection can precipitate SLE.

### Self-assessment question

Which of the following statements are true of SLE? Select **true** or **false** for each.

**A** ▷ May present in teenagers as growing pains or migraine
**B** ▷ The oral contraceptive pill should be avoided in SLE
**C** ▷ ESR is usually normal but CRP is raised
**D** ▷ Patients usually have joint erosions

**ANSWERS**

**A** ▷ *True* ▶ SLE can also present as persistent 'glandular fever' in teenagers
**B** ▷ *False* ▶ Most women can have the oral contraceptive pill apart from those with a history of thrombosis, a positive lupus anticoagulant test or the APS
**C** ▷ *False* ▶ Usually active SLE is associated with a raised ESR and a normal CRP. If the CRP is raised, a possible infection should be suspected
**D** ▷ *False* ▶ SLE is classically a non-erosive polyarthropathy

---

Box 14.2 ○ *Case study 2*

Mrs Hayward, a 45-year-old teacher, comes to see you because she has had pleuritic chest pain for a few days. She has had SLE for over 20 years and is on a small dose of oral prednisolone (5 mg daily) to control her symptoms.

Take a moment to consider what other information you need to elicit. The questions you should consider asking include:

▶ Are there any symptoms of respiratory tract infection, e.g. cough, sore throat, nasal congestion or purulent sputum?

▶ Is there any haemoptysis, calf swelling, pain or tenderness?

▶ Is she on the oral contraceptive pill, is she a smoker and is there any past history of thromboembolism, including miscarriages?

▶ Is there any associated thoracic back pain or pain associated with movement?

▶ Is there any history of a fall or local rib tenderness?

▶ Is there any family history of osteoporosis?

## Self-assessment question

Which of the following would be characteristic causes of pleuritic pain in a patient with SLE? Select **one or more** options from the list below:

A ▷ Pleurisy associated with her SLE
B ▷ Lower respiratory tract infection
C ▷ Pulmonary embolus
D ▷ Osteoporotic fracture of rib or thoracic spine
E ▷ Acid reflux
F ▷ Shingles

### ANSWER

Pleurisy associated with SLE, lower respiratory tract infection, pulmonary embolus (especially if the patient has a history of thromboembolism or ASP) and osteoporotic fracture of rib or thoracic spine are characteristically associated with pleuritic chest pain.

Shingles would typically give constant chest pain in a dermatome for several days prior to onset of a vesicular rash. Although acid reflux can cause retrosternal chest pain, it would not be pleuritic.

If Mrs Hayward's pain was not pleuritic, other causes of acute chest pain to consider would include:

▷ acute pericarditis (can be pleuritic or non-pleuritic)
▷ angina
▷ costochondritis (can be pleuritic or non-pleuritic)
▷ fibromyalgia
▷ gastritis/reflux
▷ osteoporotic vertebral collapse
▷ pulmonary embolism (can be pleuritic or non-pleuritic)
▷ renal vein thrombosis.

## How would you manage the patient?

If Mrs Hayward had symptoms and signs consistent with a respiratory tract infection and her observations are satisfactory, she could be managed in primary care with antibiotics, an increase in her oral corticosteroids, and monitoring with a chest X-ray, blood tests and regular follow-up as required.

On examination, the patient has a tachycardia, feels short of breath and is in considerable pain despite analgesia.

## What should you do?

Mrs Hayward should be referred to secondary care for further investigations, especially to exclude a pulmonary embolus.

The patient was admitted to hospital, where investigations showed no pulmonary embolus, but X-rays showed a crush fracture of T6 vertebra. She was discharged.

## Self-assessment question

How would you manage her now? Select **one** or **more** options from the list below.

A ▷ Adequate analgesia
B ▷ Increased corticosteroid dose
C ▷ Starting bisphosphonate with calcium and vitamin D
D ▷ Advising a vigorous exercise regimen
E ▷ Referral for a DXA scan
F ▷ Discussing risk factors for osteoporosis

### ANSWER

It would be correct to:

▷ ensure she has adequate analgesia
▷ start bisphosphonate with calcium and vitamin D immediately, assuming no contraindications (e.g. peptic ulceration or impaired renal function)[7]
▷ discuss osteoporosis and any possible preventable risk factors, e.g. diet, exercise, alcohol intake and smoking history, reduction of corticosteroid dose
▷ refer for a DXA scan, if available.

Corticosteroids are the main contributory factor in her developing a crush fracture.[8] She should be maintained on the minimum dosage required to control her SLE. Although exercise is beneficial in the long term for preventing osteoporosis, it is not appropriate in this situation and could exacerbate the pain from her crush fracture.

## Antiphospholipid syndrome

APS (or Hughes syndrome) is an important cause of recurrent arterial and venous thrombosis and miscarriages, and the syndrome is associated with antiphospholipid antibodies.

The laboratory tests for antiphospholipid antibodies are:

▷ anticardiolipin antibodies
▷ lupus anticoagulant.

### Clinical features

The following conditions are all associated with APS:

▷ venous thromboses, e.g. deep-vein thrombosis or pulmonary embolus
▷ arterial thromboses, e.g. strokes and transient ischaemic attacks
▷ fetal death beyond 10 weeks' gestation with confirmed normal fetal morphology
▷ recurrent miscarriages before 12 weeks
▷ premature birth due to severe placental insufficiency, pre-eclampsia or eclampsia before 34 weeks' gestation
▷ livedo reticularis.

On investigation, there is often thrombocytopenia and haemolytic anaemia.

The treatment is anticoagulation, probably for life, with ongoing management of cardiovascular risk factors. Pregnant patients should be closely monitored. In patients with CTD who are seeking contraceptive advice, there is no evidence that the combined oral contraceptive pill engenders any greater risk, unless the patient has a positive lupus anticoagulant or cardiolipin antibodies, in which case it should be avoided.

## Systemic sclerosis

Systemic sclerosis (SS) is divided into a number of subsets depending on the degree of skin involvement, including *diffuse* scleroderma when the trunk as well as the face and limbs are affected, and *limited* scleroderma with no truncal involvement.

The characteristic skin changes of scleroderma include tightening and thickening of the skin, dermal atrophy, telangiectases and variable pigmentation. **CREST** syndrome is one of the commonest forms of limited scleroderma and patients often have calcinosis in the fingertips, which resemble gouty tophi (see Figure 14.5 on p. 480). CREST stands for:

▷ **C**alcinosis
▷ **R**aynaud's phenomenon
▷ **E**sophageal hypomobility
▷ **S**clerodactyly
▷ **T**elangiectases.

Diagnosis of the CREST syndrome is based upon patients having at least three of these features.

### Self-assessment question

**Q** ▷ How can you distinguish between calcinosis and gouty tophi?

### ANSWER

You can distinguish between calcinosis and gouty tophi by looking at X-rays (see Figure 14.6 on p. 480):

▷ tophi are radiolucent
▷ calcific nodules are radio-opaque.

### Clinical features of systemic sclerosis

For patients with SS, Raynaud's phenomenon usually precedes other symptoms by many years. Patients usually have non-specific symptoms, such as fatigue, weight loss and arthralgia. Depression occurs in 50% of patients.[9] However, the main problem is restriction of movement and muscle atrophy, due to scleroderma.

Specific symptoms presented by patients with scleroderma include:

▷ respiratory symptoms, e.g. dyspnoea on exertion and chronic cough, due to interstitial fibrosis and pulmonary hypertension (especially in CREST syndrome)
▷ congestive cardiac failure, in late disease.

Scleroderma crisis occurs in SS as a result of rapidly increasing hypertension associated with deteriorating renal function, progressing to acute renal failure.

Frequent monitoring of blood pressure in SS patients and early intervention with ACE inhibitors is essential to prevent a crisis.

### Diagnosis – laboratory tests

Patients will often have a positive ANA and positive anticentromere antibodies. Other antibodies sometimes found in SS are anti-ThRNP, anti-topo-1, anti-RNA polymerases and anti-U3RNP.

### Treatment of systemic sclerosis

Unfortunately there is no curative treatment for SS; therapies are supportive and aim to treat the sequelae of the disease, such as pulmonary hypertension.

## Polymyositis and dermatomyositis

These conditions are similar in presentation to each other. Profound muscle weakness occurs in polymyositis and dermatomyositis, and is bilateral and symmetrical, affecting the proximal muscles of the shoulder and pelvic girdles.

The conditions are diagnosed by finding a raised creatine kinase, indicating muscle damage, positive ANA and positive anti-Jo1 in the ENAs test. Electromyography (EMG) also shows a characteristic appearance. It is possible to distinguish between polymyalgia rheumatica, which also causes muscle pain, and polymyositis (see Table 14.1):

Table 14.1 ○ *Differences between polymyalgia rheumatica and polymyositis*

|  | Polymyalgia rheumatica | Polymyositis |
|---|---|---|
| Pain | +++ | +++ |
| Tenderness | + | +++ |
| Weakness | None | +++ |
| Creatine kinase | Normal | Raised |

Dermatomyositis is associated with a distinctive purplish rash, mainly on the face and hands. Periorbital oedema is also often present. In dermatomyositis, Gottron's papules are erythematous flat skin lesions that develop over the interphalangeal joints.

In the elderly with dermatomyositis, there is an increased risk of malignancy of about 30%.

## Sjögren's syndrome

Sjögren's syndrome is classically associated with:

▷ keratoconjunctivitis sicca (or dry-eye syndrome)
▷ xerostomia (dry mouth)
▷ parotid gland enlargement
▷ arthritis, usually non-erosive
▷ Raynaud's phenomenon.

Sjögren's can also be associated with:

▷ RA
▷ SLE

and there is an increased risk of lymphoid malignancy.

**348**

**Practical tip** ▶ if there are marked symptoms of arthralgia with associated pain and stiffness but little objective evidence of clinical synovitis, think of CTD.

### Tests for Sjögren's

The ESR is usually very elevated with a normal CRP. Auto-antibodies are common, e.g. positive rheumatoid factor and ANA. Positive anti-Ro and anti-La will be present in the ENAs test.

A Schirmer's test identifies reduced tear secretion (see Figure 14.7 on p. 481). A strip of paper is placed in the eyelid and the absorption of tears is measured in millimetres.

### Treatment for Sjögren's

Treatment of the sicca syndrome is with artificial tear drops and salivary substitutes and stimulants. Systemic corticosteroids and immunosuppressive drugs are used for severe systemic disease.

**Practical tip** ▶ patients with Sjögren's syndrome often have fatigue and joint pain, which is difficult to manage. They can be wrongly diagnosed as having fibromyalgia.

### Dry-eye syndrome (keratoconjunctivitis sicca)

Dry-eye syndrome is caused by a reduction in lacrimal gland secretion and is a common, benign condition in the elderly. It can also be associated with nearly all CTDs, especially Sjögren's syndrome, and can occur in other chronic diseases, e.g. sarcoidosis, and in human immunodeficiency virus (HIV) infection and hepatitis C infection.

Symptoms of dry eye include:

▷ dryness, soreness or irritation
▷ sensation of a foreign body
▷ photophobia
▷ discomfort and sometimes pain.

There may be mild conjunctival infection, and diagnosis is by Schirmer's test or by fluorescein staining for punctuate dry spots on the cornea. Patients are more vulnerable to infection and corneal ulcers.

**349**

### Malignancy

GPs need to be aware of the increased risk of malignancy associated with some CTDs, particularly in Sjögren's syndrome, SS and dermatomyositis.

GPs need to retain a high index of suspicion in patients who develop a myositis and have risk factors such as a strong family history of malignancy, especially ovarian. These patients should be screened on presentation.

Alveolar cell carcinoma of the lung can occur in SS and is usually associated with pulmonary fibrosis.

Immunosuppressive treatment may be associated with malignancy, e.g. cyclophosphamide with carcinoma of the bladder, or azathioprine with non-Hodgkin's lymphoma.

Conversely, *occult malignancy*, especially lung and breast, can present with a polyarthropathy or a polymyalgia-like syndrome.

**Practical tip** ▶ if a patient complains of shoulder-tip pain without any signs of a musculoskeletal problem, consider malignancy. Both thoracic and intra-abdominal malignancy can give shoulder-tip pain and a full examination, chest X-ray and an ultrasound abdominal examination may be required.

## Investigations

The advantage for GPs is that the diagnosis of CTD is usually made on clinical grounds and investigations often add very little. Tests should only be ordered if there is reasonable clinical evidence to suspect a CTD rather than performing an 'autoimmune screen' in patients who are just unwell. *This is because up to 15% of healthy women of middle age or older will have a positive ANA.*

### Self-assessment question

Which investigations would you request if a CTD is suspected from the clinical picture?

#### ANSWER

The investigations that should be requested include:

### Inflammatory markers

ESR and C-reactive protein (CRP) are fairly non-specific tests that indicate the presence of inflammation and are useful to monitor disease activity as well as in the diagnosis of inflammatory joint disease. However, you should bear in mind that:

▷ normal results for these two tests can occur in SLE and other CTDs, such as SS
▷ ESR can be elevated in conditions such as gout, or pseudogout in osteoarthritis, and in normal individuals
▷ ESR tends to rise with age, and women over 80 years can often have an ESR of about 40 mm/h
▷ ESR can be markedly elevated in temporal arteritis and in Sjögren's syndrome, with levels of over 100 mm/h occurring frequently.

### Full blood count

Many patients with SLE will have a mild neutropenia and lymphopenia, which suggest the need for further investigations in the arthralgic patient. Anaemia of chronic disease is common and may improve with control of disease activity. Other anaemias can occur, such as haemolytic anaemia in SLE.

**Practical tip** ▶ it is important to remember that not all anaemia is due to the disease process, e.g. all non-steroidal anti-inflammatory drugs (NSAIDs) can cause upper and lower gastrointestinal bleeding and may be a cause of occult blood loss resulting in an iron-deficiency anaemia.

### Auto-antibody tests

ANA is the best screening test for CTD, although it is not specific and is often positive in low titre in the healthy elderly.

### Extractable nuclear antigens

Most good immunology laboratories will test ENAs in all patients with a high-titre ANA. It is not necessary to request a specific ENA such as anti-Ro. Give as much clinical information as possible on the request form and the lab will endeavour to perform the most relevant tests.

### Rheumatoid factor

This can be positive in all the CTDs and also in the healthy population and, therefore, are of little use in diagnosis.

### Urinalysis

The simple tests are often the best!

**Practical tip** ▶ if a patient whom you suspect of having CTD has dip test haematuria and proteinuria, exclude infection. If negative for infection, seek the advice of your local renal physician.

### Synovial fluid aspiration

This can be helpful in the differential diagnosis of other conditions such as osteoarthritis and gout, as well as excluding septic arthritis.

**Practical tip** ▶ radiology may be useful to distinguish erosive arthropathy from the non-erosive arthropathy of SLE.

### Self-assessment question

Which of the following statements are true of ESR? Select **true** or **false** for each.

A ▷ An ESR of 40 mm/h in an elderly woman is indicative of polymyalgia rheumatica

B ▷ An ESR is usually normal in Sjögren's disease but raised in RA

C ▷ A normal ESR can occur with inflammatory rheumatic disease

D ▷ A raised ESR and normal CRP in SLE means that there is minimal disease activity or it is in remission

### ANSWERS

A ▷ *False* ▶ The ESR is a non-specific test that is raised in a number of inflammatory conditions. Although an ESR over 40 mm/h is common in polymyalgia rheumatica, it rises with age and it is not uncommon for a woman over 80 years to have an ESR of about 40 mm/h

B ▷ *False* ▶ The ESR is usually raised in RA but is often markedly elevated (over 100 mm/h) in Sjögren's

C ▷ *True* ▶ The ESR can often be normal in the presence of synovitis, radiographic progression of joint destruction and increasing disability

D ▷ False ▶ SLE may be active with a raised ESR and normal CRP

---

## Treatment

Treatment of CTD is usually initiated in secondary care and includes:

▷ NSAIDs
▷ corticosteroids
▷ immunosuppressants.

### Non-steroidal anti-inflammatory drugs

All NSAIDs are now thought to increase cardiovascular risk, and GPs should try to avoid using them in hypertensive patients, patients with poor renal function and elderly patients at risk of heart failure.

**Practical tip** ▶ although NSAIDs are often useful in SLE they can cause deteriorating renal function or neuro-psychiatric symptoms.

For patients on NSAIDs the GP should:

▷ use the lowest dose for the shortest time
▷ check for over-the-counter NSAIDs self-treatment
▷ co-prescribe a proton pump inhibitor
▷ avoid co-prescribing with low-dose aspirin and ACE inhibitors
▷ monitor at least annually the patient's blood pressure, full blood count, renal and liver function
▷ consider that better control of the disease activity with immunosuppressives may enable reduction in NSAIDs dosage.

### Corticosteroid therapy

GPs should ensure that patients are carrying a steroid card and co-prescribe bisphosphonates and calcium with vitamin D if indicated. GPs should also monitor patients for the development of infections and diabetes, and heart failure in the elderly.

**Practical tip** ▶ avoid live vaccines but ensure these patients have pneumo-coccal vaccination and an annual influenza vaccination.

### Immunosupressants

The main side effects of immunosuppressive therapy are:

▷ gastrointestinal, e.g. stomatitis and nausea with methotrexate, which can often be resolved by folic acid treatment, except on the day that methotrexate is taken
▷ bone marrow suppression, which can occur with all immunosuppressives, therefore requiring regular blood counts to be mandatory, especially with a dose increase
▷ hepatic toxicity, meaning that patients on methotrexate should be advised not to drink alcohol
▷ drug interactions, with many drugs increasing the toxicity of immunosuppressives – all co-prescribing must be carefully monitored
▷ pulmonary involvement, e.g. a pneumonitis caused by methotrexate can be fatal if untreated. All patients on methotrexate who develop a persistent cough or dyspnoea must be investigated.

Also, the GP should ensure that women use contraception when taking immunosuppressants because they can be teratogenic.

GPs could also use the following symptom-specific treatments:

▷ **photosensitivity** ▶ can be minimised by prescribing sunblock creams for exposed parts

▷ **Sjögren's syndrome** ▶ dry eyes can be helped by artificial tears. Dry mouth is helped by deliberately salivating and good dental care is also important

▷ **Raynaud's phenomenon** ▶ all patients should be advised to stop smoking and to keep their hands warm. Beta-blockers should be stopped if possible. Drug treatment includes calcium channel blockers (e.g. nifedipine) and prazosin.

### Self-assessment questions

Which of the following statements are true about what NSAIDs can cause? Select **true** or **false** for each.

**A** ▷ Gastrointestinal symptoms
**B** ▷ Polycythaemia
**C** ▷ Headaches, confusion and giddiness
**D** ▷ Deterioration of renal function

**ANSWERS**

**A** ▷ *True* ▶ Any patient starting a NSAID should also be co-prescribed a PPI
**B** ▷ *False* ▶ NSAIDS can cause an iron-deficiency anaemia due to occult blood loss from the upper OR lower gastrointestinal tract
**C** ▷ *True* ▶ Can often be mistaken for dementia in the elderly or a deterioration in the CTD
**D** ▷ *True* ▶ Renal function should be monitored at least yearly and NSAIDs should be avoided in patients with poor renal function

Which of the following statements about methotrexate are true? Select **true** or **false** for each.

**A** ▷ Should be given as a weekly dose only
**B** ▷ Should be monitored regularly for FBC, renal and liver function
**C** ▷ Nausea can be controlled by giving folic acid 5 mg at the same time as the weekly methotrexate dose
**D** ▷ A flare-up in one joint should be treated by increasing the methotrexate dose

**ANSWERS**

**A** ▷ *True* ▶ It is essential that prescribing protocols are in place to avoid any possibility of methotrexate being taken daily, which could be fatal

**B** ▷ *True* ▶ Monthly monitoring of FBC and liver and renal function would be usual, but more frequent monitoring should be undertaken during dosage increases

**C** ▷ *False* ▶ Folic acid interferes with methotrexate metabolism and should be given on any day apart from the day methotrexate is taken

**D** ▷ *False* ▶ A flare-up in one joint raises the suspicion of septic arthritis and should be investigated accordingly

---

## Conclusion

Most CTDs are chronic, lifelong diseases with exacerbations and relapses. GPs and primary care teams are ideally placed to support patients with these conditions; good communication, robust management plans and teamwork between primary and secondary care are essential. GPs, primary care nurses, clinical nurse specialists and other allied professionals provide support for these patients in the community, but rapid access to secondary care during crises and relapses is also essential.

GPs and other primary care professionals have a critical role in educating patients and directing them to other sources of information and support. Empowerment of the patients to manage their own diseases is a vital part of their education and the essence of the NHS Expert Patient Programme (EPP).

Such programmes and support groups are not just about managing the practical aspects of living with a chronic disabling condition. They also enable patients and families to acknowledge, express and explore their fears and concerns, and enable them to maximise their control over their condition. Through partnership with the patient and by adopting a holistic approach, practitioners can enable patients to achieve the optimum quality of life.

### *Key points*

▶ Raynaud's phenomenon can be diagnosed and treated in primary care but may be secondary to a CTD.

▶ SLE is a multisystem disease that can present with a non-erosive arthritis and miscellaneous symptoms such as skin rashes, proteinuria, pleurisy and thromboses.

▶ Malignancy can mimic CTDs in presentation but there is also an increased risk in some conditions, e.g. Sjögren's, dermatomyositis.

▶ Holistic management is vital – GPs should assess the cardiovascular risk, osteoporosis risk and mental state of all patients with CTD.

Having read the chapter GPs should be able to:

▷ describe how CTDs present and the main differences between them

▷ recognise common CTDs including SLE, Sjögren's syndrome and Raynaud's phenomenon

▷ identify when to consider an underlying CTD in a patient, red-flag symptoms and indications for investigation and referral to specialist care

▷ clarify the GP and practice team's role in the monitoring of treatment for CTDs

▷ describe the options for managing CTD patients holistically in primary care.

## References

1 • Bakst R, Merola J F, Franks A G Jr, *et al.* Raynaud's phenomenon: pathogenesis and management *Journal of the American Academy of Dermatology* 2008; **59(4)**: 633–53.

2 • Hay E M, Huddy A, Black D, *et al.* A prospective study of psychiatric disorder and cognitive function in systemic lupus erythematosus *Annals of the Rheumatic Diseases* 1994; **53(5)**: 298–303.

3 • Bacon P A, Stevens R J, Carruthers D M, *et al.* Accelerated atherogenesis in autoimmune rheumatic diseases *Autoimmunity Reviews* 2002; **1(6)**: 338–47.

4 • Symmons D, Bruce I. Management of cardiovascular risk in R A and SLE *Hands On: arc reports on the rheumatic diseases* 2006; **5(8)**.

5 • Kwak B, Mulhaupt F, Myit S, *et al.* Statins as a newly recognized type of immunomodulator *Nature Medicine* 2000; **6(12)**:1399–402.

6 • Wajed J, Ahmad Y, Durrington P N, *et al.* Prevention of cardiovascular disease in systemic lupus erythematosus: proposed guidelines for risk factor management *Rheumatology* (Oxford) 2004; **43(1)**: 7–12.

7 • Guidelines Writing Group. *Glucocorticoid-Induced Osteoporosis: guidelines for prevention and treatment* London: Royal College of Physicians, 2002.

8 • Lukert B P, Raisz L G. Glucocorticoid-induced osteoporosis: pathogenesis and management *Annals of Internal Medicine* 1990; **112(5)**: 352–64.

9 • Roca R P, Wigley F M, White B. Depressive symptoms associated with scleroderma *Arthritis and Rheumatism* 1996; **39(6)**: 1035–40.

# Hypermobility

## 15

*Jean Oliver*

## Definition of hypermobility

When used in relation to a joint, hypermobility (HM) indicates its ability to move beyond the normal range of movement expected for that particular joint. The age, gender and ethnic background of the individual[1] need to be taken into account, as joint movement diminishes with age, and females usually display a greater range of movement than males. (The patient in this article will therefore be referred to as 'she'.) However, the incidence of HM in Europe is unknown; Asians are considered to have the greatest range of joint movement, and Europeans the least.[2] Forty-three per cent of a West African tribe scored > 3/9 on the Beighton scale.[3]

HM is not, however, confined to joints. It is the outward manifestation of a disorder of the fibrous proteins in connective tissue, and is mainly genetically determined. Grahame describes it as being indistinguishable from, if not identical to, the hypermobility type Ehlers–Danlos syndrome (formerly Ehlers–Danlos type III).[4] The tensile strength of this connective tissue is impaired, causing increased flexibility but also increased fragility. Ligaments and articular capsules are affected in particular; they are more easily injured, with healing usually taking longer than average. Dislocations and sprains occur more frequently in these patients. Adults affected by HM often mistakenly attribute their increased flexibility to having played a lot of sport or done a lot of stretching.

## Symptomatology

For many people, such as gymnasts, dancers, swimmers and musicians, HM may in fact be an asset, enabling them to perform to advantage. It may not necessarily cause problems or require treatment.

However, a significant number of people suffer ill effects – some severe – from HM. Symptoms vary enormously from patient to patient and from day to day, depending to some extent on whether a single joint is affected or whether more joints/soft tissues are involved, including the internal organs.

However, even if only one joint is affected, e.g. in the lower limb, if it is left untreated for too long the other lower-limb joints will also succumb to trauma surprisingly quickly.

The main clinical features are:

▷ pain and/or a *feeling* of stiffness in one or more joints or musculotendinous areas, exacerbated by: prolonged periods of sitting or standing; preceding menstruation, pregnancy; sudden weight gain; repetitive movements; malalignment; cold weather; unsupportive footwear
▷ impaired joint proprioception and balance; history of 'going over' on ankles [5,6]
▷ in children, 'growing pains' and problems with writing because of difficulties in gripping thin writing implements
▷ anxiety because relatively few doctors (including many rheumatologists) [7] take HM patients seriously or know what is wrong with them.

HM patients fall into one of two groups:

---

## Group 1: overuse/malalignment

Initially, a single joint/soft tissue may cause symptoms. The patient may report minor trauma, although often there appears to be no obvious cause for a joint to become painful and, sometimes, swollen. On further investigation, however, usually the patient will remember overusing a joint/s through, for example, working long hours at a computer or attending a music camp.

In the lower limb, malalignment (i.e. suboptimal alignment) of the hip (such as femoral anteversion) or foot (e.g. overpronation) will often give rise to symptoms. These are not always in those particular joints, but are often in the low back or knee. If diagnosed and treated early, good results will ensue; if not, the problem will appear to 'spread' with alarming speed to other joints in the lower limb in their unsuccessful attempt to compensate for the first painful joint.

---

## Group 2: joint hypermobility syndrome

Kirk, Ansell and Bywaters defined the hypermobility syndrome (HMS) as generalised joint laxity with associated musculoskeletal complaints in the absence of any systemic disease.[8] The name has been modified to the 'joint hypermobility syndrome' (JHS). Arthralgia is a common feature of this syndrome, the lax connective tissue also affecting the skin, eye, skeleton and heart.

For the more severely affected patients in this group, life can be a daily struggle against pain and injury.[9]

---

## Diagnosis of hypermobility

In my general musculoskeletal practice, I see far more problems related to *hyper*-than *hypo*-mobility, probably because I now routinely screen every patient for it. It is still tragically underdiagnosed, and because of the importance of early diagnosis and treatment, screening for it should form part of every clinical assessment. If spotted in an adult, the children should also be screened.

While *hypo*mobility is easy to recognise, *hyper*mobility is often less obvious for several reasons. First, the patient does not look ill and, second, once an HM joint has become painful, it will stiffen up and then appear to have an average range of movement. Also, one patient may present with different symptoms from another. Not surprisingly, in the past these patients have been mistaken for malingerers. For example, a patient may say she *feels* stiff and yet easily be able to touch the floor with her fingertips, keeping her knees straight. Her 'normal' range of movement would permit her to get her hands flat on the floor. Very often the patient will not volunteer the information that she has HM of joints as more often than not she will either not realise that she has, or will not realise the significance of this. Hence, carefully questioning the patient about her family history and flexibility in her teens can often yield more information than examining the patient's joints.

Affirmative answers to some of the following questions lead one to suspect a diagnosis of HM:

▷ Were you very supple in your teens? e.g. Did you do ballet, gymnastics or competitive swimming?
▷ Did you have any knee problems in your teens, such as patellofemoral pain or subluxation of the patella (often an indication of malalignment)?
▷ Were you ever able to get your hands flat on the floor when your knees were straight?
▷ Did you 'go over' on your ankles?
▷ Did you have 'growing pains' in your legs?
▷ Do your joints click?
▷ Did you fidget as a child?
▷ Do you find it difficult to sit or stand still for any length of time?

(Because of difficulty in stabilising their joints due to a proprioceptive deficit in them, coupled with ligamentous laxity, some HM patients find it unbearable to sit still in classrooms and lectures, even avoiding going to lectures or the cinema because of this.)

## Summary of diagnostic pointers to hypermobility

1 ▷ History of suppleness in teens (see above) and possibly subluxations or dislocations.
2 ▷ The patient may be otherwise healthy (Group 1) or may feel tired and depressed (Group 2).
3 ▷ Pain (often latent) in one or more joints or entheses (Group 1); widespread pain (Group 2).
4 ▷ A subjective feeling of stiffness in her joints that, in a younger patient, may be at variance with her range of joint movement.
5 ▷ The joints feel looser than average on passive testing.

## Scoring systems for hypermobility

Original scoring systems were based on assessing the number of joints involved; the more recent system incorporates organic dysfunction. The *Beighton score* is a 9-point scale based on the Carter and Wilkinson scoring system.[10] One point is given for each manoeuvre that the patient can carry out, up to a maximum of 9 points.

Table 15.1 ○ *Brighton revised diagnostic criteria for benign joint hypermobility syndrome, 1998*

| The ability to: | Right | Left |
|---|---|---|
| **1** Passively dorsiflex the fifth metacarpophalangeal joint to >90° | 1 | 1 |
| **2** Passively appose the thumb to the volar aspect of the forearm | 1 | 1 |
| **3** Passively hyperextend the elbow to >10° | 1 | 1 |
| **4** Passively hyperextend the knee to >10° | 1 | 1 |
| **5** Actively place hands flat on the floor without bending the knees | 1 | |
| Total | | 9 |

*Source*: Grahame R, Bird HA, Child A. The revised (Brighton 1998) criteria for the diagnosis of benign joint hypermobility syndrome (BJHS).[11]

Figure 15.1 ○ *Beighton score tests*

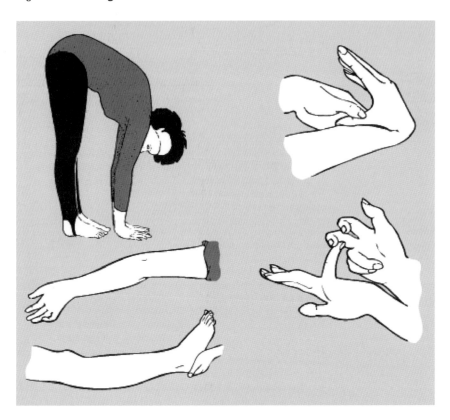

*Source*: www.arthritisresearchuk.org/files/6019_HYPER_05-3_01032010140241.pdf. Illustration reproduced by kind permission of Arthritis Research UK (www.arthritisresearchuk.org/).

This score was designed for epidemiological studies and should be used with caution in a clinical setting. Some HM patients, especially older ones, may have a low Beighton score, yet show excessive mobility in other directions, e.g. lateral flexion of the spine, or internal rotation of the hips.

Some may have a high Beighton score but no joint arthralgia, excluding them from having JHS.

The 1998 Brighton revised diagnostic criteria for benign joint hypermobility syndrome build on the Beighton score and are a useful aid in diagnosis (note that the word 'benign' is now not used with this syndrome). However, the importance of questioning older people about their previous flexibility should not be forgotten.

## Presentation of joint problems caused by hypermobility

Although not unique to HM patients, the following pathology occurs more frequently in them (see Table 15.2).

Table 15.2 ○ *Common pathology in HM patients*

| | Pathology | Physical signs/symptoms |
|---|---|---|
| Feet | Recurrent ankle sprains, OA of the first metatarsophalangeal joint or bunions, calcaneal spurs, plantar fasciitis | Excessive calcaneal eversion; flat feet (occasionally high arches), hallux abducto valgus |
| Knees | Medial or lateral knee strain, chondromalacia patellae, anterior cruciate ligament rupture, joint effusions | Knee hyperextension |
| Hips | Clicking hip; trochanteric bursitis | Anteversion (excessive internal rotation of the hip); 'squinting patellae' when standing – associated with low-back/pelvic pain and inability to stand for long periods |
| Pelvis | Sacroiliac joint instability or *hypo*-mobility, especially during pregnancy; symphysis pubis diastasis; uterine prolapse | Weakness of pelvic floor muscles |
| Lumbar spine | Low-back pain; lower two lumbar levels show disc narrowing and facet joint arthrosis at an earlier age than average, pars defects/spondylolisthesis due to ligamentous insufficiency, spinal stenosis | Increased lumbar lordosis/hollow back, difficulty in standing and sitting still |
| Thoracic spine | Scoliosis and stiffness | The thoracic spine is often the first area to stiffen up; kyphosis in old age |
| Neck | Acute wryneck episodes; susceptible to whiplash injuries; headaches; low cervical disc with nerve root entrapment | Tight ligamentum flavum band on neck flexion, associated with headaches; forward head posture |

|  | Pathology | Physical signs/symptoms |
| --- | --- | --- |
| Temperomandibular joint | Clicking and subluxation/dislocation | |
| Hands | OA of the first metacarpophalangeal joint; repetitive strain | Excessive thumb abduction and wrist flexion |
| Elbows | Tennis elbow (lateral epicondylitis); golfer's elbow (medial epicondylitis) | Hyperextension |
| Shoulders | Rotator cuff tendonitis; subluxation/dislocation of glenohumeral joint | Hyperextension, excessive internal and external rotation; crepitus on scapular movement because of its abnormal tracking |

## Investigations

X-rays and magnetic resonance imaging (MRI) scans are usually negative in the acute stage, but may show premature OA in patients in early middle age.

## Principles of management

Reassurance is vital; the patient will be relieved that a diagnosis has been made at last. From the outset, the importance of self-management should be stressed, but with guidance and some initial monitoring of the patient and sometimes her family. Periodic treatment for acute episodes may be necessary. An increasing number of physiotherapists are gaining expertise in treating HM, but it is easy to exacerbate the patient's symptoms if the therapist is not familiar with the condition. The Hypermobility Syndrome Association can be recommended for the more severely affected patients (www.hypermobility.org). However, at present some of the information on the internet relating to JHS can alarm the patients who fall into group 1 (overuse/malalignment).

## Rest

For acute episodes of soft-tissue lesions, rest is necessary in the short term. However, these patients do not do well on prolonged bed rest.

## Alignment check/correction

This is essential for both groups. A physiotherapist or podiatrist skilled in biomechanics (not all are) should be consulted, and correction given using a heel raise and orthotics (if necessary) and exercises. Correct foot alignment is usually the key to relieving pain associated with HM in the knee, hip and low back.

## Physiotherapy

Physiotherapy forms the mainstay for treatment for these patients in teaching self-management and back care.

### Exercise

This forms the basis of treatment, and should be designed to avoid injury to joints. Of particular value are exercises to re-educate the deep stabilizing muscles of the affected joints and pelvic floor muscles (core stability). Some patients may be able to progress to joining a Pilates exercise class, while others fare better with swimming/hydrotherapy or gym ball exercises. Aerobics are often contraindicated.

### Pacing of activities

This is essential because HM patients often do not get warning signs of overuse and suffer a delayed reaction to overactivity.

### Stretching

After warm-up, gentle stretching of the superficial muscles to the end of the patient's hypermobile range is in fact pain relieving. Overstretching is to be avoided. Hatha (gentle) yoga helps patients with minor problems. Stretching before going to bed will help relieve morning stiffness.

### Proprioception training

It is becoming clear that proprioception training (wobble boards, tai chi) plays an important role in protecting hypermobile joints from injury.

### Passive mobilisation

Passive mobilisation, both by the physiotherapist and the patient using self-help equipment, can give symptomatic relief, especially to areas that are difficult for the patient to reach, such as the thoracic spine. Repeated manipulation is harmful and creates dependency on the therapist.

### Ergonomic advice

This is especially appropriate for patients who work with computers or who play musical instruments.

### Posture correction

This is usually routinely given by physiotherapists, but the Alexander Technique (which works through sensory feedback) can be invaluable for the more reflective type of patient. This is best taught when the patient is pain free. The Society of Teachers of the Alexander Technique (STAT) provides a directory of local teachers.

## Medication

The usefulness of drugs in controlling pain in HM patients is limited.

### Analgesics

Paracetamol with or without codeine are the first choices. Non-steroidal anti-inflammatory drugs (NSAIDs)/COX-2s should be reserved for situations where inflammation is suspected, especially in view of the recent European Medicines Agency (EMEA)[12] review of COX-2s and ongoing NSAIDs review. Opioid matrix patches are an alternative to simple or compound analgesics but should only be used with caution and not as first-line therapy.

### Local steroid injections

These may be useful, especially for trochanteric pain in patients with hypermobile hips. Knees should be injected as little as possible to decrease the risk of dependency and to reduce the theoretical risks of weakening collagen. However, removing large effusions is usually worthwhile.

## Pain management and self-management

Most Primary Care Organisations employ or will soon appoint pain management nurses. HM patients may well benefit from a consultation.

## Prognosis

The earlier the diagnosis of HM is made, the more effective are treatment outcomes. Many symptoms from hypermobile joints (especially if there is associated malalignment) can be successfully managed with early diagnosis if the patient complies with weight reduction, alignment correction, exercise, and lifestyle modifications. However, after injury the rate of healing is slower than average; this is particularly noticeable after road traffic accidents and WRULS (work-related upper-limb syndrome). It is likely that HM predisposes to premature OA.[12] This may be due to a combination of diminished protective proprioception and microtrauma caused by joint instability. A minority of patients (from group 2) will have severe arthrosis in many joints because JHS appears to worsen with age.

---

Box 15.1 ○ *Case study*

Kate was brought along to the GP by her mother. Kate is 13 years of age and is complaining of a painful hip and back. She had recently started karate sessions and after each session was in so much pain that she limped about for a few hours. She was also in pain if she did any prolonged walking or weightbearing. The problem was impinging on her ability to take part in sports at school and she was beginning to get anxious about her karate sessions.

There had been no real history of nocturnal pain and Kate was otherwise well.

The GP took a family history and discovered that Kate's father had suffered from Perthes' disease as a child and still walks with a limp. Kate was very worried about developing a disability similar to her father.

When the GP examined Kate's hip, he was looking for a reduced range of movement, which would support a diagnosis of a dysplastic hip. Fortunately, he did not find this and, if anything, her hip had an extended range of movement. Her back movements were similarly very good and Kate could easily touch the floor when bending forward and put her palms flat on the floor.

### *Analysis of case study with respect to the six domains of* Being a GP

▷ Using *primary care management and clinical management,* the GP was able to recognise that Kate showed some features of a HM syndrome, but he did not know very much about it.

▷ With *specific problem-solving skills,* he was able to access web resources during the consultation and find a patient leaflet from Arthritis Research UK (www.arthritisresearchuk.org/) about HM, which defined the Beighton score and Brighton criteria.

▷ The GP went back to examine Kate and found that she did in fact have a Beighton score of 6 and had two other minor features of HM, which were back pain for more than three months and a Marfanoid body shape, and therefore had features of the (benign) *joint hypermobility syndrome.*

▷ In *making a diagnosis,* the GP used *person-centred care* to explain the findings to Kate and her mother. The GP used empathetic language and communication skills to ascertain if Kate had understood his findings. He gave them a copy of the patient leaflet.

▷ The GP felt that it was important to exclude hip dysplasia, especially with the family history of hip problems (*data-gathering and interpretation*); after the consultation had finished, he spoke to one of the local radiologists (*working with colleagues and in teams*) who agreed to sanction a pelvic radiograph. It was important to speak to the radiologist, as a routine hip radiograph on a child carries a significant exposure to radiation and the benefits had to outweigh the risks of the investigation.

▷ The GP was able to ring Kate's mother to give her the good news that the X-ray was normal (*primary care administration and IMT*).

▷ Kate's mother was happy for her daughter to see a physiotherapist and the GP arranged a home visit by the local paediatric therapy team (*working with colleagues and in teams*). He wrote a referral letter explaining the history, family history and features of HM (*communication skills*).

▷ Three months later, Kate and her mother returned to surgery for a review (*holistic care and managing medical complexity and promoting health*) at the GP's request. Kate was feeling much better. She had undergone a programme of core stability and strengthening exercises. She undertook different forms of exercise, rather than just karate. Swimming in particular had been beneficial. She was careful not to attend too many karate sessions per week and she was no longer in pain. She was also less anxious about the future and understood the importance of continuing with her exercises.

## Scoring systems for hypermobility

**Beighton score** ▶ Beighton P, Solomon L, Soskolne C L. Articular mobility in an African population *Annals of the Rheumatic Diseases* 1973; **32(5)**: 413–18.

**Brighton criteria** ▶ Grahame R, Bird H A, Child A. The revised (Brighton 1998) criteria for the diagnosis of benign joint hypermobility syndrome (BJHS) *Journal of Rheumatology* 2000; **27(7)**: 1777–9.

## Further reading

▷ Bird H A. Joint hypermobility in children *Rheumatology* (Oxford) 2005; **44(6)**: 703–4.

▷ Ferrell W R, Tennant N, Sturrock R D, *et al.* Amelioration of symptoms by enhancement of proprioception in patients with joint hypermobility syndrome *Arthritis and Rheumatism* 2004; **50(10)**: 3323–8.

368

**References**

1 • Keer R, Grahame R. *Hypermobility Syndrome: recognition and management for physiotherapists* London: Butterworth-Heinemann, 2003.

2 • Beighton P, Grahame R, Bird H. *Hypermobility of Joints* (3rd edn) London: Springer-Verlag, 1999.

3 • Birrell F N, Adebajo A O, Hazleman B L, *et al.* High prevalence of joint laxity in West Africans *British Journal of Rheumatology* 1994; **33(1)**: 56–9.

4 • Grahame R. Editorial: the need to take a fresh look at criteria for hypermobility *Journal of Rheumatology* 2007; **34(4)**: 4.

5 • Mallik A K, Ferrell W R, McDonald A G, *et al.* Impaired proprioceptive acuity at the proximal interphalangeal joint in patients with the hypermobility syndrome *British Journal of Rheumatology* 1994; **33(7)**: 631–7.

6 • Hall M G, Ferrell W R, Sturrock R D, *et al.* The effect of the hypermobility syndrome on knee joint proprioception *British Journal of Rheumatology* 1995; **34(2)**: 121–5.

7 • Grahame R, Bird H. British consultant rheumatologists' perceptions about the hypermobility syndrome: a national survey *Rheumatology* (Oxford) 2001; **40(5)**: 559–62.

8 • Kirk J A, Ansell B M, Bywaters E G. The hypermobility syndrome: musculoskeletal complaints associated with generalized joint hypermobility *Annals of the Rheumatic Diseases* 1967; **26(5)**: 419–25.

9 • Gurley-Green S. Living with the hypermobility syndrome *Rheumatology* (Oxford) 2001; **40(5)**: 487–9.

10 • Beighton P, Solomon L, Soskolne CL. Articular mobility in an African population *Annals of the Rheumatic Diseases* 1973; **32(5)**: 413–18.

11 • Grahame R, Bird H A, Child A. The revised (Brighton 1998) criteria for the diagnosis of benign joint hypermobility syndrome (BJHS) *Journal of Rheumatology* 2000; **27(7)**: 1777–9.

12 • Jonsson H, Valtysdottir S T. Hypermobility features in patients with hand osteoarthritis *Osteoarthritis and Cartilage* 1995; **3(1)**: 1–5.

# Polymyalgia rheumatica and giant cell arteritis

# 16

*David Walker*

## Aims of this chapter

The aim is to give a practical view of the diagnosis and management of these conditions up to the point of referral to secondary care.

### Key learning points

▶ These two conditions represent a spectrum of involvement and cannot be neatly separated.

▶ Occurrence is predominantly in elderly Northern Europeans.

▶ There are typical symptoms and response to treatment.

▶ They may mimic and be confused with a variety of systemic and painful conditions that may also respond to steroids.

▶ They must be treated promptly with steroids.

▶ They are usually self-limiting over a few years.

## Definition

Both polymyalgia rheumatica (PMR) and giant cell arteritis (GCA) are forms of arteritis that cause a spectrum of disorders.

A study in Olmsted County in the USA identified peaks of incidence of PMR every seven years, which may suggest an infective cause.[1] There is a familial occurrence[2] that has not been quantified and there is a genetic association with HLA-DR4.[3]

Involvement of a variety of vessels can affect vision. Pathology is distinctive with a panarteritis with giant cell granuloma formation.[4] It has been postulated that sunlight damage to the internal elastic lamina of superficial arteries is the cause.[5]

## Diagnosis

Both PMR and GCA occur in the same population of people and are best regarded as a spectrum with muscular pains at one end and inflamed arteries at the other. They can occur together or separately, and arteritis has been found on biopsy in 10–15% of arteritis symptom-free individuals with PMR.[6] People with diagnosed PMR may later go on to develop GCA, and myalgic symptoms may precede, follow or coincide with GCA.[7]

They occur predominantly in Northern European white people over the age of 50 (mean 70 years) with a 2:1 female to male ratio.[8]

### *Diagnostic criteria for PMR*

▷ Pain and stiffness in the proximal muscles of the shoulder and pelvic girdles, more often starting in the shoulders, is the cardinal symptom that should make you consider the diagnosis.

▷ Constitutional symptoms of fatigue, weight loss, fever and depression are common. The pain and stiffness tend to be worse at night and first thing in the morning. Morning stiffness usually lasts more than 45 minutes.

▷ Weakness is rare and if present should raise the possibility of a myositis (a condition with true inflammation in the muscles).

▷ A degree of synovitis in the joints is also reportedly common,[9] which can make differentiation from an inflammatory arthritis difficult. It may take the evolution of the disease and response to treatment to tease apart. Tenderness of the muscles is not usually pronounced and if prominent should raise the possibility of fibromyalgia syndrome (FMS). This is a syndrome where there is association of poor sleep, fatigue, widespread pain in muscles and widespread muscle tenderness.

### *Diagnostic criteria for GCA*

▷ The symptoms of GCA are often headache, fatigue, visual disturbance and muscular pain in the jaw on chewing (jaw claudication).

▷ This is associated with tenderness of the scalp; inflamed arteries may be visible.

▷ Other symptoms and signs depend on the arteries involved and the degree of involvement.

▷ The headache is usually in the temple region and may be aggravated by touching, such as with brushing the hair.

▷ Visual symptoms are reported in up to half of the patients, but visual loss probably occurs in fewer than 10%.[10] There are subtle differences in the symptoms depending on the actual arteries involved, but sudden-onset permanent blindness is the most serious feature. Fear of blindness is a major driver for prompt steroid use on diagnosis.

▷ There are diagnostic criteria for both PMR and GCA but these are primarily for classification of disease for research, rather than a help in the clinic.[11]

▷ Investigations nearly always reveal an acute-phase response with a high ESR.[12] However, occasionally this will be normal. The presence of symptoms with a normal ESR is a common reason for referral to secondary care. Other investigations are done to help differentiate the diagnosis, for example a high creatine kinase (CK) may suggest a true myositis.

## Temporal artery biopsy

A positive biopsy is very helpful to justify what are potentially toxic doses of steroids, but it is not always possible. A negative biopsy is far less useful as the arterial involvement is not uniform and there may be skip lesions.[13] Organising the biopsy is not always possible and, because of the danger of visual loss, treatment cannot be delayed. A biopsy must be done within a few days of starting the steroids if the histology is likely to be helpful. In some areas ophthalmologists offer a service for temporal artery biopsy. It is worth identifying the correct referral pathway for your locality.

Ultrasound of affected arteries is abnormal[14] and studies are currently underway to determine the reliability of this test for diagnosis and directing the biopsy to an affected area. It may well be that this will become the investigation of choice.

The classically dramatic response to modest doses of prednisolone is the most useful diagnostic test. If nothing else it indicates symptoms for which steroids are a satisfactory treatment, which is often nearer to a diagnosis than myalgia of unknown cause. It makes sense to give a trial of prednisolone 15 mg per day for two weeks on suspicion of the diagnosis. Unless there are severe contraindications to steroids then the risks of this dose are very small, and the rewards are dramatic in terms of patient symptoms and satisfaction with their medical management.

## Differential diagnosis

The differential diagnosis that catches out both GPs and specialists is proximal rheumatoid arthritis, which seems more common in the elderly age group who get PMR. They may present with very similar symptoms and patients do of course respond to prednisolone 15 mg. The response is not usually as 'dramatic' or as complete, but it may be sufficient to cause doubt. The truth will become apparent with time, usually 6 to 12 months, either because the peripheral joints become involved or that more arthritic symptoms become apparent as the dose of prednisolone is reduced. A positive rheumatoid factor may aid diagnosis, but it is frequently negative in this situation.

A genuine myositis will usually present with more weakness, more systemic symptoms and a hugely elevated CK, which should be checked if in doubt.

FMS will normally occur in a much younger age group and with a much more obvious distress that will alert the clinician. There is a much greater tenderness of the muscles and the two are rarely confused. Response to steroids can be the final arbiter if necessary.

Occult malignancy can occasionally present with symptoms similar to PMR and a detailed history of other symptoms is necessary. There may also be a response to steroids that has led to the suggestion that there is an association between PMR and malignancy. Again, it will be the passage of time and the development of other symptoms that will lead to the diagnosis. It is not usually worth screening PMR patients for malignancies in the absence of symptoms directing the area of search.

Other forms of vasculitis may affect the cranial arteries and this would usually be found because of involvement of other arteries or on biopsy. Similarly, other arteries can be affected by cranial arteritis.

## Treatment of PMR

Steroids are a mandatory treatment for PMR. Often there is not a lot of evidence to indicate what dose should be used. A dose of prednisolone 15 mg/day is recommended [12] as it is sufficient to produce the characteristic dramatic response, but not sufficient to make a dramatic difference to an arthritis that is the main differential.

On confirmation by this response at two or three weeks, the steroids may be reduced. The patient should be informed that he or she will be on the steroids for at least a year and probably two years, and bone protection should be introduced with something like alendronate 70 mg/week with calcium and vitamin D.

The rate of reduction is a matter of trial and success. The British Society for Rheumatology (BSR) guidelines for reduction of dose is shown in Box 16.1.[15] A common practice is to reduce to 12.5 mg per day for two weeks and then to 10 mg/day. The patient is then asked to reduce the dose by 1 mg a month, provided their symptoms remain under control. At the first sign of recurrence of symptoms the patient is advised to return to the previous dose for another month and then try to reduce again as before. It seems quite common for the patient to experience this sort of problem at around 6 to 8 mg. People also have problems reducing below 1 or 2 mg, which seems a trivial dose. In this circumstance bridging the gap with alternate-day dosing is worth a try.

---

**Box 16.1** ○ *BSR guidelines for prednisolone dose reduction*

**The suggested regimen is:**

▶ daily prednisolone 15 mg for three weeks

▶ then 12.5 mg for three weeks

▶ then 10 mg for four to six weeks

▶ followed by reduction by 1 mg every four to eight weeks or alternate-day reductions (e.g. 10/7.5 mg alternate days etc.).

Usually one to three years of treatment is needed.

---

A small group of patients will have problems stopping the steroids and will remain on a small dose of steroids long term, and occasionally this has to be accepted provided the dose is low. The risk benefit is only usually in favour of 'sparing' the steroid with another drug if the dose is 10 mg or above. Under this circumstance the patient will usually have been referred to secondary care and the diagnosis reconsidered. The most commonly used drugs are azathioprine and methotrexate, and the aim is to get the steroid dose comfortably below 10 mg. Comfortable for the clinician!

---

## Problem situations

There may sometimes be a conflict between the symptoms the patient has and the ESR that may be used to monitor response. This is a not infrequent reason for referral. A GP may be inclined to treat the patient's symptoms and ignore the ESR once other causes of the raised ESR have been excluded. This may be uncomfortable for the GP, so discussing and sharing care with a local rheumatologist is probably a good idea.

Another problem is the patient who responds initially and then seems to require an increase in steroids. This should prompt a review of the diagnosis and a search for complications, such as infections or malignancy, and probably requires onward referral to rheumatology if not already done. A myriad of complicated disease scenarios have emerged in this situation and all require complex investigation and treatment, usually in hospital. BSR guidelines suggest when referral to hospital is necessary (Box 16.2).

---

Box 16.2 ○ *BSR guidelines for hospital referral*

**Atypical features or features that increase likelihood of a non-PMR diagnosis:**

▶ younger than sixties

▶ chronic onset

▶ lack of shoulder involvement

▶ lack of inflammatory stiffness

▶ 'red flag' features – prominent systemic features, weight loss, night pain, neurological signs

▶ features of other rheumatic disease

▶ normal or very high acute-phase response.

**Treatment dilemmas such as:**

▶ incomplete, poorly sustained or non-responsive to corticosteroids

▶ inability to reduce corticosteroids

▶ contraindications to corticosteroid therapy.

---

## Treatment of GCA

Again, steroids are mandatory in order to preserve vision. The starting dose will be much higher at 40–60 mg prednisolone/day and the reduction will be slower according to response.[15] Reductions of 5 mg every two to four weeks are worth using initially, but the rate of reduction will diminish as the dose becomes smaller, for example 2.5 mg reductions between 20 mg and 10 mg. Eventually, reducing by 1 mg a month below 10 mg can be used, as for PMR. Bone protection, again as for PMR, is also necessary. This whole process will take much longer and will be limited by the recurrence of the original symptoms, often headache and scalp tenderness. The reassurance of a positive biopsy can be very helpful at this time if the reduction is slow, but as above is not always available.

<table>
<tr><td>

Box 16.3 ○ *Case study*

A 76-year-old woman presented to her GP complaining of pains across both shoulders, which had come on suddenly ten days before. There were no precipitating events and it was most severe at night, disturbing sleep. Her pains were making it impossible for her to enjoy any social activities and had stopped her bowling. She felt terrible and had some night sweats. She was having difficulty coping with her husband, who had Parkinson's disease and had very limited mobility.

</td></tr>
</table>

### Analysis of case history with respect to the six domains of Being a GP

She decided to visit her GP and managed to get an appointment the next day, after her call had been triaged by the practice nurse (*primary care administration and IMT*).

Her GP questioned her about her presenting symptoms and it became clear that she also had some pain in her thighs. PMR was suspected (*clinical management*) and blood was taken by the practice phlebotomist, who was able to see the patient as an extra at the request of the GP (*primary care administration and IMT*); her ESR was 56. She was started on 15 mg of prednisolone.

Fortunately, the GP knew the patient well and was aware of the problems with her husband. He arranged for the Rapid Response District Nursing team to visit later that day and offer care for her husband (*working with colleagues and in teams; managing medical complexity and promoting health; person-centred-care*).

When seen two weeks later, the patient had had a dramatic response to treatment, the day after she started the steroids, and was feeling 'normal'. She was most grateful and impressed. The District Nursing support had allowed her time to rest and to take a break from caring for her husband. She had also been put in touch with a local carers' association and was receiving emotional support as well (*practising holistically*).

The prednisolone was reduced to 12.5 mg for two weeks and then 10 mg. She was also commenced on bone protection with alendronate 70 mg/week with calcium and vitamin D. She was given the Arthritis Research UK booklet on PMR (www.arthritisresearchuk.org/arthritis_information/arthritis_ types__symptoms/polymyalgia_rheumatica_pmr.aspx) (*primary care management*).

When she was seen a month later she still felt 'wonderful'. She was instructed to reduce her steroids by 1 mg/month but told that she should return to the previous dose if she had any recurrence of her myalgia.

When next seen three months later she was on 8 mg and still feeling fine. Three days after going from 7 mg to 6 mg later she started to get a recurrence of her shoulder pains, which she recognised as being the same as her initial symptoms, though much milder. She increased the dose up to 7 mg and was fine in two days.

One month later she tried to reduce again with exactly the same effect and had to go back to the 7 mg. This process continued over the months. At six months from onset she managed to get down to 6 mg and by a year she was on 2 mg.

At this point she developed pain in the right knee, worse on use and associated with brief morning stiffness. This was thought to be osteoarthritis of the knee and she responded to paracetamol and celecoxib, which she took intermittently when her pain was severe.

Stopping the last 1 mg of prednisolone also caused some recurrence of the pains, so she was eventually asked to take 1 mg on alternate days. This worked and she was able to stop prednisolone completely at a total of 22 months after presentation. She has had no recurrence of her myalgia over the past four years.

Her husband was now in a nursing home and she visited him every day; the osteoarthritic knee was causing her some problems with the walk from the bus stop to the nursing home and she was thinking of seeing her GP again about this problem.

Her GP would have to speak to her about the weight she had gained from taking the steroids for nearly two years and would need to refer her for physiotherapy to improve the strength of her quadriceps muscles (*managing medical complexity and promoting health*).

---

## Summary

These are diseases that may be difficult to diagnose, where a trial of 'treatment on suspicion' can be justified and where a satisfactory outcome is expected.

### References

1 • Salvarani C, Gabriel S, O'Fallon W, *et al*. Epidemiology of polymyalgia rheumatica in Olmsted County, Minnesota 1970–1991 *Arthritis and Rheumatism* 1995; **38(3)**: 369–73.

2 • Liang M, Simpkin P, Hunder G, *et al*. Familial aggregation of polymyalgia rheumatica and giant cell arteritis *Arthritis and Rheumatism* 1974; **17(1)**: 19–24.

3 • Gonzalez-Gay M, Garcia-Porrua C, Rivas M, *et al*. Epidemiology of biopsy proven giant cell arteritis in northwestern Spain: trend over an 18 year period *Annals of the Rheumatic Diseases* 2001; **60(4)**: 367–71.

4 • Amouroux J. Pathology of giant cell arteritis *Annales de médecine interne* 1998; **149(7)**: 415–19.

5 • Cimmino M. Genetic and environmental factors in polymyalgia rheumatica *Annals of the Rheumatic Diseases* 1997; **56(10)**: 576–7.

6 • Alestig K, Barr J. Giant cell arteritis: a biopsy study of polymyalgia rheumatica including one case of Takayasu's disease *Lancet* 1963; **1(7293)**: 1228–30.

7 • Hunder G. Giant cell arteritis and polymyalgia rheumatica. In: WN Kelley, ED Harris, S Ruddy, *et al*. (eds). *Textbook of Rheumatology* Philadelphia, PA: WB Saunders, 1981, pp. 1123–32.

8 • Gran J, Myklebust G. The incidence of polymyalgia rheumatica and temporal arteritis in the county of Aust Agder, south Norway: a prospective study 1987–1994 *Journal of Rheumatology* 1997; **24(9)**: 1739–43.

9 • Marzo-Ortega H, Rhodes L A, Tan A L, *et al*. Evidence for a different anatomic basis for joint disease localization in polymyalgia rheumatica in comparison with rheumatoid arthritis *Arthritis and Rheumatism* 2007; **56(10)**: 3496–3501.

10 • Hayreh S S, Podhajsky P A, Zimmerman B. Ocular manifestations of giant cell arteritis *American Journal of Ophthalmology* 1998; **125(4)**: 509–20.

11 • Hunder C, Bloch D, Michel B, *et al*. The American College of Rheumatology 1990 criteria for the classification of giant cell (temporal) arteritis *Arthritis and Rheumatism* 1990; **33(8)**: 1122–8.

12 • Kyle V, Cawston T, Hazleman B. Erythrocyte sedimentation rate and C reactive protein in the assessment of polymyalgia rheumatica/giant cell arteritis on presentation and during follow up *Annals of the Rheumatic Diseases* 1989; **48(8)**: 667–71.

13 • Klein G, Campbell R, Hunder G, *et al*. Skip lesions in temporal arteritis *Mayo Clinic Proceedings* 1976; **51(8)**: 504–10.

14 • Schmidt W, Kraft H, Völker L, *et al*. Colour Doppler sonography to diagnose temporal arteritis *Lancet* 1995; **345(8953)**: 866.

15 • Dasgupta B, Borg FA, Hassan N, *et al*. *BSR and BHPR Guidelines for the Management of Polymyalgia Rheumatica* Oxford: Oxford University Press, 2009; www.rheumatology.org. uk/includes/documents/cm_docs/2009/m/management_of_polymyalgia_rheumatica.pdf [accessed October 2011].

# Musculoskeletal problems in children and adolescents

# 17

*Helen Foster*

---

### Aims of this chapter

This chapter covers topics that are important to trainees in primary care and focuses on the following:

▶ clinical assessment
▶ normal variants in musculoskelelal (MSK) development
▶ knowledge of common and medically significant conditions
▶ indicators that warrant prompt detection and referral
▶ investigations to consider
▶ shared care for the child with chronic rheumatic disease.

---

### Learning points

▶ MSK complaints in children are common, often benign and self-limiting. However, they can be presenting features of significant, severe and potentially life-threatening conditions.
▶ Making a diagnosis rests on competent clinical skills, knowledge of normal variants, knowledge of common clinical scenarios, 'red flags' to suggest severe conditions and judicious use and interpretation of investigations.
▶ Common clinical scenarios include the limping child, 'growing pains', back pain and knee pain.
▶ Juvenile idiopathic arthritis (JIA) is the most common cause of chronic arthritis in children and, in the absence of sepsis or trauma, the most likely cause of a single swollen joint in a child.
▶ Making a prompt diagnosis of JIA and referral to specialist care is key to optimal outcome.
▶ The management of MSK conditions involves a multidisciplinary approach.
▶ Many children with chronic rheumatic disease will require potent immunosuppressive medicines with increased risk of opportunistic infection and impact on immunisation schedules.

▶ Many chronic conditions that begin in childhood will continue into adult life, and the GP has an important role in shared care.

## Introduction

MSK conditions are common complaints in children and adolescents,[1] the majority being self-limiting, often trauma related, and will not need referral to secondary care. However, MSK presentations may have a broad spectrum of causes (see Table 17.1) including potentially life-threatening conditions, such as cancers, infection and non-accidental injury. They may also be a feature of many chronic diseases, such as JIA, inflammatory bowel disease and cystic fibrosis.

In the UK, most children with MSK complaints, other than instances of acute trauma, will present initially to their GP. It cannot be overstated that the GP has an important role as gatekeeper to secondary care, and is key to appropriate triage, management and referral. This process relies primarily on careful clinical assessment, with judicious use of investigations, appropriate knowledge of common and medically significant conditions, and knowledge of local referral pathways. In many cases explanation and reassurance alone may suffice, along with advice on when to bring the child back for review. A further important role of the GP is shared care of the child with chronic rheumatic disease, and providing valuable support for the growing child, the family and transition into adulthood.

## Clinical assessment

Taking a history and performing a physical examination are integral to making a diagnosis. The clinical assessment requires knowledge of normal development, clinical presentations at different ages and indicators to warrant investigation or referral. In children the MSK clinical assessment may differ from that of an adult in several ways: the history is often given by the parent or carer; may be based on observations and interpretation of events made by others (such as teachers or friends); and may be rather vague and illocalised, with non-specific complaints such as 'my child is limping' or 'my child is not walking quite right'. The examination may be difficult with a fractious child, and may necessitate an opportunistic approach. The parent or carer will undoubtedly have anxieties and concerns about the child, will often fear severe illness, and will have an expectation of referral and investigations.

It is a common pitfall in making a diagnosis to inappropriately attribute a child's problem to trauma given that the latter is a common event in the life

Table 17.1 ○ ***Common ('not to be missed') significant causes of limping according to age***

| Preschool | Early school-aged (4–10 years) | Adolescence |
|---|---|---|
| Mechanical (trauma and non-accidental injury) | Mechanical (trauma, overuse injuries, sport injuries, trampoline injuries) | Mechanical (trauma, overuse injuries, sport injuries) |
| Congenital/developmental problems (e.g. developmental dysplasia of the hip, talipes) | Reactive arthritis/transient synovitis ('irritable hip') | Slipped capital femoral epiphysis |
| Neurological disease (e.g. cerebral palsy, neurological syndromes) | Infection (septic arthritis, osteomyelitis) | JIA |
| Infection (septic arthritis, osteomyelitis) | Legg–Calvé–Perthes disease | Infection (septic arthritis, reactive) |
| JIA | JIA | Inflammatory muscle disease (e.g. juvenile dermatomyositis) |
| Metabolic disease (rickets) | Metabolic disease (rickets) | Tarsal coalition (painful non-mobile flat feet) |
| Malignant disease (e.g. leukaemia, neuroblastoma) | Tarsal coalition (painful non-mobile flat feet) | Complex diffuse/regional pain syndromes |
| Inflammatory muscle disease (e.g. inherited myopathies) | Inflammatory muscle disease (e.g. juvenile dermatomyositis) | Malignant disease (leukaemia, lymphoma, primary bone tumour) |
| | Malignant disease (leukaemia) | Metabolic disease (rickets) |
| | Complex diffuse/regional pain syndromes | |

*Source*: adapted from Foster HE, Boyd D, Jandial S. 'Growing pains': a practical guide for primary care.[2]

of all children. Admittedly, taking a history can be challenging; it is worth considering open questions to explore the problem in more detail (Table 17.2), teasing out features that may suggest mechanical or inflammatory pathology (Table 17.3) and seeking any suggestion of 'red flags' (Box 17.1). Red flags raise concern about infection, malignancy or non-accidental malignancy, and warrant urgent referral. It is always worth remembering the concept of referred pain, e.g. the knee pain may be referred from hip disease or hip pain referred from the spine.

Table 17.2 ○ *Key elements of the clinical assessment in the child with 'aches and pains'*

| Questions to parent/carer | Points to check for | Comments |
|---|---|---|
| What have you or anyone else noticed? | Behaviour, mood, joint swelling, limping, bruising | *Limping*, whether intermittent or persistent, *always* warrants further assessment. Deterioration in school performance (sport, schoolwork, handwriting) is always significant |
| What is the child like in him/herself? | Irritable, grumpy, 'clingy', reluctant to play, systemic features (e.g. fever, anorexia, weight loss) | *Systemic features* including 'red flags' to suggest malignancy or infection always warrant urgent referral. Young children may not verbalise pain but present with behavioural change such as irritability |
| Where is the pain? (Ask the child to point.) What is it like? | Asymmetry, locality and pattern, pain in joints or muscles, involvement of arms, legs or other sites | *Asymmetrical involvement* is always a cause for concern – although growing pains can affect more one side than another at times, they must involve both legs symmetrically. *Referred pain* from the hip may present with non-specific pain in the thigh or knee and must be considered. *Pain in unusual sites* (such as upper limbs or back) is not characteristic of growing pains and requires further assessment |
| How is the child in the mornings and during the day? | Diurnal variation and daytime symptoms (e.g. limping, any difficulty walking, getting dressed, toileting, or on stairs) | Characteristically the child with growing pains is well with no daytime symptoms (other than fatigue after interrupted sleep), and no change in physical abilities or performance in sport, play or school. *Pain on waking* or daytime symptoms suggestive of *stiffness or gelling* (after periods of inactivity) are indicative of inflammatory joint (or muscle) disease |
| What is the child like with walking and running? Has there been any change in the child's activities? | Motor milestones (any suggestion of delay or regression of achieved milestones) and enquiry about speech and language | *Regression of achieved motor milestones* or functional impairment (including play, sport or handwriting) are more suggestive of inflammatory joint or muscle disease. An assessment of global development is indicated with any suggestion of delay or regression in speech, language or motor skills) |
|  | Avoidance of activities that were previously enjoyed (e.g. sport, play) | *'Clumsiness'* is a non-specific term but may mask significant MSK or neurological disease. Referral for assessment is required if acquired or progressive, with or without delay or regression in developmental milestones |

384

| Questions to parent/carer | Points to check for | Comments |
|---|---|---|
| How is the child at school/nursery? | School attendance (any suggestion of school avoidance, bullying) | *Behavioural problems* in the young child may manifest as non-specific pains (headaches, stomach aches or leg pains) and sometimes sensitive questioning can reveal stressful events at home or issues around school, including bullying |
| Does the child wake at night with pain? | Pattern of night waking (any predictability of waking) | Night waking is a common feature of growing pains. As a general rule, however, the pattern of night-time waking in growing pains is intermittent, and often predictable after periods of activity the preceding day or evening (although this may not be immediately obvious to the parent until this is explored). Conversely, persistent night waking, especially if there are other concerns (such as unilaterality, limping, unusual location or systemic features), necessitates further investigation and referral |
| Can you predict when the pains may occur? | Relationship to physical activity (including during or after sporting activities) | Growing pains tend to be worse later in the day, evenings and often after busy days |
| What do you do when the child is in pain? | Response to analgesics, massages, and reaction of parent | Lack of response to simple analgesia is a concern. Vicious circle of reinforced behaviour can occur |
| What is your main concern? | Sleep disturbance, anxiety about serious disease (arthritis, cancer, family history), pain control | *Family history of muscle disease, arthritis or autoimmune disease* may indicate a predisposition to muscle or joint disease |

### Examination

| | | |
|---|---|---|
| Observe child in the room | Mood, play, chatter, parent/carer interaction with child | The happy, playful, mobile child is unlikely to have serious disease |
| Examination of joints | A pGALS screen as a minimum with a more detailed examination based on the 'look, feel, move' approach as indicated | A normal pGALS screen is to be expected in growing pains. Normal variants (e.g. mobile flat feet) are often observed. Many children with growing pains have some features of *hypermobility* (generalised or localised to the hands or feet), although not all children with hypermobility are symptomatic |

*continued overleaf*

| Questions to parent/carer | Points to check for | Comments |
|---|---|---|
| General examination (chest, abdomen, ears, throat, temperature, urinalysis) | The 'unwell' child (fever, pallor, apathy), pattern of bruising, organomegaly, lymphadenopathy, rashes (including psoriasis) | A normal pattern of bruising is expected in the healthy, active child (i.e. different size and ages of bruises over the anterior shins). Sources of infection must be looked for and any evidence to suggest malignancy |
| Growth | Height and weight and evidence of asymmetrical growth (e.g. leg length) | A normal growth pattern for height is an indicator of good general health. Asymmetrical leg length often associates with scoliosis and may be a feature of established joint disease |

*Source*: adapted from Foster HE, Boyd D, Jandial S. 'Growing pains': a practical guide for primary care.[2]

Table 17.3  ○  **Distinguishing mechanical from inflammatory musculoskeletal presentations**

| | Mechanical | Inflammatory |
|---|---|---|
| Pain | Worse on weightbearing and after activity such as walking | Often eased by movement and may be seemingly absent in young children, who manifest it as behavioural change or avoidance activity |
| Joint swelling | Usually mild and may be transient | Tends to be persistent |
| Morning stiffness or gelling after rest | Usually absent | Often marked |
| Instability (giving way) | May be present | Usually absent |
| Locking | May be present | Usually absent |
| Loss of full movement | May be present | Often present |

---

Box 17.1  ○  **Red flags**

---

▶ Fever, systemic upset.

▶ Bone/joint pain with fever.

▶ Weight loss, sweats, persistent night waking.

▶ Incongruence between history and presentation/pattern of physical findings.

---

The young child may deny having pain when asked directly, but this should not be taken to mean the child does not have any pain. Alternatively, the child in pain may present with changes in behaviour or mood (e.g. irritability or poor sleeping), decreasing ability or interest in activities, regression in hand motor skills (e.g. drawing or painting) or regression of achieved motor milestones. *Delay* in major motor milestones warrants MSK assessment as well as considering a global neuro-developmental approach. Conversely, in acquired MSK disease such as JIA, a history of *regression* of achieved milestones is often more significant, e.g. the child who was previously happy to walk unaided but has recently been asking to be carried. Clues in the history to suggest inflammatory MSK disease can be subtle or may need to be teased out with direct questioning (see Box 17.2).

---

Box 17.2  ○  **Suspected inflammatory joint disease (JIA) – practical tips**

---

▶ The lack of reported pain does not exclude arthritis.

▶ There is the need to probe for symptoms such as

  ▷ gelling (e.g. stiffness after long car rides)

  ▷ altered function (e.g. play, handwriting skills, writing, regression of milestones)

  ▷ deterioration in behaviour (irritability, poor sleeping).

▶ There is the need to examine all joints as joint involvement may often be 'asymptomatic'.

---

Swelling is always significant but can be subtle and easily overlooked by the parent (and even healthcare professionals!), especially if the changes are symmetrical. Rather than describing stiffness, the parents may notice the child is reluctant to weightbear, limps in the mornings or 'gels' after periods of immobility (e.g. after long car rides or sitting in a classroom). Systemic upset and the presence of bone rather than joint pain may be features of MSK disease and are 'red flags' that warrant urgent referral. Indolent presentations of chronic MSK disease can impact on growth (either localised or generalised) and muscle wasting. It is important to assess height and weight, review growth charts in the parent-held record where available, share concerns with other healthcare professionals (e.g. the school nurse or health visitor) and look for evidence of disproportionate growth (e.g. asymmetrical leg length) or muscle wasting.

A child in pain, frightened or very shy can result in physical examination being a challenge for everyone present. Many children are put at ease by the availability of paper and crayons. While taking the history from the parent, it is valuable to observe the child at play, moving around the room and interacting with its carer. *The well-looking child who is chatty and happily plays with toys is much less likely to have serious underlying disease.*

The *pGALS screening assessment* is a simple evidence-based approach to MSK assessment based on the adult GALS (Gait, Arms, Legs, Spine) screen and has been shown to have high sensitivity to detect significant abnormalities.[3] Key to distinguishing normal from abnormal is a knowledge of ranges of movement in different age groups and ethnicity. The GP should look for asymmetry and carry out a careful examination to identify any subtle changes. pGALS incorporates a series of simple manoeuvres and takes an average of two minutes to perform; there are some simple, practical tips to facilitate the examination (see Box 17.3). pGALS is primarily aimed at the school-aged child, but younger children will often comply with pGALS, especially if they copy the examiner and see this as a game. The pGALS screen includes three questions relating to pain and function, although a negative response does *not* exclude significant MSK disease. At a minimum an MSK screening examination should be done in all clinical scenarios where MSK disease is a concern (see Box 17.4). It is essential to perform all parts of the pGALS screen as symptoms may not be localised, and it is important to check for verbal and non-verbal clues of joint discomfort such as facial expression or withdrawal of a limb. The information needs to be interpreted in the context of examination elsewhere (e.g. chest, abdomen, neurological examinations) and, in the case of a pyrexia or unwell child, common sources of infection (such as ears, throat and urine).

---

Box 17.3 ○ *Performing the pGALS screening examination – practical tips*

▶ Get the child to copy you doing the manoeuvres.

▶ Look for verbal and non-verbal clues of discomfort (e.g. facial expression, withdrawal).

▶ Do the full screen becasue extent of joint involvement may not be obvious from the history.

▶ Look for asymmetry (e.g. muscle bulk, joint swelling, range of joint movement).

▶ Consider clinical patterns (e.g. non-benign hypermobility and Marfanoid habitus or skin elasticity, and association of leg length discrepancy and scoliosis).

---

Box 17.4 ○ *When to perform pGALS in the assessment – practical tips*

▸ Child with muscle, joint or bone pain.

▸ Unwell child with pyrexia.

▸ Child with limp.

▸ Delay or regression of motor milestones.

▸ The 'clumsy' child in the absence of neurological disease.

▸ Child with chronic disease and known association with MSK presentations.

---

The components of pGALS are given in Table 17.4, with more detail about pGALS available as free educational resources (www.arthritisresearchuk. org/arthritis_information/order_our_publications.aspx). Following the screening examination, the observer is directed to a more detailed examination of the relevant area, based on the *'look, feel, move'* principle, as in the adult Regional Examination of the Musculoskeletal system (called REMS,[4] www.arthritisresearchuk.org/arthritis_information/information_for_medical_profes/medical_student_handbook.aspx). An evidence-based approach to a children's regional examination (to be called pREMS) is being developed.

---

Table 17.4 ○ *The pGALS musculoskeletal screen*

**Screening questions:**

Do you (or does your child) have any pain or stiffness in your (their) joints, muscles or back?
Do you (or does your child) have any difficulty getting yourself (him/herself) dressed without any help?
Do you (or does your child) have any problem going up and down stairs?

| Screening manoeuvres | What is being assessed? |
| --- | --- |
| Observe the child standing (from front, back and sides) | Posture, habitus, skin rashes, deformity – such as leg length inequality, leg alignment (valgus, varus), scoliosis, joint swelling, muscle wasting, flat feet |
| Observe the child walking and **'Walk on your tip-toes'** and then **'Walk on your heels'** | Ankles, subtalar, midtarsal, and small joints of feet and toes. Foot posture and presence of longitudinal arches of feet |
| 'Hold your hands out straight in front of you' | Shoulders forward flexion, elbow extension, wrist extension and extension of small joints of fingers |

*continued overleaf*

| Screening manoeuvres | What is being assessed? |
| --- | --- |
| 'Turn your hands over and make a fist' | Supination of wrists and elbows, flexion of small joints of fingers |
| 'Pinch your index finger and thumb together' | Manual dexterity and co-ordination of small joints of index finger and thumb |
| 'Touch the tips of your fingers' | Manual dexterity and co-ordination of small joints of fingers and thumbs |
| Squeeze the metacarpophalangeal joints for tenderness | Metacarpophalangeal joints |
| **'Put your hands together palm to palm' and 'Put your hands together back to back'** | Extension of small joints of fingers, extension of wrists, flexion of elbows |
| **'Reach up, touch the sky' and 'Look at the ceiling'** | Extension of elbows and wrists, abduction of shoulders and extension of neck |
| 'Put your hands behind your neck' | Abduction and external rotation of shoulders, flexion of elbows |
| Feel for effusion at the knee (patella tap or cross-fluctuation) | Knee effusion |
| Active movement of knees and feel for crepitus | Knee flexion and extension |
| Passive movement (full flexion, internal rotation of hip) | Hip |
| **'Open wide and put three [child's own] fingers in your mouth'** | Temporomandibular joints |
| 'Try and touch your shoulder with your ear' | Cervical spine |
| 'Bend forwards and touch your toes' | Thoraco-lumbar spine |

*Source*: Foster HE, Jandial S. pGALS: a screening examination of the musculoskeletal system in school-aged children. *Hands On* 2008. Copyright© Arthritis Research UK. Used with permission.[5]

*Note*: Manoeuvres in bold are additional to the adult GALS screening examination.

*Hypermobility* may be generalised or limited to peripheral joints such as hands and feet. Generally speaking, younger female children and those of non-Caucasian origin are more flexible than adults. Benign hypermobility is suggested by symmetrical hyperextension at the fingers, elbows, knees, and flat, pronated feet with normal arches on tiptoe; such children may present with mechanical aches and pains after activity (and hypermobility is a common feature of growing pains as outlined below). It is important, however, to consider and exclude inherited collagen disorders associated with hypermobility, e.g. Marfanoid syndromes. These, although rare, associate with retinal and cardiac complications, and may be suggested by family history, tall habitus with long, thin fingers, and high, arched palate.

## Normal variants in musculoskeletal development

It is important that GPs are aware of normal variants in gait, leg alignment and normal motor milestones (see Tables 17.5 and 17.6, and Box 17.5) as these are a common cause of parental concern, especially in the preschool child, and often can be managed with explanation and reassurance. There is considerable variation in the way normal gait patterns develop – these may be familial (e.g. 'bottom-shufflers' often walk later) and subject to racial variation (e.g. black African children tend to walk sooner and Asian children later than average).

Table 17.5 ○ *Motor milestones in normal development*

| | |
|---|---|
| Sit without support | 6–8 months |
| Creep on hands and knees | 9–11 months |
| Cruise/or bottom shuffle | 11–12 months |
| Walk independently | 12–14 months |
| Climb up stairs on hands and knees | Approx. 15 months |
| Run stiffly | Approx. 16 months |
| Walk down steps (non-reciprocal) | 20–24 months |
| Walk up steps, alternate feet | 3 years |
| Hop on one foot, broad jump | 4 years |
| Skipping | 5 years |
| Balance on one foot, 20 seconds | 6–7 years |

*Source*: Foster HE, Jandial S. pGALS: a screening examination of the musculoskeletal system in school-aged children. *Hands On* 2008. Copyright© Arthritis Research UK. Used with permission.[5]

Table 17.6 ○ ***Common normal variants in gait and leg alignment***

| | |
|---|---|
| *Toe walking* | Habitual toe walking is common in young children up to three years |
| *In-toeing* | Can be due to:<br><br>▶ *persistent femoral ante version* (characterised by child walking with patellae and feet pointing inwards; common between the ages of 3–8 years)<br><br>▶ *internal tibial torsion* (characterised by child walking with patellae facing forwards and toes pointing inwards; common from onset of walking to three years)<br><br>▶ *metatarsus adductus* (characterised by a flexible 'C-shaped' lateral border of the foot; most resolve by six years) |
| *Bow legs (genu varus)* | Common from birth to early toddler, often with out-toeing (maximal at approximately one year of age); most resolve by 18 months |
| *Knock knees (genu valgus)* | Common and are often associated with in-toeing (maximal at approximately four years of age); most resolve by age of seven years |
| *Flat feet* | Most children have a flexible foot with normal arch on tiptoeing and resolve by seven years |
| *Crooked toes* | Most resolve with weightbearing |

*Source*: Foster HE, Jandial S. pGALS: a screening examination of the musculoskeletal system in school-aged children. *Hands On* 2008. Copyright© Arthritis Research UK. Used with permission.[5]

---

Box 17.5 ○ ***Indications for referral – practical tips***

▶ Persistent changes (beyond the expected age ranges).

▶ Progressive or asymmetrical changes.

▶ Short stature (especially short limbs) or dysmorphic features.

▶ Painful changes with functional limitation.

▶ Flat feet if fixed (i.e. non-mobile) or painful.

▶ High, fixed foot arches.

▶ Regression or delayed motor milestones.

▶ Abnormal joint examination elsewhere.

▶ Suggestion of neurological disease.

## Common and medically significant conditions with musculoskeletal presentations

### Growing pains

This is a lay term often used to describe children with non-specific MSK pains. Growing pains are a common clinical entity experienced by many healthy young children with equal gender preponderance, characterised by aches and pains poorly localised in the calves, shins, feet and ankles, and not always localised to the joint.[6] Typically, parents report no obvious swelling or bruising; the pains are often relieved with massage or simple analgesics, and are often predictable to occur later in the day, in the evenings and after periods of activity. There is no clear association with growth, but the term is embedded in medical literature and reflects our poor understanding of this condition. Undoubtedly, growing pains cause distress to the child and sleep disturbance and misery for the whole family due to their presence in the evening and at night. The important message is that growing pains are a recognised clinical syndrome with clear parameters for making the diagnosis and guiding management. Given that there is no specific test to positively confirm the diagnosis, it is important to be aware of the 'rules of growing pains' (see Box 17.6), to elicit indicators of concern based on the potential differential diagnoses (see Table 17.1) and to use open questions to explore the problem further (see Table 17.2). The case history on p. 402 (Liam) highlights the importance of the clinical assessment and of exploring the issues with the other healthcare professionals involved.

393

---

Box 17.6 ○ **The 'rules of growing pains'**

▸ Pains *never* present at the start of the day after waking.

▸ Child does not limp.

▸ Physical activities not limited by symptoms.

▸ Pains symmetrical in lower limbs and not limited to joints.

▸ Physical examination normal (with the exception of joint hypermobility).

▸ Systemically well.

▸ Gross motor milestones normal.

▸ Age range 3–12 years.

---

A suggested approach to management and an information leaflet for parents about growing pains (see Figure 17.1 on p. 395) is available as a free educational resource (www.arthritisresearchuk.org/pdf/6541_informationsheet.

pdf). It is important to give the family clear instructions when to seek medical attention again so that potentially serious disease is not overlooked. Indicators for referral would be that the 'rules of growing pains' have been 'broken', such as limping, joint swelling, one leg being affected, pains elsewhere (e.g. fingers) or daytime symptoms. Furthermore, children who are particularly hypermobile or who fail to respond to the above simple approach warrant a referral (to paediatric rheumatology or orthopaedics) to confirm the diagnosis and facilitate a biomechanical assessment from an experienced paediatric physiotherapist, who may advise about footwear, exercises, and occasionally orthotics, although the latter are not always necessary. An experienced physiotherapist, often with a play therapist present, can provide valuable insight into problems in the family, behavioural concerns or parental coping with the situation. The physiotherapist will also contact other healthcare professionals to facilitate the multidisciplinary approach that may be needed. In the vast majority of cases, however, the symptoms settle with no long-term sequelae, but may fluctuate over several months and sometimes years before settling.

### The 'limping child'

This is a common presentation, with a spectrum of age-related causes (see Table 17.1) and the site of the problem may be broad (from a foreign body in the sole of the foot to a tumour in the spine), necessitating a comprehensive assessment. This will include an abdominal examination, pGALS as a minimum MSK assessment, and checking for infection (i.e. ears, throat, chest and urine).

Many 'limping child' protocols focus on hip disorders but it is important to exclude pathology at other joints also. JIA, for example, presents commonly with a limping child and rarely involves the hip in isolation. The most common joint involvement is the knee or ankle and changes are often overlooked, especially if the history is vague. However, orthopaedic conditions at the hip are common and important; early detection and management will improve the outcome. The pGALS screen at the hip checks for internal rotation and flexion with the child lying supine. If there is suspected hip disease, it is advised that the *hip rotation test* be performed as part of the regional examination (i.e. the hip is examined with the child *prone*, allowing the legs to flex at the knees and 'flop' outwards; a loss of internal rotation, particularly asymmetrical, is more apparent this way).

### Sepsis

Sepsis (septic arthritis or osteomyelitis) must always be considered in the ill, febrile, acutely non-weightbearing child with reluctance to move the leg;

Figure 17.1 ○ *Arthritis Research UK leaflet on growing pains*

## Information Sheet (HO1)

# 'GROWING PAINS'
## ADVICE TO PARENTS AND CARERS

## What are growing pains?

- They are common and can be distressing to the whole family.
- They appear to be more common in children who are physically active.
- The cause is not known but children are otherwise completely healthy.
- They do not increase the risk of developing arthritis.
- In most cases no tests are needed to confirm the diagnosis, although sometimes your doctor may request a blood test or an x-ray for your child.
- There is no clear relationship between growing pains and growth problems.
- The term 'growing pains' is a popular, non-technical term but easier to remember than the medical name, 'benign idiopathic nocturnal limb pains of childhood'!
- Most growing pains settle completely with time, although this can take months.

## How can I help my child with growing pains?

- Reassure your child that the pains do not mean serious illness but that you understand the pains do really exist.
- Keep a diary of when the pains tend to occur and what sort of activities tend to bring on the pains – do tell your doctor as this may help him/her to suggest ways to help.
- Check that your child's footwear is supportive and well fitting. Trainers are ideal. It is important that shoelaces should be tied and that shoes with Velcro are fastened firmly.
- Many trainers come with arch supports and these may be helpful. Very occasionally, specially made insoles (called orthotics) may be advised, but check with your doctor.
- By keeping a diary you may be able to tell when the pains may happen (e.g. after your child has had a busy day). To prevent pains from starting and to prevent night waking, try giving your child a dose of painkillers (such as paracetamol or ibuprofen) before physical activities or at bedtime. *(Make sure you use sugar-free medicines to look after his or her teeth!)*
- If your child does get pain, try massaging the muscles and joints. You can give more painkillers if necessary (check the packaging for the right dose or, if you are not sure, ask your pharmacist or doctor).

## What should I look out for and when should we go back to see the doctor?

If you notice any of the following, make an appointment for the doctor to check your child:

- Joint swelling
- Pains in one leg rather than both
- Pains affecting arms or back rather than just legs
- Fever, loss of appetite or weight loss
- Waking every night with pain
- Reluctance to walk or limping, especially in the mornings
- Reluctance to take part in sports or play because of pains
- Missing school owing to pains.

---

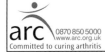

0870 850 5000
www.arc.org.uk
Committed to curing arthritis

*This information sheet can be downloaded as a separate PDF file via www.arc.org.uk/arthinfo/medpubs/6541/6541.asp.*

*'Hands On'* Autumn 2008 No 1. **Medical Editor** Louise Warburton, GP, GPwSI in Rheumatology and Musculoskeletal Medicine. **Production Editor** Frances Mawer (**arc**). Published by the Arthritis Research Campaign, Copeman House, St Mary's Court, St Mary's Gate, Chesterfield S41 7TD. Registered Charity No. 207711.

*Source:* Foster HE, Boyd D, Jandial S. 'Growing pains': a practical guide for primary care. *Hands On* 2008. Copyright© Arthritis Research UK. Used with permission.[5]

urgent referral is warranted. However, the clinical presentation of *transient synovitis* or '*irritable hip*' is similar to that of septic arthritis. In young children it presents as acute onset of fever, limp and reluctance to weightbear; there is limited hip movement, especially internal rotation. Urgent *same-day* referral for orthopaedic assessment is required (with full blood count, acute-phase reactants and radiographic and ultrasound imaging as a minimum). Sepsis is more likely in the ill child, with raised inflammatory markers and white cell count, necessitating joint aspiration and prolonged antibiotics. Transient synovitis tends to respond to rest and analgesia; it resolves over a few days with no long-term sequelae.

### Legg–Calvé–Perthes disease

Legg–Calvé–Perthes disease (avascular necrosis of the femoral head) sometimes follows a transient synovitis (< 5% of cases) and may be suspected if a mild synovitis persists or the limp recurs after settling. In the older child (often overweight) an acute (or subacute) presentation of a well, albeit limping, child and limitation of hip movement raises the possibility of *slipped upper femoral epiphysis*. It is important to request radiographs of both hips with 'frog views' to detect subtle changes that can be masked in standard views. In the very young child it is important to consider *developmental dysplasia of the hip*, which may have been missed in early hip screening. Clues would include a well-looking child with a more persistent limp, asymmetrical skin creases, leg length discrepancy and limited hip movement.

### Knee pain

This is common in children and adolescents, with a spectrum of age-related diagnoses. Adolescent boys who are physically active (taking part particularly in football or basketball) are prone to osteochondritis of the patellar tendon insertion at the knee (such as *Osgood–Schlatter's disease*), which commonly presents with knee pain after exercise, localised tenderness and sometimes swelling over the tibial tuberosity. *Meniscal injury* may be suggested by acute severe pain, often with a clear history of injury, with joint swelling and a history of instability (i.e. locking or giving way). More indolent and persistent knee pain in the physically very active adolescent, with localised tenderness over the femoral (usually lateral) condyles and joint line, is suggestive of *osteochondritis dissecans* (segmental avascular necrosis of the subchondral bone); most cases settle with rest although the lesions may progress, produce a loose fragment and cause instability and ultimately require surgery. *Anterior knee pain* is a common cause of mechanical knee pain, predominantly adolescent females with pain worse on stairs or after exercise. It is often associated with hypermobility and flat feet, suggesting a biomechanical component to the aetiology. The concept of *referred pain* from the hip or thigh, for example, must be sought in situations where the child has knee pain but there is no evidence of localised disease at the knee. *Malignant bone tumours* are most common in the distal thigh and upper tibia, most often in the older child and adolescent, and may present with joint swelling (often the knee) as well as bone pain and tenderness with or without systemic features. Persistent night waking and asymmetrical leg pain relieved by NSAIDs is a characteristic presentation for *osteoid osteoma*, a benign bone tumour presenting in childhood and most commonly in the thigh (or spine).

In the absence of sepsis and trauma, JIA is the most likely diagnosis in the child with a single swollen joint and, although this is a relatively uncommon occurrence in the clinical workload of a GP, the prevalence of JIA is the same as diabetes or epilepsy in children (1 in 1000).[7] JIA most commonly affects the knee although other joints are frequently involved but often overlooked, especially in young children (such as fingers, toes, feet and ankles). The most common presentation of JIA is a well-looking child, often of preschool age, female and with a swollen knee and intermittent limp. Verbalised pain may be absent. These children have the highest risk of *chronic anterior uveitis*, a potentially blinding condition that is invariably asymptomatic (i.e. without redness, pain or visual blurring) in the early stages and only detected by slit-lamp examination by an experienced ophthalmologist. If there is suspicion of inflammatory joint disease (JIA), then *prompt referral* to paediatric rheumatology is required to confirm the diagnosis, minimise disability through rapid access to medical treatments and facilitate access to eye screening for chronic anterior uveitis.

### Back pain

This warrants concern, especially in the pre-adolescent as described in the case study (Angie). Invariably, back pain requires referral, although in many cases it is deemed *mechanical*, with contributory factors such as poor posture, physical inactivity or abnormal loading (such as carrying heavy school bags on one shoulder). 'Red flags' for urgent referral for a child with back pain include a painful scoliosis, night pain, persistence of pain, neurological symptoms suggestive of nerve root entrapment or cord compression and systemic features to suggest *malignancy* or *sepsis*. Localised tenderness is helpful and, in the very young (infant), pain and distress on spine flexion (such as in nappy changing) along with systemic upset and a fever raises suspicion of *discitis*. Inflammatory back pain in the adolescent may be a late feature of *enthesitis-related arthritis* (a subtype of JIA) with a strong association with expression of HLA-B27 and a family history of ankylosing spondylitis. Certain sporting activities such as cricket bowling or gymnastics pose an increased risk of back pain, with possible consequences such as *spondylolysis* and *spondylolisthesis*, which present as acute, or acute on chronic pain, with pain on spine extension and also with localised tenderness. *Scheuermann's disease* results from vertebral wedging due to an osteochondosis of the thoracic spine and may or may not be symptomatic (i.e. may be a coincidental finding on radiograph), although it can result in thoracic kyphosis, and warrants referral to orthopaedics.

### Systemic diseases

Widespread myalgia, arthralgia and fatigue are features of *anaemia*, thyroid disease (especially *hypothyroidism*) and also *viral infections and post-viral syndromes*. In the context of failure to thrive, irritability, generalised aches and pains, and joint swelling (often wrists), *osteomalacia* must be considered, especially with non-Caucasian ethnic background, poor socioeconomic status, certain diets (e.g. vegan) and certain chronic diseases (such as renal disease or malabsorption syndromes). *Inflammatory muscle disease* can be indolent and the photosensitive rash of juvenile dermatomyositis can be subtle and easily missed. *Systemic lupus erythematosus (SLE)* is rare but must be considered in the child or adolescent with non-specific aches and pains and systemic upset, especially if non-Caucasian and female. *Leukaemia and other malignancies* (such as neuroblastoma in the preschool child) need to be considered with any suggestion of 'red flags'. Systemic diseases are unlikely to be misdiagnosed as growing pains as clearly the presentations are not compatible with the 'rules of growing pains', and investigations and referral are warranted.

### Complex regional pain syndromes

Complex regional pain syndromes (CRPS, previously called idiopathic pain syndromes) may present with aches and pains but, unlike growing pains, invariably appear in older female children (often adolescents). Patients are markedly debilitated by pain and fatigue, with an accompanying poor sleep pattern, symptoms during the day, and there is often school absenteeism. The pain can be extreme and incapacitating, affect any region, including arms, legs or back, and patients may present to clinic in a wheelchair. The child or adolescent with CRPS is otherwise well and physical examination is usually normal; the characteristic tender points that are found in adults with fibromyalgia may be absent or fewer in number in children. The aetiology of CRPS is unknown but affected children often have significant associated stresses in their lives, such as in the family or at school, which may trigger or exacerbate the syndrome (e.g. parental disharmony, family bereavement, bullying or abuse). They may also be high achievers, for example in sport or academia. Some potential stressors may only be uncovered by interviewing teachers and other family members.

### When to consider investigations?

In the majority of cases, with a typical presentation consistent with the 'rules of growing pains', no investigations are necessary. When the presentation warrants investigation as outlined above, the clinical scenario determines the tests required, with those most helpful listed (see Box 17.7). *If there is clinical concern, however, then referral should not be delayed while arranging investigations in primary care – referral to general paediatrics, paediatric orthopaedics or rheumatology is appropriate depending on the local referral pathways.*

---

**Box 17.7 ○ *Investigations that may be indicated in primary care***

▶ Full blood count (and film).

▶ Acute-phase reactants (ESR, CRP).

▶ Biochemistry (with bone biochemistry and vitamin D).

▶ Thyroid function tests.

▶ Muscle enzymes.

▶ Growth chart (parent-held record).

▶ Radiograph (both limbs for comparison) and, if hips are to be examined, include request for frog views to help detect early changes (e.g. slipped capital femoral epiphysis).

---

In most cases, a full blood count (with a blood film) and acute-phase reactants (ESR, CRP) will help to exclude anaemia, infection and inflammatory conditions. Biochemistry and vitamin D, thyroid function and muscle enzymes may be indicated and, if in doubt, then it is worth discussing with hospital colleagues. Laboratory tests are seldom diagnostic, but help to exclude other diagnoses; they are used to monitor disease activity and help to predict complications. Auto-antibodies must be interpreted in the clinical context; although antinuclear antibodies (ANA) are positive in many patients with JIA and SLE, they also occur transiently in viral illnesses, non-rheumatic diseases and healthy children. Rheumatoid factor is a poor diagnostic test and is often negative in JIA, but its presence in a child with polyarticular JIA indicates a guarded prognosis. Uric acid assay is not necessary. Urinalysis is often over-looked but in the adolescent with aches and pains, where SLE is suspected, evidence of haematuria or proteinuria suggests nephritis and prompts blood pressure checks and urgent referral to secondary care. In the young child with unilateral leg pain and limp, hip pathology must be suspected and it is important to request radiographs of both hips with 'frog views' to detect subtle changes. Back pain usually warrants radiographs but again, if there is clinical concern, the referral should not be delayed while awaiting imaging.

### The child with chronic rheumatic disease and the role of the primary care team

The GP and the primary care team are integral to the multidisciplinary man-agement of the child with chronic inflammatory rheumatic disease (Box 17.8). The medical management is often complex, with increasing use of potent immunosuppressive agents to optimise outcome. Many children with JIA, for example, are likely to require joint injections, but many will progress to methotrexate, often in high doses and by parenteral route on a weekly basis, often for several years. Systemic corticosteroids are sometimes required and, in accordance with strict national guidelines, children with severe disease progress to 'biologic' agents such as etanercept. Children with vasculitis are often treated with cyclophosphamide and other agents such as mycopheno-late mofetil, often in addition to steroids. Many children are treated with medicines that are home administered (such as methotrexate and etanercept). Children need regular blood tests to assess for efficacy and side effects, and are frequently reviewed in the paediatric rheumatology clinics.

An important aspect of care of these *immunosuppressed children* is *education and support* (e.g. about the safe handling and storage of medicines at home, the need for vigilance regarding infections, avoidance of live vaccines and the impact on having to carry medicines on holiday). Healthy children, especially the very young starting nursery and school, acquire several infec-tions (usually viral) each year, and in the immunosuppressed child it can be difficult to distinguish self-limiting infections (such as a flu-like illness or a common cold) from flares of disease or septicaemia (as classical features of severe invasive infections may be less obvious). Furthermore, the immuno-suppressed child may decompensate quickly and is at risk of opportunistic infection with potentially life-threatening consequences.

The GP and the primary care team need to be regularly informed about the child, its medications and given guidance on managing the febrile child (and

Box 17.8 ○ *Shared-care issues for the GP with the child with chronic rheumatic disease and taking immunosuppressive agents*

▶ Avoid live vaccines.

▶ Promote regular immunisation schedules and booster programmes (avoidance of live vaccines).

▶ Promote annual flu vaccine.

▶ Promote pneumococcal immunisation (current advice is five-yearly).

▶ Vigilance regarding infections in the immunosuppressed (e.g. varicella and shingles, opportunistic infections such as listeriosis, pneumocystis pneumonia).

▶ Advice regarding travel abroad and medicines.

▶ Generic health issues (e.g. contraception, safe-sex practice, alcohol advice).

▶ Travel insurance.

▶ Benefits and allowances.

▶ Support for the family.

▶ Communication between health agencies, education and social services.

▶ Information regarding immunosuppressive agents and monitoring, as well as family information sheets, are available (www.arthritisresearchuk.org/arthritis_information/arthritis_drugs__medication.aspx and www.bspar.org.uk/pages/clinical_guidelines.asp).

401

when to refer), action in the event of *varicella* infection (shingles or primary infection), and the impact on *normal immunisation schedules* for children. It is advocated that children on immunosuppressive drugs receive annual *flu vaccine* and five-yearly *pneumovax immunisation*. Live vaccines are contraindicated and, increasingly at presentation of JIA, all children are checked for varicella status. If non-immune, they are offered varicella vaccine (unless urgent immunosuppressive treatment is needed, in which case the vaccine is contraindicated, advice on varicella exposure is given and non-immune siblings are advised to be vaccinated in order to protect the immunosuppressed child). Many of the current guidelines and information sheets for families and GPs are available online (www.bspar.org.uk/pages/clinical_guidelines.asp), with paediatric rheumatology teams having local variations for shared-care protocols for drug monitoring.

The older child and adolescent require access to appropriate *generic health information*, but there are additional concerns with the impact of the chronic disease and treatments. Pregnancy is contraindicated for patients in the majority of immunosuppressive agents used in rheumatology (biologics and methotrexate) and excess alcohol is contraindicated in patients taking methotrexate. The GP has an important role in supporting the young person growing up with his or her chronic disease, and facilitating him or her taking on responsibility for their health as part of the transition process towards transfer to adult services. Dealing with a new diagnosis of rheumatic disease in a child and the impact on family life is invariably very stressful. Parents will often seek support from their GP, who may have known the family for a long time. The GP and primary care team are integral to facilitating links between community and social services, as well as co-ordinating the various teams involved in the child's care.

---

Box 17.9 ○ *Case study 1 – growing pains*

Liam, aged 5 years, is brought by his mother to see the GP. She is concerned that he frequently complains of pains in his legs, and cries with the pains sometimes, occasionally during the night. Otherwise he is well. He has been complaining of pains in his legs on and off for a few weeks but the problem seems to be getting worse. She is concerned because a cousin on her side of the family has a 'muscle disease' and thinks that Liam may have something similar.

On further enquiry, it transpires that the pains occur mostly in the evenings. Liam is not systemically unwell, is fine in the mornings and is active during the day, including taking part in PE at school. There has been no limping observed. She says he points usually to his knees and shins, and the pains are sometimes worse in one leg, but can affect both. He wakes occasionally at night but goes back to sleep quite readily after some analgesia (paracetamol). He has previously been well and the mother says he was an early walker at 11 months. The mother is a single parent and the health visitor has had considerable input regarding parenting skills.

The GP examines him and finds that he does have flat, mobile feet with normal arches on tiptoes, and this is deemed a normal variant. Otherwise he looks well (i.e. is not pale or febrile), albeit is very shy and sits close to his mother as the GP examines his joints (pGALS negative), abdomen, chest, ears and throat (all normal). His muscle bulk is normal (calf hypertrophy evident in some muscular dystrophies) and after some coercion he shows that he can jump quite easily (a good indicator that he does not have proximal muscle weakness or hip pathology). It is important to consider the family history and mum's concerns about the possibility of an inherited muscle disease (such as a muscular dystrophy), but this is unlikely as he was an early walker and has always been physically active, with no recent difference in his mobility and no limping observed. The GP appropriately concludes that the presentation is consistent with the rules of growing pains, reassures the mother, gives advice on pain relief and suggests she brings him back to in two weeks or sooner if she has further concerns.

In the mean time, the GP talks to the practice's health visitor, who knows the family well and has supported the mother after Liam's father died in a road traffic accident just before he was born. The mother does not have close family nearby and has been anxious to leave Liam with relatives or friends.

## Analysis of case study 1 with respect to the six domains of Being a GP

This case history can be reviewed with regard to the six domains of *Being a GP*. This allows an analysis of events to be made.

### DOMAIN 1: PRIMARY CARE MANAGEMENT

A history was taken and there were already many possible differential diagnoses. The GP assessed the history, looking for 'red flag' signs that would encourage immediate referral. In this case, no real red flags were present, so management could continue within primary care.

### DOMAIN 2: PERSON-CENTRED CARE

The GP used communication and consultation skills to ascertain the key points in the history, including the mother's concern about a cousin with a muscle disease and the fact that this is a single-parent family. This would be a good opportunity to explore the mother's beliefs and concerns.

### DOMAIN 3: SPECIFIC PROBLEM-SOLVING SKILLS

Using specific problem-solving skills, the GP made an assessment and proceeded to an examination. It was appropriate to assess Liam's musculoskeletal system, and pGALS was suitable for this assessment.

Using the expertise of the primary care team, the GP then discussed Liam's case with the health visitor, who was able to provide useful background information about the family circumstances and the death of Liam's father.

### DOMAIN 4: A COMPREHENSIVE APPROACH

Liam's case presents many problems and ramifications that must be addressed. There is the issue of bereavement and a possible family history of a muscle disease. The GP may need to involve other members of the practice team such as the school nurse to help manage the problem. Should Liam be referred at this stage of presentation? Or are there simple measures that can be instituted now? With help from the school nurse and perhaps some family support at home, will reassurance work?

**DOMAINS 5 AND 6: COMMUNITY ORIENTATION, A HOLISTIC APPROACH**

Community orientation and a holistic approach will help the GP to see what impact Liam's joint pains are having on his family and school. Does Liam's mother need medical help? Is she depressed and not coping with the situation? How is she interacting with neighbours, friends and family?

The mother returns after two weeks, saying Liam is worse and being sent home early from school due to leg pains. He cries in the evenings and cannot sometimes be consoled. The mother is upset and concerned that something has been 'missed'. The GP enquires further. Liam is physically active in the day and there are no systemic features, with no history of a limp or a joint swelling. The symptoms are as before, affecting both legs and rather poorly localised to his knees and shins. He is waking only occasionally at night but the mother admits that, when he wakes, she tends to sleep with him to help him get off to sleep again.

On examination he is again unremarkable. He has a normal pGALS screen, is not pale or febrile and his general examination seems normal. The daytime symptoms and having to leave school early, however, are a concern. Appropriately, the GP decides to refer him as the 'rules of growing pains' do not apply. He arranges for a full blood count and ESR, and for his muscle enzymes to be checked (all normal). Liam is seen in the paediatric rheumatology clinic two weeks later. The assessment confirms flat, mobile feet and peripheral hypermobility, but otherwise he was unremarkable. However, it was commented on that Liam was difficult to engage with, even with a play therapist present. His symptoms were deemed not to be explained by hypermobility alone and there were concerns about his behaviour in clinic. The paediatric physiotherapist subsequently assessed him on another day and gave advice on footwear and keeping him active with swimming. The mother disclosed that school had referred them to an educational psychologist due to concerns about profound separation anxiety behaviour in Liam. Both the mother and Liam were subsequently referred to the clinical psychology services, with input from the paediatric physiotherapist and support from the health visitor.

In summary he was deemed to have 'growing pains' but the main issue was behavioural, and the tendency was to ascribe all his symptoms to pain rather than separation anxiety. It is clear, therefore, that Liam's pains were not a simple case of 'growing pains'. There is much scope for the GP to help in this situation and provide support to this vulnerable family. A holistic and comprehensive approach has revealed the underlying psychological co-morbidities and allowed more beneficial treatment to be undertaken.

---

Box 17.10 ○ *Case study 2 – back pain in an adolescent*

Angie, aged 12, is a keen dancer and attends classes at least three times per week. Her mum brings her to see the GP. Angie has a three-week history of intermittent low-back pain that is worse after her exercise sessions but which responds to simple analgesics. She is well otherwise.

---

### Analysis of case study 2 with respect to the six domains of Being a GP

The GP enquiry focuses on the exclusion of serious pathology (i.e. infection, tumour, trauma, prolapsed disc). She asks about the pain locality (low back with no radiation), exacerbation with coughing or straining (there is none) and any systemic upset such as fever, night waking or malaise (there is none). Enquiry is made about family circumstances and how Angie is performing at school, and the GP asks how much exercise she takes. Using appropriate *communication skills* she explores Angie and her mother's concerns about the nature of the pain and their expectations of management and treatment. If deemed appropriate, the GP may involve members of the wider multidisciplinary team (MDT), such as the school nurse, to glean more information about Angie.

#### DOMAIN 3: SPECIFIC PROBLEM-SOLVING SKILLS

The GP decides that a musculoskeletal examination would be appropriate and seeks permission and consent from Angie and her mother. She enquires about whether they would like a chaperone.

General examination is unremarkable and she looks well with no fever; abdominal examination is normal. Angie's pGALS screen is negative other than joint hypermobility of her peripheral joints; she is able to touch her toes quite easily. A more detailed examination of her back reveals no scoliosis on forward bending; there is no tenderness of her spine and she can stand on one leg and extend her back without pain (a good indicator that local pathology is unlikely).

#### DOMAINS 4 AND 6: A COMPREHENSIVE APPROACH, A HOLISTIC APPROACH

The GP assessment concludes that there are no indicators of serious pathology and that her symptoms are likely to be related to minor trauma and may settle. The GP explores Angie's concerns (which are that she may miss out on the opportunity for a role in a local show in two months' time) and suggests a fortnight of rest from the gym. She recommends swimming instead to keep up her fitness. Angie should use simple analgesia and return in two weeks for review. This comprehensive approach has revealed possible reasons for the presentation at this point in time and the GP decides to use time as a factor in allowing rest and healing.

She returns, however, just after a week, with increasing pain in her back, which is there most of the time and has meant she has been unable to get to school today. She has had some night waking in the last few days. Otherwise she is well, with no systemic upset; the pain is again localised to the lower back without radiation or cough impulse. On examination, her pGALS screen demonstrates that her forward bending is reduced and she complains of pain on bending. A more detailed examination demonstrates that standing on one leg reproduces her pain and she has a positive straight-leg raise test. She is tender over her lower lumbar spine but neurological examination is normal.

## DOMAIN 1: PRIMARY CARE MANAGEMENT

The GP is concerned about the worsening symptoms and the physical findings. It is decided to refer Angie for urgent assessment, and the GP appropriately contacts the local orthopaedic department by phone and the patient is seen the next day at the orthopaedic clinic (*knowledge of local consultant colleagues and clinics, and how to refer quickly into the local secondary care system*).

This case highlights the emergence of important localising signs and symptoms that warrant urgent referral without need to arrange a radiograph or blood tests beforehand. Angie was investigated (radiographs and subsequent MRI) and found to have a mild spondylolisthesis (a fracture of the pars interarticularis that can allow forward slippage of the vertebra, which often results from a defect and may be congenital). She did not require surgical intervention but was kept under orthopaedic review. She responded well to a period of rest and subsequently began a much reduced and less competitive dancing regime.

The GP received the letter from the hospital clinic stating that the problem was a 'spondylolisthesis'. The GP was not aware of this spinal pathology and decided to spend time searching the web to discover more about spondylolisthesis in adolescents and its management. The GP recorded this as a patient's unmet need (PUN) and doctor's educational need (DEN) in her appraisal documents (*fitness to practice; issues of maintaining good medical practice*). She also decided to discuss this case with her practice team at one of their clinical meetings, to educate and inform her colleagues about this spinal problem (*working with colleagues and teams*).

Sporting activities involving repeated extension of the spine predispose patients with a spondylolysis to spondylolisthesis, which presents typically with acute or acute on chronic exacerbation of pain, often with limited straight-leg raise – although the rest of the neurological examination is often normal. Standing on one leg (the stork test) and pain on extension of the back are indicators of local pathology but may be absent. Further differential diagnoses include prolapsed disc and tumour, even without systemic symptoms.

Back pain in adolescents is a cause for concern, although in many cases it will be ascribed to mechanical factors such as poor posture. It is increasingly common in sedentary and overweight individuals. However, all cases must be taken seriously and the clinical assessment is important. A painful scoliosis is an indication for urgent same-day referral.

### Online and DVD resources

▷ A full demonstration of the pGALS screen is available as a free DVD and as a web-based resource, **www.arthritisresearchuk.org/arthritis_information/order_our_publications.aspx**.

▷ *Hands On* articles, **www.arthritisresearchuk.org/arthritis_information/information_for_medical_profes/hands_on,_syn_and_topical_revi.aspx**.

▷ Regional Examination of the Musculoskeletal System for Medical Students DVD, **www.arthritisresearchuk.org/arthritis_information/information_for_medical_profes/medical_student_handbook.aspx**.

### Further reading

▷ Adebajo A. *ABC of Rheumatology* (4th edn) Chichester: Wiley-Blackwell, 2009.

▷ Jandial S, Foster HE. Examination of the musculoskeletal system in children: a simple approach *Current Paediatrics* 2008; **18(2)**: 47–55.

**References**

1 • Yeo M, Sawyer S. Chronic illness and disability *British Medical Journal* 2005; **330(7493)**: 721–3.

2 • Foster HE, Boyd D, Jandial S. 'Growing pains': a practical guide for primary care *Hands On* 2008; **1**: 1–6.

3 • Foster HE, Kay LJ, Friswell M, *et al*. Musculoskeletal screening examination (pGALS) for school-age children based on the adult GALS screen *Arthritis and Rheumatism* 2006; **55(5)**: 709–16.

4 • Coady D, Walker D, Kay L. Regional Examination of the Musculoskeletal System (REMS): a core set of clinical skills for medical students *Rheumatology* 2004; **43(5)**: 633–9.

5 • Foster HE, Jandial S. pGALS: a screening examination of the musculoskeletal system in school-aged children *Hands On* 2008: **15**: 1–7.

6 • Peterson HA. Leg aches *Pediatric Clinics of North America* 1977; **24(4)**: 731–6.

7 • Ravelli A, Martini A. Juvenile idiopathic arthritis *Lancet* 2007; **369(9563)**: 767–78.

# Pre-hospital emergency care and the management of burns

# 18

*Alastair Wass and Brian Fitzsimons*

## Pre-hospital emergency care: introduction

In today's general practice, pre-hospital care can take place not only in the GP surgery but also in a community hospital or a walk-in centre. Patients often have a choice of access for emergency care other than their local A&E department. Modern GPs are more likely to come across minor injuries and emergencies because of portfolio careers, and the increased likelihood that they will be working as salaried GPs in walk-in centres and in out-of-hours co-operatives, rather than spending their working lives within one general practice.

Many minor injuries are *musculoskeletal* in nature. Weekend sporting activities are on the increase. Sports injuries and musculoskeletal sprains and strains are presenting much more commonly to general practice than to A&E, and it is important that today's GPs can recognise when to refer these injuries on for imaging and further management.

This chapter will discuss some of the commoner minor musculoskeletal injuries that present to general practice.

It will also discuss pre-hospital care in an emergency situation and draw on some of the expertise of the British Association for Immediate Care (BASICS UK/BASICS Scotland).

## Safety

In all situations, safety is of vital importance. Always consider:

### *Personal safety*

An injured doctor becomes an additional casualty – or worse!

So, if called out to an incident, stay calm. Ascertain where you are going, and to what type of incident you are being called. Plan your journey. Put on your personal protective equipment (PPE). Drive carefully, concentrating on the road, not on what you may face. Use permitted emergency warning devices as necessary. Park the car safely on arrival.

If you are first on the scene, use the fend-off position: 30–100 m from the scene, at an angle of 40° towards the verge, wheels angled in to the verge. If the emergency services are in attendance, park so as not to disrupt the flow of vehicles, and at the direction of the police officer directing traffic.

Then, approach the scene carefully.

### Scene safety

Safety is four-dimensional: left and right; up and down; back and front; over time. With the four dimensions in mind, make a **SAFE** approach:

▷ **S**hout for help
▷ **A**ssess the scene
▷ **F**ree from danger
▷ **E**valuate the casualty.

So, how does one assess the scene? A simple checklist can help, for example:

▷ Is it safe to approach?
▷ Are there specific hazards present?
▷ Is additional help needed?
▷ Are any specialist resources needed?
▷ Who needs to be treated, and in what order?
▷ Is everyone accounted for?
▷ Where do we send the casualties?

#### CASUALTY SAFETY

It is not uncommon for the casualty to be unable to give a history. Additionally, on arrival in hospital, the casualty may be packaged up on a spinal board with full immobilisation applied. The receiving doctors then have no direct indication of potential injuries from the casualty's presentation. It is essential to glean as much information as possible from the scene, to inform your assessment of the casualty.

Learn to 'read the scene', looking for the mechanism of injury. Examine the wreckage for pointers towards expected injuries. Witnesses to the event, and members of the Emergency Services already in attendance, can also add crucial information. Finally, the casualty him or herself, even when unable to communicate, may possess additional information, e.g. medical alert bracelets, steroid treatment cards, or prescription drugs.

In entrapment situations, the clinician will need to decide on the urgency of extrication. Hazards from the scene, and the clinical state of the casualty, will inform this decision.

## Triage

The triage sieve is a quick, reproducible tool to assess the priority of a casualty, and is essential when the number of casualties may swamp the available resources. The four accepted priority categories are shown on Table 18.1.

Table 18.1  ○  *Priority categories*

| P1 | Red | Immediate priority |
| --- | --- | --- |
| P2 | Yellow | Urgent priority |
| P3 | Green | Delayed priority |
| P4 | White | Dead |

The triage sieve (Figure 18.1) is simple, quick and reproducible. It incorporates the ability to walk with the basic A, B, Cs of Airway (with C-spine control), Breathing (with supplementary oxygen) and Circulation (with haemorrhage control). It is a dynamic process that needs to be reviewed and repeated on an ongoing basis.

After completing the initial assessment, it is crucial that correct information is relayed back to the Emergency Medical Dispatch Centre (EMDC) at Ambulance HQ. Again, there is a very useful mnemonic to aid this process, **METHANE**:

▷ **M**y designation, and **M**ajor incident standby/declared (where relevant)
▷ **E**xact location
▷ **T**ype of incident
▷ **H**azards present
▷ **A**ccess and egress routes
▷ **N**umber of casualties
▷ **E**mergency services on scene or required.

This is not time wasted. It is essential that you are safe, that you make a full assessment, and that you pass accurate information back to the EMDC in order that the necessary help is summoned and arrives without delay. This will give the casualty the best chance of survival.

Figure 18.1 ○ *Triage sieve*

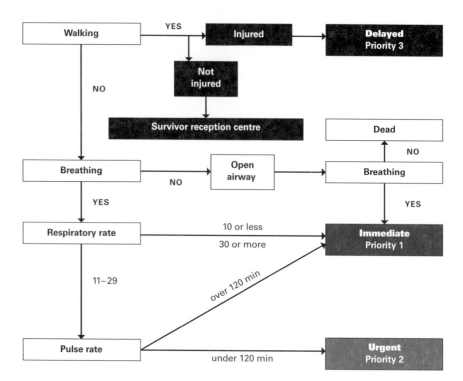

*Note*: capillary refill test (CRT) is an alternative to pulse rate, but is unreliable in the cold or dark. If used, a CRT of >2 seconds indicates **Priority 1**.

## Treatment

**Rule 1** ▶ *anxiety provokes memory loss, so learn a system and stick to it.*[1] A good template for the assessment and management of all emergencies is:

▷ SAFE approach
▷ primary survey with interventions
▷ secondary survey with treatment
▷ definitive treatment.

The system to adopt for the primary survey is:

▷ **C** ▶ Catastrophic, life-threatening haemorrhage – stop it
▷ **A** ▶ Airway with cervical spine stabilisation
▷ **B** ▶ Breathing with supplementary oxygen
▷ **C** ▶ Circulation with control of haemorrhage
▷ **D** ▶ Disability of the central nervous system (CNS)
▷ **E** ▶ Exposure appropriate to allow for clinical examination.

The primary survey is also a dynamic process. The casualty needs to be continually reassessed, especially after any intervention, as his or her condition can change rapidly.

### Catastrophic haemorrhage

This will kill before you have a chance to move to A, B, Cs. Arrest it quickly, and move on.

### Airway with C-spine

An unconscious casualty cannot maintain his or her airway, and one must assume cervical spine injury. The airway takes priority, even when it cannot be maintained without some movement of the neck. The definite risk of hypoxia and death is greater than the potential risk of spinal cord damage.

The common causes of airway obstruction are: the tongue; aspiration of blood or vomit; foreign bodies; tissue swelling within or around the upper airway; and trauma to face, neck and larynx.

A compromised airway should be opened initially using, as appropriate, either head tilt or jaw thrust. An oropharyngeal or nasopharyngeal airway can then be utilised to maintain it. Oropharyngeal airways tend to be only tolerated in the absence of a gag reflex, i.e. in the profoundly unconscious patient, whereas a nasopharyngeal airway tends to be well tolerated even in the semi-conscious.

When these interventions fail, more invasive methods need to be used. Laryngeal mask airways (LMAs) are simple devices to learn to use, and can quickly secure a definitive airway. Where the skill is possessed, and maintained, endotracheal intubation will also secure a definitive airway. However, this is a skill that is quickly lost unless used regularly, whereas LMA insertion is not.

Manual control of the C-spine should be maintained, even with the use of a hard cervical collar, until the casualty is properly secured on either a spinal board with blocks/sand bags or a vacuum mattress. A collar alone will not prevent rotational movement of the neck. Once the casualty is properly secured, the collar should be loosened, to avoid raising intracranial pressure.

### Breathing with oxygen

Brain cells do not tolerate hypoxia. Proper assessment of breathing includes assessment of the structures used for the purpose. Therefore, the neck and chest need to be properly examined.

A simple mnemonic for examining the neck is **TWELVE**:

▷ **T** ▶ Trachea; deviation suggests an underlying pneumothorax
▷ **W** ▶ Wounds; these can threaten both airway and circulation
▷ **E** ▶ Emphysema; suggests pneumothorax or disrupted airway
▷ **L** ▶ Larynx; misalignment or crepitus suggest serious damage
▷ **V** ▶ Veins; engorgement suggests either a tension pneumothorax or cardiac tamponade
▷ **E** ▶ check these *every time*.

Chest examination must include assessment of the rate and depth of breathing. Look for cyanosis, and examine chest movement. Then assess for signs of injury, e.g. bruising, penetrating wounds, or flail segments. Remember, the chest has a front and back. It may not be possible to fully examine both sides, but slipping gloved hands gently behind and down the 'hidden' side can yield essential clues, e.g. blood on the gloves, tenderness, or crepitus. Finally, percussion and auscultation, where the conditions allow, complete the examination.

Rule 18 states that 'all trauma patients are dying for oxygen'.[1] High-flow oxygen delivered though a non-rebreathable Hudson mask with reservoir bag, or by bag-valve-mask with reservoir bag where ventilation needs to be supported, is a must with significant trauma, even when dealing with patients who have chronic obstructive pulmonary disease. Trauma causes hypoxia, and chronic lung disease compounds this. If respiration does become suppressed, ventilation can be supported. The British Thoracic Society's guideline[2] for the use of oxygen is only applicable once the situation is stable, and must be adapted for use in the immediate, pre-hospital environment.[3]

Emergency decompression of any tension pneumothorax will need to take place at this stage, before moving on to assessing circulation.

### Circulation

Protecting the central organs, especially the brain, from hypoxia, is the prime directive in pre-hospital care. Thus, the aim is to maintain adequate circulating volume and avoid shock, which is a physiological response to hypoxia – not a disease. Treatment must concentrate on cause, and not signs and symptoms. The body has excellent compensatory mechanisms. Only after a loss of 1500 ml (one quarter of the adult blood volume) does blood pressure begin to drop.

Even in a trauma situation, one must consider all the causes of shock: cardiogenic, neurogenic, septicaemic, anaphylactic and hypovolaemic.

Why? The bee sting caused anaphylaxis resulting in collapse behind the wheel. The resulting road traffic collision (RTC) caused spinal cord damage plus significant bleeding from lacerations. All of this compromised the already ischaemic heart. Treating only hypovolaemia would clearly be insufficient in this disastrous scenario!

### Treatment

**Remember the A, B, Cs** ▶ Treat the underlying cause where possible. Initiate fluid resuscitation if indicated. Transport rapidly to the appropriate hospital. Pre-alert the receiving hospital with all relevant details.

In the case of hypovolaemia, when looking for causes remember the rule: *blood on the floor and four more*. That is, look for obvious external haemorrhage, then remember to look for signs of internal haemorrhage in the:

▷ chest
▷ abdomen
▷ pelvis
▷ long bones

as these can all be the location of significant hidden blood loss.

To relate the systolic blood pressure to a palpable pulse:

▷ **radial pulse palpable** ▶ systolic BP at least 80 mmHg
▷ **femoral pulse palpable** ▶ systolic BP at least 70 mmHg
▷ **carotid pulse palpable** ▶ systolic BP at least 60 mmHg.

In the case of hypovolaemic shock, consensus opinion on pre-hospital fluid resuscitation has established some guiding principles for fluid replacement.[4]

▷ All trapped patients should be cannulated. However, attempts at cannulation should not extend the on-scene time.
▷ Limit to two attempts, using large, obvious veins where possible. Intraosseous needles provide alternative means to secure access to the central circulation.

**415**

▷ Administer fluids to maintain a radial pulse – hypotensive resuscitation – irrespective of age (a brachial pulse is more practical if < 1 year old). In significant head injury a higher BP (around 100 mmHg) will be needed to maintain cerebral perfusion; in penetrating cardiac injury a lower BP – sufficient to maintain a central pulse – will be needed.

▷ Crystalloid is the fluid of choice.

▷ In adults, normal saline in 250 ml boluses up to a maximum of 2 L is titrated to maintain the desired pulse. In paediatric resuscitation, the bolus used is 20 ml/kg in medical causes, 10 ml/kg in controlled haemorrhage and 5 ml/kg in uncontrolled haemorrhage.

▷ In cold weather, pre-warm the fluids to avoid hypothermia.

### Disability

Repeatedly monitor A, B, C – a brief neurological assessment can be made using **AVPU**. This is simpler to administer and easier to remember in pre-hospital care:

▷ **A** ▶ Alert

▷ **V** ▶ responding to Verbal commands

▷ **P** ▶ responding to Pain

▷ **U** ▶ Unresponsive.

Pupils should also be assessed for size, equality and light reaction. Assessment of blood sugar via BM measurement would be appropriate in an unconscious patient at this stage. Remember, a patient scoring **P** or **U** cannot protect his or her own airway! Definitive management of the A, B, Cs, and correction of hypoglycaemia, are all that can practically be done to address disability in the pre-hospital environment. This is unless the clinician is skilled in, and equipped for, rapid sequence induction, where clinically indicated.

### Exposure

In order to allow a proper secondary survey, this is the final step in management. This may not be achievable in the pre-hospital situation. It is important to remember the risk of hypothermia, and to protect the casualty's modesty as much as possible.

Though a full secondary survey and treatment is unlikely to take place in the pre-hospital environment, a brief skeletal survey and assessment for other injuries, and possibly a more detailed CNS assessment using the Glasgow Coma Scale, is achievable. The pre-alert to the receiving hospital should include a list of suspected injuries and problems based on the brief secondary survey.

On scene after any intervention, and during transport, constantly reassess the A, B, Cs and manage the dynamic situation as appropriate.

---

## Specifics

### *Fractures*

Patients with suspected fractures are a common presentation in general practice. One can come across this in the sometimes harsh conditions of an incident in the community, or in the relative warmth and security of the consulting room. When the diagnosis is uncertain, there are proven pointers that can help.

This is by no means an exhaustive list, but is instead a brief look at the injuries that can cause uncertainty and anxiety about missed diagnoses.

### CERVICAL SPINE

A young, fit, healthy male presented in the surgery having rolled his 4×4 in heavy snow at 40 m.p.h. five hours previously. He has been complaining of neck pain since the incident, and of increasing stiffness and paraesthesia down his arms. He was reluctant to move his head and neck, and had central C-spine tenderness from C4–7.

Given that he had extricated himself from the scene, and then waited five hours before presenting, how should he be managed?

What are the problems of missed diagnosis?

There are no effective treatments for spinal cord injuries. A missed fracture can displace, causing pain and neurological damage. Estimates suggest that 26% of spinal cord injuries after spinal fracture are avoidable with correct handling. Ten to 15% of neck fractures are diagnosed late, resulting in persistent pain, deformity and disability. Late reconstruction is difficult and complex. Litigation, in such circumstances, is not uncommon![5,6]

Can we reduce the level of uncertainty?

Combining the Canadian C-Spine Rules and the NEXUS Guidelines, NICE has produced a guideline that can assist the pre-hospital practitioner.[7] This guideline identifies which patients need X-rays. They can thus guide the pre-hospital practitioner in determining which casualty needs to be treated as a potential C-spine injury. X-rays are needed when:

▷ neck pain or midline tenderness is present, together with:
  □ age ≥65 years

□ dangerous mechanism of injury. (A dangerous mechanism of injury is considered to be: a fall from a height of at least a metre or five stairs; an axial load to the head (for example during diving); a motor vehicle collision at high speed (>100 km/h) or with rollover or ejection; a collision involving a motorised recreational vehicle; or a bicycle collision. A simple rear-end motor vehicle collision excludes: being pushed into oncoming traffic; being hit by a bus or a large truck; a rollover; and being hit by a high-speed vehicle)

▷ it is not considered safe to assess movement in the neck for reasons other than those above

▷ it is considered safe to assess movement in the neck, and on assessment the patient cannot actively rotate the neck 45° to the left and right. Safe assessment can be carried out if the patient:

□ was involved in a simple rear-end motor vehicle collision

□ is comfortable in a sitting position

□ has been ambulatory at any time since injury with no midline cervical spine tenderness

□ has delayed onset of neck pain

▷ a definitive diagnosis of cervical spine injury is needed urgently (for example before surgery).

Using the NICE guideline, the aforementioned patient merited C-spine X-rays due to:

*a dangerous mechanism of injury, midline neck pain, unsafe to assess neck movements and the presence of worrying symptoms. After discussion with a local Emergency Department Consultant, he was fully immobilised and transported for assessment and imaging. Fortunately, the C-spine was intact.*

### Scaphoid

A man in his late twenties was admitted to A&E after a serious RTC – a head-on collision with a bus. X-rays excluded serious injury. However, the patient complained of pain in the left wrist overlying the anatomical snuffbox. There was no visible fracture on X-ray. How should this patient be managed?

What are the problems of missed diagnosis?

Poor healing of the scaphoid can result in malunion, leading to limited wrist motion, decreased grip strength and pain. Delayed union or non-union and possible avascular necrosis can lead to arthritis, particularly in the radioscaphoid joint, but also in surrounding joints. Carpal collapse can also occur. This may occur 4–5 years, or more than 20 years, after injury!

Timely diagnosis, appropriate immobilisation and referral, when indicated, can decrease the likelihood of adverse outcomes. Ninety per cent of all acute scaphoid fractures heal if treated early.

Can we reduce the level of uncertainty?

The scaphoid is the most commonly fractured carpal bone and occurs most often in young men aged 15 to 30. It is rare in young children and the elderly because of the relative weakness of the distal radius in these age groups. The primary mechanism of injury is a fall on to the outstretched hand. Wrist extension and radial deviation result in extreme dorsiflexion and compression to the radial side of the hand. The force is transmitted through the scaphoid. A collision whilst gripping the steering wheel tightly can produce such forces in the wrist, with resulting scaphoid fracture.

**EXAMINATION**

Remember – compare the injured wrist with the uninjured. The patient will often complain of a deep, dull pain in the radial side of the wrist, worsened by gripping or squeezing. There may be swelling, bruising, and possibly fullness in the anatomic snuffbox.

Classically, anatomical snuffbox tenderness on examination is a highly sensitive predictor of a fracture. It is best tested for by pronation of the wrist followed by ulnar deviation. However, it is non-specific. For example, accidentally pressing on the radial nerve sensory branch, as it passes through the snuffbox, can cause pain. Pain on compressing the scaphoid tubercle (extending the patient's wrist with one hand and applying pressure to the tuberosity at the proximal wrist crease with the other hand) has a similar sensitivity to that of anatomic snuffbox tenderness, but is more specific to scaphoid fracture. The scaphoid compression test (axially/longitudinally compressing the thumb along the line of the first metacarpal) can also be helpful in identifying a scaphoid fracture. Absence of tenderness with these manoeuvres makes a scaphoid fracture highly unlikely.

Focally tender wrists need X-raying.

The patient from the RTC fulfilled the age/sex criteria. The mechanism of injury was highly suggestive: clinical examination, with swelling and pain, all pointed to a possible scaphoid fracture. X-ray was negative. However, management with plaster of Paris immobilisation followed by review at 14 days confirmed a fracture, which successfully healed with conservative management.

### Knee

A 37-year-old postman attended an emergency appointment with an acute effusion of his right knee, and pain on weightbearing. He had been playing five-a-side football the previous evening, and clashed whilst tackling an opponent. From his description, he had suffered a forced valgus, external rotation injury. There was an obvious, large effusion with patellar tap, and positive anterior drawer test on this side. He was struggling to weightbear.

How should he be managed? What are the problems of missed diagnosis?

Possibly the commonest missed diagnosis in the knee is not a fracture but an anterior cruciate ligament (ACL) rupture. This injury often requires surgical repair and results in prolonged injury.[8] Permanent disability, and the risk of premature arthritis, can result.

Can we reduce the level of uncertainty?

There really is no substitute for thorough history taking and good clinical examination. Mechanism of injury can often be determined from the history, and can inform the examination. Look for signs of injury – bruising and effusions, range of movement, bone and ligament tenderness – and stress the ligaments. The menisci should be assessed using McMurray's and Apley's tests, and by looking for joint line tenderness.

The Ottawa Knee Rules can be useful in determining whether there are sufficient grounds for X-rays. In addition, applying the Pittsburgh Decision Rules is helpful.[9] These can be summarised as follows:

### Ottawa Knee Rules

▷ Age ≥ 55 years.
▷ Tenderness at head of fibula.
▷ Isolated tenderness of patella.
▷ Inability to flex knee to 90°.
▷ Inability to walk four weightbearing steps immediately after the injury and in the Emergency Department.

### Pittsburgh Decision Rules

▷ Blunt trauma or a fall as mechanism of injury plus either of the following:
  □ age ≤ 12 years or ≥ 50 years
  □ inability to walk four weightbearing steps in the Emergency Department.

Ligament injuries are usually diagnosed by effective history taking and clinical examination. There are currently no validated rules for the use of radiography in such injuries.

Mr Postman had limited knee movement because of a massive, immediate effusion – highly suggestive of an acute haemarthrosis. He fell outwith the age range of concern, and there was no history of blunt trauma to the knee itself, or of a significant fall. His knee was tender and, although he was limping badly, he could weightbear. He did not fit the criteria for referral for X-ray. However, he had clearly suffered a significant injury – probable acute ACL rupture and meniscal tear. After discussion with the on-call orthopod, he was seen urgently for assessment and ultimately underwent surgery for these very injuries.

### Ankle

A teenage girl presented to her father, a GP, having jumped up to 'high five' a friend, landing on the edge of the kerb and sustaining an inversion injury. She complained of pain, and had swelling and tenderness over the anterior talofibular ligament and down over the base of the 5th metatarsal. Because of the lateness of the hour, and distance to the district general hospital, X-ray was not easily obtainable.

How should this be best managed?

Can we reduce the uncertainty?

The Ottawa Ankle and Foot Rules have been shown to be effective instruments in diagnosing or excluding fractures in these regions. Application of these should reduce the number of unnecessary radiographs.[9]

Figure 18.2 ○ *Lateral and medial view of the ankle*

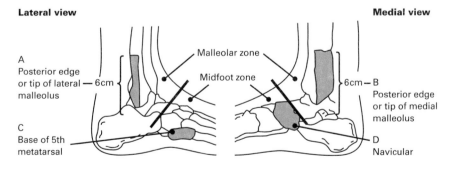

*Source*: Bachmann LM, Kolb E, Koller MT, *et al*. Accuracy of Ottawa ankle rules to exclude fractures of the ankle and mid-foot: systematic review.[10] Copyright© *British Medical Journal*. Used with permission.

### Ottawa Ankle Rules

An ankle X-ray is required only if there is any pain in the malleolar zone and any of these findings (letters refer to Figure 18.2):

▷ bony tenderness at the lateral malleolar zone A (from the tip of the lateral malleolus to include the lower 6 cm of posterior border of the fibular)
▷ bony tenderness at the medial malleolar zone B (from the tip of the medial malleolus to the lower 6 cm of the posterior border of the tibia)
▷ inability to walk four weightbearing steps immediately after the injury and in the Emergency Department.

### Ottawa Foot Rules

A foot X-ray is required if there is any pain in the mid-foot zone and any of these findings:

▷ bone tenderness at navicular bone (C)
▷ bone tenderness at base of the 5th metatarsal (D)
▷ inability to weightbear both immediately and in the Emergency Department.

The RICE mnemonic (Rest, Ice, Compression, Elevation) was applied, and NSAIDs were taken. By the following morning, the swelling had significantly reduced, although the pain remained over the 5th metatarsal. Remembering GMC guidelines that one should not look after one's own family except in exceptional circumstances, the GP telephoned a colleague in the Emergency Department, and it was decided that she should attend. Having examined her, the mechanism of injury – a forced inversion injury, pain on weightbearing, and specific tenderness over the base of the 5th metatarsal – suggested the need for X-ray, which excluded a fracture.

In finishing off this section, it would be useful to review the case of another ankle that the author had to treat!

An 18-year-old female was kicking a football on wet grass when she slipped down a steep bank causing rotational stress to her ankle. The local ambulance and the GP were asked to assist. She had sustained a severe fracture dislocation of her ankle, with external rotation. The talus had slipped posteriorly; the whole foot was rotated almost 180°. The foot, some five minutes after injury, was cold and dusky blue; there were no palpable pedal pulses.

What are the dangers of such an injury? How should it best be treated?

This was clearly a complex injury – a mixture of a trimalleolar fracture dislocation, plus a subtalar dislocation. A trimalleolar fracture of the ankle involves the lateral, medial and posterior malleoli (which is the latter distal posterior aspect of the tibia). These three parts articulate with the foot's talus bone. In actuality there are only two malleoli (medial and lateral) and the term 'trimalleolar' is a misnomer.

The complications of severe ankle fractures include: neurovascular compromise, chronic pain (including complex regional pain syndrome), DVT and pulmonary embolism, non-union of the fracture and malunion of the fracture – both of which can result in joint instability, osteonecrosis, and post-traumatic arthritis. In subtalar dislocation alone, 15% develop symptomatic arthritis, 89% radiographic subtalar arthritis, 72% radiographic mid-foot arthritis. Arthrosis frequently occurs and is the most common long-term complication. It must be remembered also, in children, ankle fractures may involve the epiphyseal plates, which can lead to chronic deformity with disturbance of limb growth.[11, 12]

Pre-hospital reduction of a fracture is not advised unless neurovascular compromise is evident (e.g. presence of a cool, dusky foot) and a significantly prolonged transport time is anticipated.[12]

Clearly in this case there was significant instability and vascular compromise; with the prospect of a two-hour ambulance journey to definitive care. There was no option but to reduce her ankle on scene. Adequate analgesia and relaxation was secured and, using firm but gentle traction and counter-rotation, the dislocations were reduced and the fractures placed in reasonable anatomical position. Immediate restoration of the circulation saved her foot. Splinting to reduce pain and bleeding, and limit further damage, maintained position and circulation till operative reconstruction could take place.

---

## The management of burns: introduction

Injuries resulting in burns are a common cause of attendance in both primary care and Emergency Departments. The majority of burns result from thermal injury. The commonest presentation within this group is with scalds, especially amongst the paediatric population. Each year approximately 250,000 minor burn injuries are assessed and treated in the community setting.[13] A further 175,000 injuries present to hospital, the majority of which do not require admission.[13] Following appropriate initial assessment and treatment, many of these injuries can be managed thereafter in the primary care setting or by the patients themselves. Annually, just over 16,000 patients with burns require hospital admission. The majority, though not all, are managed by Plastic Surgery or Burns Units.[13] Approximately 300 patients die each year as a result of burn-related injuries.[13]

## The role of primary care

Patients who sustain 'major' burns are extremely unlikely to present initially to primary care. They require aggressive resuscitation with urgent assessment of the airway, possible ventilatory support and aggressive fluid replacement, followed by an extended period of continued specialist in-patient care. However, primary care can reasonably be expected to undertake the following:

▷ provide patient education regarding accidents and appropriate sunburn prevention
▷ undertake confident initial assessment and treatment (including analgesia) of minor superficial burns that present to primary care
▷ facilitate and encourage self-care where appropriate following minor thermal injury
▷ initiate urgent secondary care referral of potentially more serious or difficult burns
▷ consider the potential for non-accidental injury (NAI) in the paediatric, elderly or institutionalised populations
▷ continue appropriate burn care after initial Emergency Department assessment (or in-patient care) following hospital discharge
▷ provide appropriate post-burn care advice
▷ consider referral for scar review when the initial functional or aesthetic outcome is a cause for concern
▷ support secondary care to provide comprehensive rehabilitation for patients (and their immediate family) following major burns, especially those with disfiguring scars
▷ be aware of the potential for long-term psychological disturbance including post-traumatic stress disorders.

## Pathophysiology

The skin is the largest organ of the human body. The cells of the outer layer or epidermis differentiate into keratinocytes as they migrate to the surface and are finally lost during desquamation. The deeper layer or dermis is made up of dense fibroelastic connective tissue containing both collagen and elastic fibres. This layer also contains not only the epidermal appendages (hair follicles, sweat and sebaceous glands) but also blood vessels and nerve endings.

The severity and depth of burn injury is dependent upon the transfer of heat from the causative agent to the skin. This will depend upon the heat capacity of the agent, initial temperature at the instant of contact, duration of contact and the tissue conductivity. Overall, skin is a relatively poor conductor of heat, providing a natural barrier to thermal injury. However, children who have underdeveloped skin and the elderly who have atrophic skin changes are more likely to sustain deeper burns.

Thermal insult may result in up to three zones of injury, namely the zones of coagulation, stasis and hyperaemia. The zone of coagulation represents the area of significant thermal contact, which results in coagulative necrosis and death of the skin. The necrotic skin is surrounded by the zone of stasis, which represents skin that is ischaemic though potentially salvageable. The outer zone is hyperaemic, as a result of inflammatory markers causing increased local blood flow, which invariably recovers unless there is severe infection or prolonged hypoperfusion.[14]

---

## Burn assessment

Burn assessment requires a detailed, focused history and careful examination. The initial clinical assessment of the depth of a burn is notoriously unreliable even if undertaken by an experienced clinician. The distinction between superficial and deep burns is not always precise, and burn wounds may not be homogenous with respect to depth (see Figure 18.3 on p. 481).[15] Therefore it is advisable to undertake burn review at 24–48 hours post-injury to reassess the burn, specifically to identify any components of the injury that appear deeper than on initial presentation. When estimating the total body surface area (TBSA) of a burn, it is common hospital practice to use Wallace's 'rule of nines' to assist the initial resuscitation of larger burns, the initial management of which is beyond the scope of primary care. Of more practical use for smaller burns is the surface area of the patient's palm (including fingers) as an approximation for 1% of TBSA.[16] Overestimation of burn size is common in both small and more major burns, though this can be minimised by remembering that erythema alone should not be included when undertaking the calculation.

Thermal injuries that remain confined to the epidermal layer, most commonly sunburn, are characterised by erythema, localised tenderness and persistent pain. Blistering is not associated with epidermal injury, which heals within a few days without residual scarring.

Partial-thickness burns extend into the dermis. These injuries are characterised by the survival at least in part of the skin appendages. Superficial partial-thickness burns classically result from scald injuries (see Figure 18.4 on p. 482) and prolonged sunburn. They involve the epidermis and superficial dermal layers, resulting in tense, extremely painful fluid-filled blisters. The underlying skin blanches and appears a bright pink/red. These burns generally heal within 14–21 days by epithelialisation, with good functional and aesthetic outcome.

Deep dermal burns (i.e. deeper partial thickness) extend into the lower layers of the dermis and heal by epithelialisation from the wound edge and the surviving epidermal appendages (see Figure 18.5 on p. 482). They may initially appear superficial and appear to blanch. However, subsequent review after 48–72 hours reveals a 'blotchy' appearance with fixed capillary staining.[17] There are fewer intact skin appendages for regeneration, which inevitably results in a delay in healing of up to 4–6 weeks. Contraction commonly occurs in association with hypertrophic scar formation.

Full-thickness burns involve the whole of the epidermis and dermis, including the epidermal appendages and the neurovascular supply. All regenerative elements within the skin are destroyed by such injuries.[17] They are commonly associated with flame, chemical and electrical burns. The skin is non-viable and usually appears white or charred, is insensate and has a 'leathery' appearance (see Figure 18.6 on p. 482). Healing occurs by contraction over an extended period of time, with inevitable residual hypertrophic scarring.

**Mechanism of injury**

Burns presenting to primary care may arise following a variety of mechanisms:[18]

*Thermal*

**Sunburn** ▶ from overexposure to direct sunlight results in painful localised erythema, though may progress to blistering in association with superficial partial-thickness injury.

**Scalds** ▶ result from exposure to hot liquids (or vapours) and account for up to 60–70% of burns in children (see Figure 18.7 on p. 483). They tend to cause superficial partial-thickness injuries.

**Flame burns** ▶ are more commonly associated with deep dermal or full-thickness injuries. These patients are at potential risk of associated inhalational injury.

**Contact burns** ▶ arise from either extremely hot objects or prolonged exposure to heat (see Figure 18.8 on p. 483). They are more common in patients with epilepsy, elderly patients who have collapsed (see Figure 18.9

on p. 484) and in those who abuse alcohol or drugs. Contact burns tend to be either deep dermal or full thickness.

### Chemical

Chemical injuries may arise either from industrial accidents or following exposure to household products. The degree of skin destruction is determined mainly by the concentration of the toxic agent and the duration of contact. The corrosive agents cause coagulative necrosis until removal is complete. Alkalis, e.g. cement, generally penetrate deeper, resulting in more extensive injury (see Figure 18.10 on p. 484). Following skin contact, the absorption of certain chemicals, e.g. hydrofluoric acid, may result in systemic toxicity.

### Electrical

Electrical injuries presenting to primary care are likely to be as a result of contact with low-voltage domestic current as opposed to 'high tension' or 'lightning strike' exposure. The hands are most commonly affected, with small, localised full-thickness burns (see Figure 18.11 on p. 484). The alternating nature of domestic electricity can predispose to cardiac arrhythmias.

### Non-accidental injury

A small percentage of paediatric burns are caused by NAI. Vulnerable adults, especially those who are institutionalised, are also at risk of such injury. Delayed presentation, changing history, a history inconsistent with the pattern or severity of injury, an unusual injury pattern, evidence of branding or cigarette contact, immersion injuries, evidence of multiple injuries (not just burns) of different ages and repeat attendances with different or suspicious injuries, should raise the possibility of NAI.

---

**Which burns require initial secondary care review?**

Referral should be undertaken in the following circumstances, after appropriate 'first aid' measures:

▷ extremes of age (< 5 or > 60 years)
▷ evidence of inhalation injury
▷ site of injury, e.g. face, eyes, neck, hands, perineum and across large joints

▷ burns across flexure creases

▷ circumferential burns

▷ superficial scalds (>1% TBSA)

▷ deep dermal burns and full-thickness burns (unless < 1 cm × 1 cm) as skin grafting is often required

▷ chemical burns

▷ electrical injury

▷ NAI

▷ any partial-thickness burn that has not healed within two weeks

▷ symptoms and signs of toxic shock syndrome (TSS).

**First aid for minor burns**

The immediate management of all burns should adhere to simple first-aid principles.[14, 19] These limit progression of the burn, which have a positive influence upon the eventual outcome.

▷ Remove the source of heat and stop the burning process.

▷ Cool the burn by either immersion in or irrigation with tepid water (avoid iced water as this causes vasoconstriction and can cause burn progression) for 10–30 minutes (there are no agreed guidelines). There are also a number of cooling gels that can be used to cover burns.

▷ Dilute any toxins with copious irrigation with tepid water for 15–30 minutes at least.

▷ Cover the burn with an appropriate dressing if the burn is to be treated locally. If referral to secondary care is required, apply cling film or a sterile towel.

▷ Provide adequate analgesia, considering opiates initially.

▷ Beware hypothermia, especially in young children, and keep the patient warm.

**Management of minor burns**

Burns suitable for management in the primary care setting throughout are usually small, superficial and do not affect the 'special' areas, i.e. face, eyes, hands or perineum. Associated injuries, pre-existent co-morbidities, e.g. diabetes and pre-existent psychosocial difficulties including home circumstances, should also be considered. The early priorities in the management of burns are pain control and infection prevention. Appropriate analgesia should be prescribed. Non-steroidal anti-inflammatory preparations or co-codamol are usually sufficient, unless the patient is elderly or there are contraindications. Ensure that tetanus prophylaxis is current. Routine antibiotic prophylaxis is not advocated even in patients with severe burns.[20] Neither prophylactic topical nor oral antibiotic preparations should be prescribed for patients with minor burns. Elevation of the burn is advised to reduce associated swelling.

A European working party of burns specialists advocates cleaning partial-thickness burns and the removal of loose non-viable skin including open blisters (see Figure 18.12 on p. 485). They acknowledge that the evidence for managing intact blisters is weak, though advise blister puncture in burns less than 2% TBSA to reduce pain.[15] It is acceptable to leave small, non-tense blisters alone. Burn dressings need to be non-adherent and maintain a moist environment to facilitate epithelialisation, yet have sufficient capacity to absorb wound exudate. The accumulation of excessive exudate can lead to skin maceration and delayed healing, and predisposes to infection. The dressing must also act as an effective barrier, accommodating local contours to prevent external contamination and reduce the risk of infection.[15] It is advisable to support the non-adherent dressing with either a padded gauze or cotton wool bandage. There are many different 'specialist' wound dressings available. The final choice should be based upon the criteria outlined above in conjunction with local availability.

Initial dressing review should be undertaken at 24–48 hours to assess for infection and to reassess burn depth. It is likely that the dressing will be soaked through at this stage. There may be new blisters that require assessment. Dead or necrotic blister skin may require removal with sterile scissors. In the absence of infection or progression of the burn, thereafter, superficial partial-thickness burns can be treated with non-adherent dressings undertaken no more frequently than every five days. More frequent dressing changes should be undertaken in association with excessive fluid loss (dressing soaked through), offensive dressing odours, contaminated dressing or signs of infection. Dressing changes are often painful for the patient and consideration with regard to appropriate analgesia should be undertaken.

Any burn treated in primary care that has not healed within 14 days should be referred for specialist advice as it is highly likely that the depth of burn may have been deeper than initially identified.

All cases of suspected NAI should be referred to the appropriate agencies following local safeguarding procedures.

## Complications associated with burns

Scarring is commonly associated with burns but is by no means inevitable. A retrospective cohort study of 337 children identified hypertrophic scarring in less than 20% of superficial scalds that healed within 21 days. However, scarring was apparent in up to 90% of burns that had taken more than 30 days to heal.[21] Even if superficial partial-thickness injuries heal without scarring, the healed skin often appears hyper-pigmented for several months before usually fading to attain colouration in keeping with the surrounding skin. Deep dermal and full-thickness burns are commonly associated with hypertrophic scarring (see Figure 18.13 on p. 485) with contractures (see Figure 18.14 on p. 486) if left to heal without early surgical intervention, hence the need for referral to secondary care. Patients of Afro-Caribbean origin are prone to develop prominent keloid scars following even minor burns (see Figure 18.15 on p. 486).

Patients should be advised that infection is a potential threat and may result in a progression in both extent and depth of the burn. Local infections in minor burns are usually staphylococcal or streptococcal in origin. Infection (see Figure 18.16 on p. 487) usually presents with increasing pain, surrounding cellulitis, lymphangitis and adjacent lymphadenopathy. Wound swabs should be taken and 'best guess' antimicrobial treatment commenced, subsequently guided by microbiological sensitivities. Increased frequency of dressing review should be undertaken until the infection has resolved. Signs of burn progression or systemic symptoms will necessitate urgent referral for hospital opinion.

TSS is a rare complication of minor burns and wounds that predominantly affects the paediatric population. The majority of burns that become infected with either staphylococcal or streptococcal organisms are easily treated with simple oral antibiotics. However, rarely, such organisms produce toxins that result in TSS. Therefore any child with an apparently superficial burn who presents with the following should be referred for urgent specialist in-patient care:

▷ generalised erythematous or blistering rash
▷ high temperature
▷ vomiting
▷ diarrhoea
▷ muscular cramps
▷ confusion
▷ dizziness
▷ signs of 'shock' including hypotension.

## Long-term follow-up

Healed burns are often dry, itchy, scaly, sensitive and abnormally pigmented. Regular application of simple moisturisers should be advised to avoid the healed skin drying out. This helps prevent cracking and splitting, and subsequently reduces the risk of secondary infection and breakdown of the skin.[22] Treatment with antipruritic agents may be required. Patients should also be advised to avoid prolonged exposure to bright sunlight and protect the healed burn with high-factor preparations (preferably total sunblock) if undertaking foreign travel to sunny climates for at least 12 months.[15]

The majority of patients who sustain burns return to their normal lifestyle within a few weeks of their injury without either physical or psychological sequelae. Those patients who survive major burns to hospital discharge, or lesser injuries (as a percentage of TBSA) resulting in significant cosmetic disability, will require not only physical but also psychosocial support during their recovery. The young, elderly, those with significant co-morbidities, pre-existent psychological disturbance, drug or alcohol dependence will need increased support and surveillance.[23] Management in conjunction with the local Burns Service must be undertaken to achieve optimal outcomes for these patients. The psychosocial difficulties encountered after burns are varied and include the following:[13,23]

▷ long-term problems with pain and itching
▷ post-traumatic nightmares and flashbacks
▷ grief and bereavement that may manifest as anger or depression
▷ functional issues with mobility and dexterity that may hamper return to work or school
▷ difficulties with decisions surrounding further reconstructive procedures
▷ impaired social interaction/integration
▷ social abuse/discrimination
▷ impaired family dynamics or difficulty with long-term relationships
▷ heightened self-awareness with issues surrounding body image
▷ concern regarding financial wellbeing.

These symptoms will require multidisciplinary support over many months and potentially years to allow the patient adjustment to his or her burn injury.

## Summary

▷ Burns are a common cause for attendance in both primary and secondary care facilities. The majority can be safely managed in primary care.

▷ Superficial partial-thickness burns usually heal within 14–21 days without residual scarring.

▷ Deep partial-thickness and full-thickness wounds, if left untreated, heal with hypertrophic scarring.

▷ Consider the possibility of NAI and initiate safeguarding procedures as appropriate.

▷ Timely first-aid measures limit progression of the burn injury.

▷ The ideal burn dressing is non-adherent, maintains a moist environment, absorbs excess exudates and prevents contamination.

▷ Ensure tetanus prophylaxis is current.

▷ Do not treat minor burns with prophylactic antibiotics; reserve these for secondary infections. Left untreated, secondary infection may result in burn progression in terms of extent and depth.

▷ Burns that have not healed within 14 days merit referral for a specialist opinion.

▷ Be aware of potential long-term complications and the potential for psychosocial disturbance following major/disfiguring burn injuries.

### References

1 • Hodgetts T, Turner L. *Trauma Rules 2. Incorporating military trauma rules* (2nd edn) Oxford: Blackwell Publishing, 2006.

2 • O'Driscoll B R, Howard L S, Davidson AG; British Thoracic Society Emergency Oxygen Guideline Group. *Guideline for Emergency Oxygen Use in Adult Patients,* www.brit-thoracic.org.uk/clinical-information/emergency-oxygen/emergency-oxygen-use-in-adult-patients.aspx, 2008 [accessed October 2011].

3 • Resuscitation Council. *British Thoracic Society Guideline for Emergency Oxygen Use in Adult Patients* London: Resuscitation Council, 2009.

4 • Porter K, Greaves I. Fluid resuscitation in prehospital trauma care: a consensus view *Emergency Medicine Journal* 2002; **19(6)**: 494–8.

5 • Paquette S. *Acute Spinal Cord Injuries,* www.slidefinder.net/a/acute_spinal_cord_injuries_scott/5598097 [accessed October 2011].

6 • Norfolk and Norwich University Hospitals. News archive: tribute for spinal team, 2006, www.nnuh.nhs.uk/News.asp?ID=231 [accessed October 2011].

7 • Wee B, Reynolds J H, Bleetman A. Imaging after trauma to the neck *British Medical Journal* 2008; **336(7636)**: 154–7.

8 • de Roeck N, Lang-Stevenson A. Meniscal tears sustained awaiting anterior cruciate ligament reconstruction *Injury* 2003; **34(5)**: 343–5.

9 • Tandeter H, Schvartzman P, Stevens M. Acute knee injuries: use of decision rules for selective radiograph ordering *American Family Physician* 1999; **60(9)**: 2599–608.

10 • Bachmann L M, Kolb E, Koller M T, *et al.* Accuracy of Ottawa ankle rules to exclude fractures of the ankle and mid-foot: systematic review *British Medical Journal* 2003; **326(7386)**: 417.

11 • http://eorif.com/AnkleFoot/SubtalarDislocation.html [accessed October 2011].

12 • http://emedicine.medscape.com/article/824224-followup [accessed October 2011].

13 • *National Burn Care Review* London: NBCR, 2001.

14 • Hettiaratchy S, Dziewulski P. ABC of burns: pathophysiology and types of burns *British Medical Journal* 2004; **328(7453)**: 1427–9.

15 • Alsbjorn B, Gilbert P, Hartmann B, *et al.* Guidelines for the management of partial-thickness burns in a general hospital or community setting: recommendations of a European working party *Burns* 2007; **33(2)**: 155–60.

16 • Enoch S, Roshan A, Shah M. Emergency and early management of burns and scalds *British Medical Journal* 2009; **338**: b1037.

17 • Papini R. Management of burn injuries of various depths *British Medical Journal* 2004; **329(7458)**: 158–60.

18 • Benson A, Dickson W, Boyce D. ABC of wound healing: burns *British Medical Journal* 2006; **332**: 649–52.

19 • Hudspith J, Rayatt S. First aid and treatment of minor burns *British Medical Journal* 2004; **328(7454)**: 1487–9.

20 • Avni T, Levcovich, Ad-El D, *et al.* Prophylactic antibiotics for burns patients: systematic review and meta-analysis *British Medical Journal* 2010: **340**: c241.

21 • Cubison T C S, Pape S A, Parkhouse N. Evidence for the link between healing time and the development of hypertrophic scars (HTS) in paediatric burns due to scald *Burns* 2006; **32(8)**: 992–9.

22 • Edgar D, Brereton M. Rehabilitation after burn injury *British Medical Journal* 2004; **329(7461)**: 343–5.

23 • Wiechman S, Patterson D. Psychosocial aspect of burn injuries *British Medical Journal* 2004; **329(7462)**: 391–3.

## Appendix: equipment for pre-hospital care

### *Protective equipment*

#### PERSONAL PROTECTION

▷ All equipment must conform to the appropriate British Standard.
▷ Fluorescent Saturn yellow waterproof, wind-resistant jacket with reflective flashes and identification placard.
▷ Overtrousers (as appropriate).
▷ Protective (Kevlar) helmet with polycarbonate.
▷ Ear defenders or earplugs (as appropriate).
▷ Splash protection goggles.
▷ Gloves.
  □ Waterproof, thermal gloves.
  □ Debris gloves.
  □ Neoprene chemical-resistant gloves (as appropriate).
  □ Disposable procedure gloves.
▷ Sturdy boots with non-slip, spark-free soles, oil and chemical resistance with toe protection.
▷ ID badge with photograph.
▷ Hand lamp and/or head light.
▷ Whistle.
▷ One-piece disposable chemical, nuclear, biological (CNB) protection suit (as appropriate).

#### VEHICLE AND SCENE PROTECTION

▷ Green or blue flashing light (as authorised).
▷ Reflective warning triangle.

#### OTHER CONSIDERATIONS

▷ Tough cut scissors.
▷ Map(s), site plans, etc.
▷ Sustenance.
▷ Radiocommunications equipment and spare batteries (as appropriate).
▷ Hazchem code card.

## Contents of a first-response satchel

### AIRWAY

▷ Hand-operated suction unit.
▷ Yankauer suction catheter.
▷ Oropharyngeal airways – 00–4.
▷ Nasopharyngeal airways with safety pins, sizes 6, 7, 8.
▷ Laryngeal mask airway, single use, sizes 3, 4, 5.
▷ Laryngoscope handle, size 3 Macintosh blade.
▷ Spare batteries and bulb for laryngoscope.
▷ Magill's forceps.
▷ Introducer (gum elastic bougie).
▷ Lubricating jelly.
▷ 50 ml syringe for cuff inflation.
▷ Set of cuffed oral tracheal tubes with connectors.
▷ Tape for securing tube.
▷ End-tidal $CO_2$ monitor.

### CERVICAL SPINE MONITOR

▷ Set of semi-rigid collars.

### BREATHING

▷ Oxygen cylinder and reservoir/flow control.
  □ Tubing.
  □ Oxygen mask with reservoir.
  □ Mask or catheter for controlled $O_2$ therapy in COPD patients.
▷ Oxygen-powered nebuliser.
▷ Pocket resuscitation mask with one-way valve, filter and oxygen port.
▷ Bag-valve-mask with oxygen reservoir.
▷ Flexible catheter mount connector.
▷ Wide-bore IV cannula.
▷ Asherman chest seal.

### CIRCULATION

▷ Wound packs.
▷ Pressure dressings.
▷ Cling film.

▷ IV giving sets ×2.

▷ IV fluids – see pharmacopoeia.

▷ IV cannulae – range of sizes.

▷ Venous tourniquet.

▷ IV dressings and tape.

▷ IV arm-immobilising splint.

▷ Specimen, X-match tubes and labels (as appropriate).

▷ Intraosseous needle.

▷ Three-way tap and extension tube.

▷ Range of IV syringes and needles.

▷ Alcohol swabs.

**DRUG POUCH DIAGNOSTIC**

▷ Stethoscope.

▷ Pen torch.

▷ Sphygmomanometer.

▷ Blood glucose analyser.

▷ Peak flow meter.

▷ Reference charts.

**PAEDIATRIC KIT**

▷ (Children's sizes of A, B, C equipment.)

▷ Paediatric sizing/dosage guide.

▷ Paediatric triage tape.

**MISCELLANY**

▷ Spare plastic gloves.

▷ Tough cut scissors.

▷ Sharps container.

▷ Set of triage cards and triage count checklist.

### Ancillary equipment

▷ Defibrillator/monitor with manual over-ride and ECG data recorder (Defib Pads, electrodes, razor, etc.).

▷ 12-lead ECG recorder.

▷ Transport ventilator.

▷ Additional oxygen cylinders.

▷ Entonox apparatus.
▷ Fluid warmer/IV insulation jacket.
▷ Pressure infuser.
▷ Immobilisation equipment.
   ☐ Rescue board (as appropriate) with head immobiliser/sandbags, tape.
   ☐ Straps.
   ☐ Extrication device (as appropriate).
   ☐ Limb splints/straps.
   ☐ Traction splint (as appropriate).
▷ Maternity/delivery pack (as appropriate).
▷ Plastic ground sheet.
▷ Blankets.
▷ Plastic bag for clinical waste.
▷ Sharps box.

▶ *Large items such as trolley cot, carry chair, vacuum mattress will be carried by the ambulance.*

*Source*: Royal College of Surgeons Faculty of Pre-Hospital Care. *Manual of Core Material*. Used with permission.

# Gout

**19**

*Edward Roddy and Michael Doherty*

---

## Aims of this chapter

▸ To recognise risk factors for the development of gout and the co-morbid association of gout with cardiovascular disease.
▸ To be able to manage acute gout.
▸ To recognise the role of both risk factor modification and pharmacological therapies in the long-term management of gout.
▸ To understand when and how to commence urate-lowering therapies such as allopurinol.
▸ To be aware of options for treatment in patients who are intolerant of allopurinol.

## *Key learning points*

---

▸ Gout is frequently associated with traditional cardiovascular risk factors and an increased risk of cardiovascular disease. Presentation with gout should be seen as a 'red flag' to screen for and treat traditional cardiovascular risk factors.
▸ First-line drugs for the treatment of acute gout are a quick-acting oral non-steroidal anti-inflammatory drug (NSAID) or low-dose colchicine (0.5 mg two to four times daily).
▸ If NSAIDs and colchicine are ineffective or poorly tolerated, corticosteroids are an effective treatment by intra-articular, intra-muscular or oral routes.
▸ Where appropriate, patients should be advised to lose weight, and reduce their consumption of alcohol (particularly beer) and purine-rich foods. If possible, diuretics should be discontinued.
▸ The main indications for allopurinol are recurrent acute attacks of gout (three or more in a 12-month period), the presence of clinically detectable tophi, and radiographic joint damage.

▶ Allopurinol should be commenced in low dose, for example 50–100 mg daily, and increased slowly with the aim of lowering serum urate to below 360 μmol/L.

▶ Concomitant NSAID or low-dose colchicine (0.5 mg once to twice daily) reduces the risk of an allopurinol-induced acute attack.

▶ Patients intolerant of allopurinol should be referred to a rheumatologist to consider uricosuric drugs, febuxostat or allopurinol desensitisation.

## Introduction

Gout is the most prevalent inflammatory arthritis and is largely managed in primary care in the UK. The unadjusted adult population prevalence of gout in the UK is approximately 1.4%.[1] The primary risk factor for the development of gout is hyperuricaemia, or elevation of serum urate levels.[2] As serum urate levels rise and exceed the physiological saturation threshold of urate (approximately 380 μmol/L), monosodium urate (MSU) crystal formation and deposition can occur in and around joints. After a period of asymptomatic hyperuricaemia, the first clinical manifestation of gout is usually an acute attack of synovitis affecting a peripheral joint, most characteristically the 1st metatarsophalangeal (MTP) joint. Acute attacks are characterised by rapid onset (less than 24 hours to reach peak intensity), excruciating pain and tenderness, redness and swelling. Other commonly affected joints are the mid-foot, ankle, knee, small finger joints, wrist and elbow (see Figure 19.1).

Axial joints such as the shoulder, hip and spine are rarely affected. Even without treatment, attacks are self-limiting and resolve completely over a two- to three-week period. The patient then enters another asymptomatic or intercritical ('between crises') period until the next attack of gout occurs. With time, recurrent attacks occur more frequently and with increasing severity, and involve an increasing number of peripheral joints. At certain sites MSU crystals may compact together to form hard nodules ('tophi'), which can cause pressure damage to cartilage, bone and other tissues. Eventually, the patient may develop 'chronic tophaceous gout', characterised by chronic joint symptoms, superimposed acute attacks and clinically evident subcutaneous tophi (see Figure 19.2 on p. 487).

Gout is traditionally classified as primary or secondary according to clinical presentation and risk factor profile (see Table 19.1 on p. 442). Primary gout predominantly affects men, presenting from the fourth decade onwards, but may also occur in older women. It is typically a disease of the lower limb with formation of clinically evident subcutaneous tophi occurring as a relatively late phenomenon. Primary gout has an important association

Figure 19.1 ○ *Distribution of joints typically affected by gout*

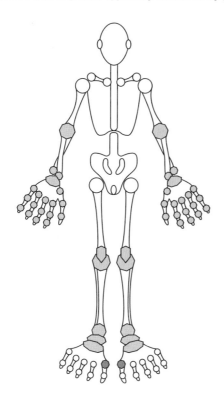

with the metabolic syndrome and its individual components – hypertension, hyperlipidaemia, insulin resistance and obesity.[1,3,4] Hyperuricaemia is thought to occur in the metabolic syndrome as a result of the inhibitory effect of hyperinsulinaemia on renal tubular urate excretion.[5] Primary gout, therefore, is associated with an excess burden of cardiovascular disease including acute myocardial infarction and fatal coronary heart disease.[6,7] The increasing prevalence of metabolic syndrome in the past few decades is probably largely responsible for the increased incidence and prevalence of gout that has been observed in many countries, occurring particularly in men but also in older women.[8-10] Other important risk factors for primary gout include family history and dietary factors such as excess consumption of alcohol, particularly beer, purine-rich foods such as red meat and seafood, fructose and sugar-sweetened soft drinks (carbonated beverages with sugar including cola).[11-13] Of alcoholic beverages, beer confers the greatest risk (owing to its high content of guanosine, a purine) followed by spirits, whereas modest wine consumption confers little risk.[12]

Table 19.1 ○ *Primary and secondary gout: clinical features and risk factors*

|  | **Primary gout** | **Secondary gout** |
|---|---|---|
| Age | Middle-aged | Elderly |
| Gender | Male | Equal gender distribution |
| Acute attacks | Common | Less common<br>May present with tophi alone |
| Distribution | Predominantly lower limb | Equal upper and lower limb |
| Risk factors | Family history of gout<br>Metabolic syndrome<br>Hypertension<br>Obesity<br>Hyperlipidaemia<br>Insulin resistance<br>Excess alcohol consumption<br>Purine-rich diet | Diuretics<br>Renal failure<br>Osteoarthritis |

Secondary gout, which most commonly arises secondary to drugs or renal disease, has a more equal gender distribution and most frequently presents from the seventh decade onwards. It affects the upper and lower limbs more equally, and may present for the first time with tophi without a history of preceding acute attacks. Important risk factors for secondary gout are diuretics and renal disease (resulting in hyperuricaemia) and osteoarthritis (which locally encourages MSU crystal formation if hyperuricaemic).[3,14]

Treatment of gout is usually considered in two separate phases: 1) the acute attack, where treatment aims to provide rapid relief from the severe pain and inflammation of acute gout; and 2) long-term management, where the aim of treatment is to lower serum urate sufficiently to prevent further crystal formation and to dissolve existing crystals, thus preventing further acute attacks and the development of irreversible joint damage.

**Management of acute gout**

The aim of treatment of acute gout is to provide rapid relief of pain by reducing inflammation and intra-articular hypertension. Ice packs can be applied safely to the affected joint to reduce pain and swelling,[15] and the joint should be rested.

The first drug of choice to treat acute gout is usually an NSAID or oral colchicine.[16] Oral NSAIDs are a highly effective treatment for acute gout. There is no clear evidence of superiority of one NSAID over any other but the chosen NSAID should be quick-acting and used at full dose. Although, historically, indometacin has had a central place in the management of gout (it was one of the first two NSAIDs to become available),[17] it is no more effective than other NSAIDs and, given its particularly bad adverse side effect profile, is best avoided. Where indicated, a proton pump inhibitor (PPI) should be co-prescribed. Alternatively, the cyclo-oxygenase-2 (COX-2) inhibitor etoricoxib has been shown to be at least as effective as indometacin, with better gastrointestinal tolerability.[18]

Colchicine is a naturally occurring alkaloid, derived from *Colchicum autumnale*, the autumn crocus. It is an effective treatment for acute gout when given orally in doses of 0.5 mg two to four times daily.[16, 19] Colchicine inhibits neutrophil phagocytosis of crystals and also cell-mediated immune responses. The most common side effects of colchicine are diarrhoea and vomiting, which very frequently occur when colchicine is used in high doses,[20] for example 1 mg immediately followed by 0.5 mg every two to four hours until pain abates or gastrointestinal side effects occur. This dosage was recommended, until very recently, in the *British National Formulary* (BNF). Such high-dose regimes are best avoided. More recent editions of the BNF have changed the dosing schedule in line with lower doses advocated above, and recent trial data confirm good efficacy with fewer side effects with a low-dose compared with high-dose schedule.[21]

Joint aspiration and intra-articular injection of corticosteroid is probably the most effective treatment for acute gout, and often brings about an immediate improvement in symptoms. Aspiration provides rapid relief of painful intra-articular hypertension, with corticosteroid subsequently reducing inflammation. Aspiration has the additional advantage that aspirated fluid can be examined under compensated polarised light microscopy for the presence of monosodium urate crystals to confirm the diagnosis of gout. However, the necessary expertise to aspirate and inject certain joints that may be affected may not be readily available in primary care.

Intramuscular or oral corticosteroids, for example oral prednisolone 20 mg daily, are an appropriate treatment for acute gout when NSAIDs or colchicine are contraindicated or poorly tolerated. They are also appropriate for oligo- or poly-articular attacks, or for mono-articular attacks that occur at sites not easily amenable to injection, such as the 1st MTP or mid-tarsal joints.

---

**Long-term management**

Long-term management of gout aims, first, to screen for important co-morbidity and hence reduce cardiovascular risk, and, second, to reduce serum urate levels with the objective of preventing further acute attacks and joint damage, and shrinking tophaceous deposits. Urate lowering is achieved most often by a combination of risk factor modification and pharmacological therapy.

### Assessment of co-morbidity and modifiable risk factors

As discussed above, gout has well-established co-morbid associations with components of the metabolic syndrome, namely hypertension, hyperlipidaemia, obesity and insulin resistance,[1,3,4] which put patients with gout at increased risk of coronary heart disease.[6,7] Presentation with gout, therefore, should be seen as a 'red flag' to screen for and treat traditional cardiovascular risk factors such as smoking, hypertension, hyperlipidaemia and diabetes mellitus.[16,22,23]

Several lifestyle factors including obesity and excess consumption of alcohol and dietary purines, sugar-sweetened soft drinks and fructose have been established as independent risk factors for the development of hyperuricaemia and gout.[3,11–13] Where appropriate, gout sufferers should be advised to lose weight, and reduce their consumption of alcohol (particularly beer) and purine-rich foods such as red meat and seafood,[16,22] with the aim of reducing serum urate levels. Useful resources on dietary modification can be found in the patient leaflet on gout produced by Arthritis Research UK (www.arthritisresearchuk.org/).

Both loop and thiazide diuretics predispose to the development of hyperuricaemia and gout, independent of the association between gout and hypertension.[3] Ideally, diuretics should be discontinued in patients with gout, although this is not always possible when the indication for the diuretic is cardiac or renal failure rather than hypertension.[16,22]

### Urate-lowering therapies

The mainstay of the long-term management of gout is urate-lowering therapy (ULT). Allopurinol, which is a non-specific inhibitor of the enzyme xanthine oxidase, is the most commonly used ULT in the UK. The indications for ULT are recurrent acute attacks of gout (three or more in a 12-month period), the presence of clinically detectable tophi, and radiographic joint damage, and, additionally for allopurinol, the special cases of urate nephropathy and renal urate stones (see Box 19.1).[16,22,24]

---

**Box 19.1** ○ *Indications for urate-lowering therapy*

- ▶ Recurrent acute attacks of gout (three or more in a 12-month period).
- ▶ Clinically detectable tophi.
- ▶ Radiographic joint damage.
- ▶ Urate nephropathy (allopurinol only).
- ▶ Renal urate stones (allopurinol only).

---

Allopurinol is usually started at a dose of 100 mg daily, then escalated in 100 mg increments every four weeks until serum urate levels are lowered below 360 μmol/L (6 mg/dL).[16] Dose escalation is guided by serum urate levels and renal function, which should be checked approximately four weeks after each dose increase. Although 300 mg is the most commonly used dose in the UK,[25] some patients require higher doses. The maximum dose of allopurinol in the UK is 900 mg, although dose reduction is required in patients with impaired renal function. In severe renal disease, allopurinol should be initiated at a dose of 50 mg and then escalated in 50 mg increments. The aim of ULT is to reduce serum urate levels below the physiological saturation threshold of urate within body tissues (approximately 380 μmol/L), thereby discouraging the formation of new MSU crystals and facilitating dissolution of existing crystals. The frequency of acute attacks and overall crystal load, for example tophus bulk, has been shown to be reduced by lowering serum urate levels below 360 μmol/L.[26–28] It should be noted that the saturation threshold of urate, which provides the physiological basis for target urate levels, lies well within the 'normal range' of urate in most clinical laboratories. Once the target serum urate level has been reached, this should be re-checked every one to two years to ensure it is maintained. Therapy with allopurinol is usually considered to be lifelong. Even when gout is very well controlled by ULT, discontinuation commonly leads to rapid-rebound hyperuricaemia with eventual recurrence of acute attacks and tophi.[29]

Allopurinol therapy is generally well tolerated but can be complicated by skin rash, hepatitis or marrow suppression. Rarely, a severe hypersensitivity reaction can occur, characterised by severe skin rash, malaise, fever and potential multiple organ failure.[30] This is almost confined to patients with renal failure and can be life threatening. If such a reaction occurs, allopurinol should be stopped immediately. Important drug interactions include increased risk of marrow suppression with azathioprine and potentiation of the anticoagulant effect of warfarin. The most common side effect of allopurinol, however, is the precipitation of an acute attack of gout. This is a direct effect of urate-lowering leading to partial dissolution of monosodium urate crystals, which are then more easily shed into the joint space, triggering an acute attack. A number of strategies exist to reduce the likelihood of such an attack occurring on initiation of ULT (see Box 9.2). First, before commencing ULT it is important to explain to the patient that this may occur and to reassure them that, if a flare occurs, it is not an indication that therapy is ineffective but, conversely, it is a sign of successful urate-lowering and crystal dissolution. ULT should not be discontinued in the event of an acute attack occurring. Second, ULTs should be started in low doses as described above and titrated up slowly until target urate levels are reached. Theoretically, gradual dose escalation should bring about smaller sequential reduction in urate levels and hence slower dissolution of crystals and less tendency to crystal shedding. Third, oral NSAID (plus PPI if indicated) or low-dose colchicine (0.5 mg once to twice daily) can be used as prophylaxis against the triggering of an acute attack until a stable ULT dose is reached, guided by individual patient profile and the risk of adverse events.[16,22,31] It is also customary to delay the initiation of ULT until an acute attack of gout has resolved. This strategy makes it easier to educate the patient about the need for ULT and reach a rational management decision once the pain of acute gout has been relieved. It may also reduce the risk of initiation of ULT exacerbating an existing acute attack.

---

**Box 9.2 ○ *Strategies to prevent triggering of an acute attack of gout following initiation of urate-lowering therapy***

▸ Patient information – explain the risk of an acute attack and reassure that this indicates successful, not unsuccessful, treatment. Advise *not to discontinue* ULT if an attack occurs.

▸ Commence ULT in low dose and escalate slowly (e.g. monthly) until therapeutic target is achieved (i.e. serum urate level < 360 μmol/L or 6 mg/dL).

▸ Prescribe concomitant NSAID (with or without PPI) or low-dose colchicine (0.5 mg once to twice daily) during dose escalation phase guided by patient profile.

---

Inability to tolerate allopurinol is infrequent, but if this occurs referral to a rheumatologist should be made to consider alternative urate-lowering strategies. These include uricosuric drugs such as sulfinpyrazone, probenecid and benzbromarone, the specific non-purine xanthine oxidase inhibitor febuxostat, and allopurinol desensitisation. Sulfinpyrazone and probenecid are less effective than allopurinol and cannot be used in patients with impaired renal function.[32,33] Benzbromarone is a more potent uricosuric drug that can be used in the presence of mild-to-moderate impairment of renal function,[34] but rarely may be associated with severe hepatotoxicity. Losartan and fenofibrate have modest uricosuric properties (not generalisable to other angiotensin II receptor antagonists or fibrates), which might make them attractive options in patients with concomitant hypertension and hyperlipidaemia, but they do not have this urate-lowering benefit in the presence of impaired renal function.[35]

Febuxostat is a specific non-purine xanthine oxidase inhibitor that at its two recommended doses (80 or 120 mg daily) appears to achieve target urate levels more frequently than allopurinol at a fixed dose of 300 mg (although comparison with the recommended regimen of upward titration of allopurinol has not yet been made).[36] It was approved in the UK by the National Institute for Health and Clinical Excellence (NICE) in December 2008 and will be available from March 2010. NICE approved febuxostat as a urate-lowering agent to consider in patients who are intolerant of allopurinol or in whom allopurinol is contraindicated (mainly patients with moderate to marked renal impairment). It is metabolised by the liver and requires no dose reduction in patients with renal impairment. In the event of a mild cutaneous reaction to allopurinol, without features of allopurinol hypersensitivity syndrome, oral desensitisation to allopurinol can be considered if the patient cannot be treated with other urate-lowering drugs. This involves commencing allopurinol at a very low dose and then escalating the dose very slowly every few days, increasing up to 100 mg daily over the course of a month.[37]

---

Box 19.3 ○ *Case study*

Mr Brown is a salesman who came to see his GP because of recurrent gout. He had suffered from gout since his mid-thirties and is now in his fifties. Mostly, he had isolated attacks affecting the 1st MTP joints, but in the previous hot summer he had been troubled by recurrent attacks in his feet and ankles. Now, he had almost permanent pain in his feet and walked with a limp. He had once tried allopurinol, but stopped it immediately when it caused an acute attack of gout.

---

The GP knew Mr Brown because he was on the practice's obesity register (*this is part of the primary care management domain of general practice: administration and information management technology, IMT*). He had successfully evaded the practice nurse when asked to attend for repeat weight checks and dietary advice. He reluctantly agreed to standing on the surgery scales and his BMI was 35! He was also classically apple-shaped with a large waist circumference. The GP and Mr Brown discussed his diet (*data gathering and interpretation*). He admitted to drinking approximately 20 pints of beer per week.

The GP explained to Mr Brown what was causing and contributing to his attacks of gout and provided him with information about gout, dietary modification and restriction of his beer consumption (*person-centred care and communication skills*).

It was likely that he had originally had primary gout, due to the metabolic syndrome. Now, he may well have developed secondary gout, as he was hypertensive and taking bendroflumethiazide.

The GP arranged blood tests to check his renal function, serum urate levels and fasting glucose and lipids. Serum urate was 484 μmol/L. The GP noted from his records (*administration and IMT*) that he previously had a raised cholesterol and triglyceride level when he had a blood test five years previously. Unfortunately, this had not been followed up and Mr Brown had failed to attend his diet sessions with the practice nurse. The GP made a reminder note on his electronic records to check that he did not default again (*administration and IMT*).

Because Mr Brown had been reluctant to address his obesity before, the GP explained carefully about the risks to his health (*holistic care and communication and consultation skills*) and encouraged him to try to exercise more. He agreed to be referred to the local gym where there was a special scheme for obese patients (*working with colleagues and in teams*). Mr Brown even agreed to take his wife, who was also overweight (*holistic care*).

The GP arranged to see Mr Brown again in two weeks to discuss the results of his blood tests. It was decided to change his medication for hypertension, from a thiazide diuretic to an ACE inhibitor (*clinical management and making a diagnosis/making decisions*). He also required treatment with allopurinol because of recurrent acute attacks of gout. Allopurinol was commenced at a dose of 100 mg daily. This was increased in 100 mg increments following monthly serum urate checks with the aim of reducing his serum urate below 360 μmol/L. An allopurinol dose of 400 mg daily was required to achieve this. His fasting glucose was raised and the GP requested an oral glucose tolerance test (*clinical management*). Mr Brown would require close follow-up from the GP and the practice nursing team over the coming months and years, to ensure that he started to lose weight and reduced his cardiovascular risk (*holistic care and a comprehensive approach, promoting health and wellbeing*).

---

### Summary

Gout is the most common inflammatory arthritis and is potentially curable, in contrast with other chronic arthropathies. Treatment of gout is tailored to the clinical phase. In acute gout, treatment with NSAIDs, low-dose colchicine or corticosteroids aims to provide rapid relief of intra-articular hypertension and inflammation. Long-term management of gout combines non-pharmacological risk factor modification (weight loss, restriction of consumption of alcohol and dietary purines, and diuretic cessation) and pharmacological ULT, most commonly allopurinol, to reduce serum urate levels below 360 μmol/L. A number of strategies exist to prevent the precipitation of an acute attack of gout on initiation of ULT, which is the most common side effect of ULT. The patient should also be screened and treated for co-morbid cardiovascular risk factors. When allopurinol is not tolerated, referral to a rheumatologist should be made to consider alternative ULT. However, most gout can be managed safely and successfully in primary care.

### References

1 • Mikuls T R, Farrar J T, Bilker W B, *et al*. Gout epidemiology: results from the UK General Practice Research Database, 1990–1999 *Annals of the Rheumatic Diseases* 2005; **64(2)**: 267–72.

2 • Campion E W, Glynn R J, DeLabry L O. Asymptomatic hyperuricemia. Risks and consequences in the Normative Aging Study *American Journal of Medicine* 1987; **82(3)**: 421–6.

3 • Choi H K, Atkinson K, Karlson E W, *et al*. Obesity, weight change, hypertension, diuretic use, and risk of gout in men: the health professionals follow-up study *Archives of Internal Medicine* 2005; **165(7)**: 742–8.

4 • Choi H K, Ford E S, Li C, *et al*. Prevalence of the metabolic syndrome in patients with gout: the Third National Health and Nutrition Examination Survey *Arthritis and Rheumatism* 2007; **57(1)**: 109–15.

5 • Ter Maaten J C, Voorburg A, Heine R J, *et al*. Renal handling of urate and sodium during acute physiological hyperinsulinaemia in healthy subjects *Clinical Science* (London) 1997; **92(1)**: 51–8.

6 • Choi H K, Curhan G. Independent impact of gout on mortality and risk for coronary heart disease *Circulation* 2007; **116(8)**: 894–900.

7 • Krishnan E, Baker J F, Furst D E, *et al*. Gout and the risk of acute myocardial infarction *Arthritis and Rheumatism* 2006; **54(8)**: 2688–96.

8 • Arromdee E, Michet C J, Crowson C S, *et al*. Epidemiology of gout: is the incidence rising? *Journal of Rheumatology* 2002; **29(11)**: 2403–6.

9 • Roddy E, Zhang W, Doherty M. The changing epidemiology of gout *National Clinical Practice: Rheumatology* 2007; **3(8)**: 443–9.

10 • Wallace K L, Riedel A A, Joseph-Ridge N, *et al*. Increasing prevalence of gout and hyperuricemia over 10 years among older adults in a managed care population *Journal of Rheumatology* 2004; **31(8)**: 1582–7.

11 • Choi H K, Atkinson K, Karlson E W, *et al*. Purine-rich foods, dairy and protein intake, and the risk of gout in men *New England Journal of Medicine* 2004; **350(11)**: 1093–103.

12 • Choi H K, Atkinson K, Karlson E W, *et al*. Alcohol intake and risk of incident gout in men: a prospective study *Lancet* 2004; **363(9417)**: 1277–81.

13 • Choi H K, Curhan G. Soft drinks, fructose consumption, and the risk of gout in men: prospective cohort study *British Medical Journal* 2008; **336(7639)**: 309–12.

14 • Roddy E, Zhang W, Doherty M. Are joints affected by gout also affected by osteoarthritis? *Annals of the Rheumatic Diseases* 2007; **66(10)**: 1374–7.

15 • Schlesinger N, Detry M A, Holland B K, *et al*. Local ice therapy during bouts of acute gouty arthritis *Journal of Rheumatology* 2002; **29(2)**: 331–4.

16 • Zhang W, Doherty M, Bardin T, *et al*. EULAR evidence based recommendations for gout. Part II: Management. Report of a task force of the EULAR Standing Committee for International Clinical Studies Including Therapeutics (ESCISIT) *Annals of the Rheumatic Diseases* 2006; **65(10)**: 1312–24.

17 • Roddy E, Mallen C D, Hider SL, *et al*. Prescription and comorbidity screening following consultation for acute gout in primary care *Rheumatology* (Oxford) 2010; **49(1)**: 105–11.

18 • Rubin B R, Burton R, Navarra S, *et al*. Efficacy and safety profile of treatment with etoricoxib 120 mg once daily compared with indometacin 50 mg three times daily in acute gout: a randomized controlled trial *Arthritis and Rheumatism* 2004; **50(2)**: 598–606.

19 • Morris I, Varughese G, Mattingly P. Colchicine in acute gout *British Medical Journal* 2003; **327(7426)**: 1275–6.

20 • Ahern M J, Reid C, Gordon T P, *et al*. Does colchicine work? The results of the first controlled study in acute gout *Australian and New Zealand Journal of Medicine* 1987; **17(3)**: 301–4.

21 • Terkeltaub R A, Furst D E, Bennett K, *et al*. High versus low dosing of oral colchicine for early acute gout flare: twenty-four-hour outcome of the first multicenter, randomized, double-blind, placebo-controlled, parallel-group, dose-comparison colchicine study *Arthritis and Rheumatism* 2010; **62(4)**: 1060–8.

22 • Jordan K M, Cameron J S, Snaith M, *et al*. British Society for Rheumatology and British Health Professionals in Rheumatology guideline for the management of gout *Rheumatology* (Oxford) 2007; **46(8)**: 1372–4.

23 • Zhang W, Doherty M, Pascual E, *et al*. EULAR evidence based recommendations for gout. Part I: Diagnosis. Report of a task force of the Standing Committee for International Clinical Studies Including Therapeutics (ESCISIT) *Annals of the Rheumatic Diseases* 2006; **65(10)**: 1301–11.

24 • Mikuls T R, MacLean C H, Olivieri J, *et al*. Quality of care indicators for gout management *Arthritis and Rheumatism* 2004; **50(3)**: 937–43.

25 • Roddy E, Zhang W, Doherty M. Concordance of the management of chronic gout in a UK primary-care population with the EULAR gout recommendations *Annals of the Rheumatic Diseases* 2007; **66(10)**: 1311–15.

26 • Li-Yu J, Clayburne G, Sieck M, *et al*. Treatment of chronic gout. Can we determine when urate stores are depleted enough to prevent attacks of gout? *Journal of Rheumatology* 2001; **28(3)**: 577–80.

27 • Perez-Ruiz F, Calabozo M, Pijoan J I, *et al*. Effect of urate-lowering therapy on the velocity of size reduction of tophi in chronic gout *Arthritis and Rheumatism* 2002; **47(4)**: 356–60.

28 • Shoji A, Yamanaka H, Kamatani N. A retrospective study of the relationship between serum urate level and recurrent attacks of gouty arthritis: evidence for reduction of recurrent gouty arthritis with antihyperuricemic therapy *Arthritis and Rheumatism* 2004; **51(3)**: 321–5.

29 • van Lieshout-Zuidema M F, Breedveld F C. Withdrawal of longterm antihyperuricemic therapy in tophaceous gout *Journal of Rheumatology* 1993; **20(8)**: 1383–5.

30 • Hande K R, Noone R M, Stone W J. Severe allopurinol toxicity. Description and guidelines for prevention in patients with renal insufficiency *American Journal of Medicine* 1984; **76(1)**: 47–56.

31 • Borstad G C, Bryant L R, Abel M P, *et al*. Colchicine for prophylaxis of acute flares when initiating allopurinol for chronic gouty arthritis *Journal of Rheumatology* 2004; **31(12)**: 2429–32.

32 • Bartels E C, Matossian G S. Gout: six-year follow-up on probenecid (benemid) therapy *Arthritis and Rheumatism* 1959; **2(3)**: 193–202.

33 • Scott J T. Comparison of allopurinol and probenecid *Annals of the Rheumatic Diseases* 1966; **25(6 Suppl)**: 623–6.

34 • Perez-Ruiz F, Alonso-Ruiz A, Calabozo M, *et al*. Efficacy of allopurinol and benzbromarone for the control of hyperuricaemia. A pathogenic approach to the treatment of primary chronic gout *Annals of the Rheumatic Diseases* 1998; **57(9)**: 545–9.

35 • Takahashi S, Moriwaki Y, Yamamoto T, *et al*. Effects of combination treatment using anti-hyperuricaemic agents with fenofibrate and/or losartan on uric acid metabolism *Annals of the Rheumatic Diseases* 2003; **62(6)**: 572–5.

36 • Becker M A, Schumacher H R, Jr., Wortmann R L, *et al*. Febuxostat compared with allopurinol in patients with hyperuricemia and gout *New England Journal of Medicine* 2005; **353(23)**: 2450–61.

37 • Fam A G, Dunne S M, Iazzetta J, *et al*. Efficacy and safety of desensitization to allopurinol following cutaneous reactions *Arthritis and Rheumatism* 2001; **44(1)**: 231–8.

# Musculoskeletal disorders and working-age health

# 20

*Nerys Williams*

## Aims of this chapter

- ▶ To understand the links between health and work.
- ▶ To understand the work-related risk factors for the development of musculoskeletal disorders (MSDs).
- ▶ To appreciate the impact of having an MSD on the ability to work.
- ▶ To understand basic concepts of vocational rehabilitation.
- ▶ To be able to complete supportive 'Fit Notes' and provide advice to aid early return to work.

## *Key learning points*

- ▶ Work is generally good for both physical and mental health.
- ▶ Early intervention is essential to help patients regain and retain their jobs.
- ▶ It is necessary to focus on what people can do rather than what they cannot.
- ▶ If vocational rehabilitation is to work, it needs work-focused health care and workplaces that are flexible and accommodating.
- ▶ There is a strong evidence base both for vocational rehabilitation and for adjusted work leading to successful return to work for patients with musculoskeletal problems.

## Introduction

MSDs are a common cause of attendance in primary care with arthritis accounting for about one in five consultations.[1] Low-back pain is the commonest musculoskeletal complaint in the working population with a lifetime prevalence of 60–80%, a point prevalence of 15–40% and an annual prevalence of 5%.[2] It is the most common cause of absence from work, accounting for 4.9 million days per year, and is the most common cause of work-related ill health.[3] It is the second most common cause of incapacity benefit.[4] Work-related upper-limb disorders are also common, with some surveys suggesting that up to 17–20% of people complain of neck–shoulder pain and 20% report hand–wrist pain in the last seven days.[2] Resolution of and recovery from both back and neck/upper-limb pain can be strongly influenced by non-medical factors. Hence, the biopsychosocial model is more applicable than the medical model of care, and a holistic approach is essential. MSDs are thus costly for the individual in terms of pain and disability, for the GP in the time taken for appropriate treatment and for the NHS in cost of prescriptions, appointments and staff sick leave.

Conventionally, the Department of Health, National Institute for Health and Clinical Excellence (NICE) in England and Wales, and the NHS have focused just on the costs of MSDs to the healthcare system, but the costs are even greater when the impact of these common conditions on the working-age population and wider society is also taken into consideration. Politicians of all parties are taking increasing interest in the health of the working-age population due to demographic challenges that will face all countries over the coming decades and the increased demands for health and social care from an ageing population.

---

### The demographics and challenges of the future

Most countries are experiencing low birth rates at a time of increased longevity. Not only are people living longer but there are also many more people living a lot longer as well. This has led to increased costs for health and social care as the number of elderly and very elderly (>85 years of age) people increases. This trend will continue to increase and over time we will experience an ongoing reduction in the number of people of working age generating income to support the growing number of older people, dependent due to their age. This is graphically seen in the projected trends for the old-age support ratio (see Figure 20.1). Over 25 years it is predicted that the number of workers compared with the number of people retired will fall from 3.2 to below 2.8. In addition to older people, the workforce will also need to support children and people of working age unable to work due to ill health.

At the same time, our working-age population is also changing and we can expect to see a growing number of older people in the workforce (Figure 20.2) and of people working past what is now considered to be a usual retirement age.

Figure 20.1 ○ *Projected old-age support ratio*

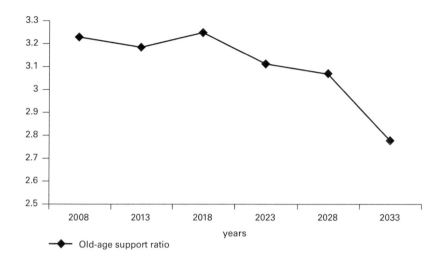

*Source*: adapted from Office for National Statistics. *Statistical Bulletin: national population projections*, 2008-based.[5]

Figure 20.2 ○ *Trends in the population of workers who are >40 years of age compared with those <40 years of age*

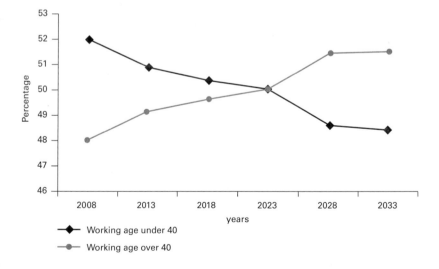

*Source*: adapted from Office for National Statistics. *Statistical Bulletin: national population projections*, 2008-based.[5]

With an increasingly older workforce we are also likely to see more workers with chronic health problems such as MSDs, so timely and supportive management will become even more essential as we strive to remain efficient and effective as an economy. We will need to support workers to stay in work for longer, both for their own physical and mental health, and that of other members of society.

## Benefits of work

Against this background of older workers and more people to support, there is a strong evidence base for the benefits of work for the majority of working-age people. Waddell and Burton's review of the evidence around several aspects of health and work was published in 2006, concluding that:[6]

▷ work is generally good for physical and mental health and wellbeing
▷ worklessness is associated with poorer physical and mental health
▷ work can reverse the adverse health effects of unemployment
▷ work can be therapeutic
▷ the beneficial effects of work outweigh the potential risks
▷ the beneficial effects of work are greater than the harmful effects
    of long-term unemployment or prolonged sickness absence.

## Working-age ill health – where we are now?

Working-age ill health has been estimated to cost the UK over £100 billion a year.[7] Around 172 million working days were lost due to sickness absence in 2007[8] with direct costs to businesses of £13 billion.[9] About two-thirds of lost time is due to common health problems such as mild/moderate mental health, musculoskeletal and cardio-respiratory conditions. The same conditions also lead to about two-thirds of incapacity benefit claims and cases of ill-health retirement. It has been estimated that back pain alone cost the UK economy an estimated £5.7 billion per year in 1995/6[10] – the equivalent of £7 billion when adjusted to 2007 prices.[11] This is clearly money that could be spent on other health care, education and social support.

There are a number of issues around work and health that need exploring:

1  ▷ Work as a cause of ill health
2  ▷ Working with a chronic health problem such as back or upper-limb pain
3  ▷ Rehabilitation, particularly vocational rehabilitation.

## Work as a cause of ill health

Badly designed work not only injures workers but also affects productivity. It is easy from a primary care perspective to accept that when a patient says that his or her work causes a musculoskeletal problem that this is in fact the truth. However, work is often only one of many factors influencing the causation of a condition and its continuation. Carpal tunnel syndrome is a common condition but so is keyboard use both at home and at work. It is likely to be more symptomatic when the hands are used, so patients may blame their job without considering that the ergonomics of their equipment at work is much better than that of their computer at home. The Health and Safety Executive estimates that there are about half a million people who have a back problem caused by work.[12] Back pain is not just associated with manual jobs but also with static and constrained postures. It can be aggravated by working without breaks and changes of posture and position. Risk factors within jobs include heavy and repeated lifting, working outside the ergonomic envelope of comfort for the joints, excessive grip and force. Other factors include cold and draughty workplaces and inappropriate protective equipment, which protects against one hazard but makes another worse (an example might be very bulky gloves, which protect against sharps injuries but reduce manipulation so the person has to grip harder). If a musculoskeletal injury results from an accident and results in significant disability then the individual may be eligible for Industrial Injuries Disablement (IIDB) under the Social Security (Prescribed Diseases) Regulations 1985,[13] which is administrated by the Department for Work and Pensions. There are also a few musculoskeletal conditions that may attract benefit – these all have an evidence base, which shows a significant excess of risk in specific occupations. Thus carpal tunnel syndrome is listed but only for workers using vibrating tools. There is insufficient evidence to pay state compensation for carpal tunnel syndrome arising in a typist for example – the strength of cause and effect is just not strong enough. MSDs and their relevant occupations for IIDB are listed in Box 20.1.

## Prevention of work-related musculoskeletal ill health

Musculoskeletal ill health can be prevented through good work design, both of the tasks undertaken and the work organisation. In the UK the Health and Safety at Work Act 1974 (HASAWA)[13] requires employers to do all that is reasonably practicable to ensure the health, safety and welfare of their employees. Employees also have duties to comply with their employers' policies and procedures, and arrangements for health and safety. The self-employed are

---

**Box 20.1 ○ *Musculoskeletal conditions that may attract IIDB***

▶ Cramp of the hand or forearm due to repeated movements, e.g. writer's cramp.

▶ Subcutaneous cellulitis of the hand, knee or elbow due to severe friction or pressure.

▶ Traumatic inflammation of the tendons of the hand or forearm, or of associated tendon sheaths – tenosynovitis.

▶ Episodic blanching affecting middle or proximal phalanges, or in the case of the thumb the proximal phalanx due to the use of hand-held percussive or powered tools.

▶ Osteoarthritis of the hip in farmers or farm workers.

▶ Osteoarthritis of the knee in miners (this is only newly prescribed).

*Source*: IIAC. www.dwp.gv.uk/directgov/industrial injuries benefit.

---

also covered and have duties, as do the manufacturers of goods and equipment. The act sets out the broad requirements but it is the regulations that provide more detail on what is required. There are several discrete pieces of legislation that are relevant to preventing MSDs.

These are:

▷ The Management of Health and Safety Regulations 1992
▷ The Manual Handling Operations Regulations 1992
▷ The Health and Safety (Display Screen Equipment) Regulations 1992.

The first of these requires employers to, amongst other duties, carry out risk assessments and identify risks to employee health. The Manual Handling Operations Regulations require them to carry out risk assessments on manual handling (pushing and pulling, as well as lifting) and the display screen equipment regulations require risk assessment of workstations and give users the right to eye and eyesight examinations. The general aim of all legislation is to lead to identification and then reduction of risks, so protecting workers' health with a hierarchy of measures. This starts with avoiding an activity if the risk is high, down to carrying out health surveillance if all that is reasonably practicable has been done to reduce risk but risk still remains. The aim of health surveillance is to allow early identification of harm and protection of both the worker and his or her fellow workers. If a patient feel that his or her health is being harmed by work, he or she can contact either the Health and Safety Executive (HSE) (www.hse.gov.uk) or the local council health and safety department, depending on which body is the relevant authority. For work in shops and offices, the local council enforces the relevant legislation, while the HSE covers factories, mines, quarries and NHS premises.

## Working with a chronic heath problem

The number of days lost through people acquiring MSDs from their work is dwarfed by the number of people who have non-work-related problems that impact on their ability to do their job. Back, neck, arm and leg pain can result in both short- (<7 days) and long-term (>4 weeks) sickness absence. NICE has recently published guidance on both the management of low-back pain [14] and long-term sickness absence [15] in its public health and clinical guidance series. The NICE guidance on long-term sickness absence encourages discussion with the patient about return to work and work issues, ideally at 2–6 weeks but certainly before 12 weeks. The NICE guideline on low-back pain [14] encourages self-management and the importance of maintaining normal activity (including work). Individuals should not need to be off work whilst attending for their exercises, acupuncture or manual-therapy treatments.

## Vocational rehabilitation

Because MSDs are so common amongst the working-age population it is very important that, when an individual develops an MSD, he or she receives the right rehabilitation at the right time in the course of his or her condition. A recently published evidence review [16] looked at the definition of vocational rehabilitation and its underlying principles, with the focus of the review being on adults of working age with common health problems including MSD.

The review concluded that vocational rehabilitation was 'whatever helps someone who has a health problem to stay at, return to and remain in work'. The authors described it as an idea and an approach as much as an intervention or a service, but it demonstrated that there is a strong scientific evidence base for many aspects of vocational rehabilitation as well as a good business case and good evidence on its cost benefits.

The concept of early intervention is central to vocational rehabilitation, because the longer anyone is off work, the greater the obstacles to return to work and the more difficult vocational rehabilitation becomes. They concluded that doing something early is simpler, more cost-effective, and helps to prevent people going on to long-term sickness absence.

Most people with common health problems can be helped to return to work by following a few basic principles of health care and workplace management, and this is often low-cost or cost-neutral. Health care and employers both have key roles – effective vocational rehabilitation depends on work-focused health care and accommodating workplaces. Both are necessary and must be co-ordinated.

There is strong evidence that structured vocational rehabilitation interventions are effective for the minority (possibly 5–10%) of people with common health problems who need additional help to return to work after about six weeks. However, there is a need to develop system(s) to deliver these interventions to all who need them.

The review identified some key messages:

---

**For employers (including GP employers)**

1 ▷ Sickness absence is a major and often underestimated cost to your business.

2 ▷ You do not need to wait until your employees are 100% symptom free. Helping them return to work as soon as their condition permits often aids their recovery and minimises your sickness absence and costs.

3 ▷ There is strong evidence that vocational rehabilitation can be effective and have major cost benefits for your business.

4 ▷ About two-thirds of long-term sickness absence and ill-health retirement is due to common health problems (mild/moderate mental health, musculoskeletal and cardio-respiratory conditions), yet these conditions should be manageable.

5 ▷ Early intervention is simple, effective and cost-effective.

6 ▷ Health care is important, but vocational rehabilitation cannot be left to health care alone.

7 ▷ The employer's role is crucial. Proactive company approaches to sickness, together with the temporary provision of modified work and accommodations, are effective and cost-effective. These are often low-cost or cost-neutral.

8 ▷ Maintaining contact with the absent worker and better communication between health care and the workplace facilitates earlier return to work.

---

**For employees**

1 ▷ You do not need to stay off work till you are completely better. Staying at work or returning to work as early as your condition permits often helps your recovery.

2 ▷ The earlier you get help the better. What you need is a combination of health care focused on getting back to work and help from your employer.

3 ▷ If necessary, temporary adjustments to your job can help you return to work earlier. Many employers are sympathetic if you explain you are keen to get back to work and take a positive and reasonable approach.

4 ▷ Staying in touch with your workplace while you are off sick and giving your doctor and employer permission to communicate with each other will help your return to work.

5 ▷ The goal is preventing long-term sickness and disability with all its social and economic consequences for you and your family.

---

**For primary care health professionals**

1 ▷ You play a key role in advising and supporting patients about (return to) work.

2 ▷ Helping patients to stay at, and return to, work is generally good for their health and can help promote recovery.

3 ▷ Routine health care for common health problems should include a focus on work, incorporating advice to remain active, reassurance, and suitable recommendations about work – based on the presumption that work is beneficial unless there is clear evidence to the contrary (e.g. occupational asthma due to occupational exposure). Emphasise what the patient can do rather than what they can't, and always consider, with the patient's permission, contacting the occupational health physician (OHP) at the place of work (if there is one). The OHP is subject to the same standards regarding consent and confidentiality as the primary care team, and is uniquely placed to be able to offer advice to allow the person to work safely.

4 ▷ Patients do not need to be totally symptom-free before returning to work. Facilitating return to work through workplace accommodations is preferable to prolonging sickness absence 'to play safe'.

5 ▷ Patients off work more than a few weeks are at risk of long-term absence. It is then important to identify and address obstacles to return to work.

6 ▷ More structured vocational rehabilitation interventions are only needed by a minority of patients.

7 ▷ Return to work should be a key outcome measure of health care.

The underlying principles identified by the review have now been incorporated into a highly practical approach to managing MSDs in primary care. Kendall *et al.* in their recent publication[17] have outlined an approach describing the psychosocial flags that impact on return to work:

These relate to:

**the person** ▶ psychosocial factors associated with unfavourable clinical outcomes and transition to persistent pain and disability (*yellow flags*, e.g. catastrophising, negative expectation of recovery, preoccupation with health)

**the workplace** ▶ perceptions about the relationship between work and health, belief that he or she has a reduced ability to work (*blue flags*, e.g. fear of re-injury, high physical job demand, low job satisfaction)

**context** ▶ the person's social setting (*black flags*, e.g. litigation, spouse with negative views about return to work, social isolation).

The authors describe an approach of stepped care and essentially of providing people with what they need at the right time but without over-medicalising management. The flags described do not indicate a diagnosis, but are a way of looking at all of the factors that may contribute to persistent absence from work.

The 'stepped care' approach involves:

1 ▷ Identifying specific obstacles to recovery, activity and work
2 ▷ Developing a plan to target these obstacles and co-ordinate input from key players (patient, GP, employer and, if available, OHP or nurse) with the goal of restoring the person to his or her normal activity, including work. This involves all players agreeing common goals
3 ▷ Finally taking action to implement the action plan so that there is optimal health care to deal with the biomedical issues, to support and not hinder a return to work, and to continually stress the importance of communication.

The key components of the medical consultation in a working-age patient with an MSD need to include:

1 ▷ Encouraging the patient to keep in contact with his or her employer
2 ▷ Stressing the need for the patient to consider what he or she is capable of, not the disability
3 ▷ Encouraging early intervention – avoiding long waits for medical treatment during which time the patient gets further and further psychologically from a return to work, and increases the risk of a patient falling out of work.

## Legal protection for people with chronic health conditions

If an individual has a chronic health condition then he or she may have a degree of legal protection against unfair practices by his or her employer if the individual is deemed 'disabled' under the Disability Discrimination Act (DDA) 1995 and its associated amendments. Conditions such as HIV, multiple sclerosis and cancer are now covered under the DDA from the time of diagnosis, and do not require any impairment of activities. However, for a person with a musculoskeletal condition to be considered disabled certain criteria must be met. It is important to note as well that only a tribunal can decide if a person meets the definition of being disabled within the meaning of the act – neither a GP nor a hospital specialist has the right to do so.

To qualify as disabled under the DDA both of the following circumstances must apply:

▷ the person has a 'physical or mental impairment', which has a
▷ 'substantial and long term negative effect on their ability to carry out day to day activities'. 'Substantial' means it is more difficult and time consuming to carry out an activity compared with someone without the impairment. 'Long term' means that the impairment has lasted or will last more than 12 months. Normal day-to-day activities involve mobility, physical co-ordination, continence, and ability to lift and carry everyday objects.

If a person is covered by the DDA then his or her employer has to make reasonable adjustments to ensure that this individual is not disadvantaged by his or her condition. These adjustments may be at the pre-employment stage (e.g. more time to sit a test), at interview (e.g. someone to sign for them if they are deaf), when they take up and do the job (e.g. more time to complete tasks) or when they are sent for training or development (e.g. be accompanied by a carer if he or she has a learning disability). Employers do not have to make all and every adjustment, but those that are deemed by the courts to be reasonable. The DDA not only applies to an individual's rights with regards to work but also education and access to goods and services. Further information on the DDA can be found at www.equalityhumanrights.com.

The Equality Act 2010 became law in late 2010 and replaced the DDA. It also provides legal protection for people with chronic health problems but the requirement for the health condition(s) to affect one of the activities of daily living has been removed, so a larger group of people are now protected than previously. One other change of interest is that employers are not able to ask prospective employees about their health until after a job offer has been made unless there are specific intrinsic requirements of the job (e.g. a pilot must have a good standard of vision). If they do ask about health then, if the person is not subsequently offered the post, the onus is on the employers to prove they did not discriminate because of the person's health condition.

---

> Box 20.2 ○ *The Disability Discrimination Act 1995 – reasonable adjustments*

> ▶ Employers need to make 'reasonable *adjustments*' to work activities in order to avoid disadvantaging those with disabilities.
>
> ▶ What constitutes 'reasonable *adjustments*' and whether a person is classified as disabled under the act are matters for tribunals.
>
> ▶ Work adaptations can be financed through the Access to Work scheme; disability employment advisers at Jobcentre Plus offices can also provide further details.

### *Examples of reasonable adjustments*

▷ A 28-year-old office clerk suffers from severe back pain after a car accident the previous year. It affects her mobility and prevents her from driving her car for more than ten minutes, although she works 50 minutes away from home at her usual travelling time. Her employer may offer her work from home for two days per week and change her hours so she avoids peak travel, for example an earlier start and finish to avoid traffic congestion.

▷ A 45-year-old supervisor, employed as a machinist, has osteoarthritis of the knees and is awaiting surgery. He finds standing for more than an hour uncomfortable. A reasonable accommodation might be to provide a high stool or support to take the weight off his knees.

▷ A 32-year-old nurse has been recently diagnosed with rheumatoid arthritis and is experiencing stiffness, which affects her ability to dress and move around in the mornings. With her agreement her employer alters her shift pattern and moves her to afternoon and evening shifts as she starts new medication.

This concept of adjustments and flexible workplaces has been shown to be effective in several studies, specifically in people with musculoskeletal conditions.[18, 19]

---

### The new 'Fit Note'

The strong evidence base for the benefits of work, the business case for vocational rehabilitation and the negative effects of unemployment on health have led to recognition that the current system of sickness certification does not meet the needs of patients, GPs or employers. In 2008 Dame Carol Black published her review, entitled *Working for a Healthier Tomorrow.*[7] In response to her recommendations the government has revised the current medical statement following discussion with healthcare professionals and after an extensive consultation period.

Completion of the new statement, *which was introduced* on 6 April 2010, is similar in many ways to the existing form but with a few key differences:

1 ▷ There is no 'fit for work' option so GPs will no longer be asked by patients or employers to certify fitness to return to work
2 ▷ There is an option of 'may be fit for work taking account of the following advice', which gives the GP the opportunity to provide clinical information on any limitations (e.g. 'cannot raise arm above shoulder height', 'cannot bend, twist or lift heavy objects') and advice (e.g.' would benefit from avoiding customer complaints work', 'would be helped by ability to stand, sit and stretch frequently')
3 ▷ There are boxes where the GP can indicate what adaptations or adjustments may facilitate a return to work. The boxes cover graded return, altered hours, amended duties and workplace adaptations.

The statement of fitness for work will continue, as with the current statement, to be advice from the GP to the patient, but the patient can use it to discuss return to work with his or her employer. The advice and recommendations made by the GP on the form are not legally binding, and if the patient and the employer cannot agree on suitable adjustments then the situation is as if the person were signed off sick. The length of the adaptations are for as long as the statement lasts – if the individual requires ongoing adjustments then these would need to be agreed by the individual with his or her employer. Sometimes employers may be able to achieve the same outcome by a different adjustment; they are able to do this and are not bound to the exact detail of the GP's advice. Thus, if a patient has anxiety that is aggravated by travelling at peak times and the GP writes on the form 'should avoid peak travelling times' and ticks the adjusted-hours box, then the employer could ensure avoidance of travel at peak times by either asking the employee to work shorter hours or work the same hours but with a later start and finish time. The employer could also suggest the person works at home. Different employers may thus approach the same request with different offers of adapted or adjusted work to suit their business needs.

More information on the Fit Note, including guidance for GPs, can be found at www.dwp.gov.uk/fitnote and more general information on health

Figure 20.3 ○ *Fit Note*

## Statement of Fitness for Work
## For social security or Statutory Sick Pay

Patient's name | Mr, Mrs, Miss, Ms

I assessed your case on: ❶ / /

and, because of the
following condition(s): ❷

I advise you that: ❸ ☐ you are not fit for work.

❹ ☐ you may be fit for work taking account
of the following advice:

If available, and with your employer's agreement, you may benefit from:

☐ a phased return to work          ☐ amended duties

☐ altered hours          ❺          ☐ workplace adaptations

Comments, including functional effects of your condition(s):

❻

This will be the case for ❼

or from ❽ / /          to / /

❾ I will/will not need to assess your fitness for work again at the end of this period.
*(Please delete as applicable)*

Doctor's signature

Date of statement | / /

Doctor's address

Med 3 04/10

*Source*: Department for Work and Pensions. *Statement of Fitness for Work*.[20]

466

and work can be found at www.dwp.gov.uk/healthcare-professional/ (see Figure 20.3).

---

Box 20.3 ○ **Case study 1**

---

Mr Hughes is a 28-year-old shop assistant with a long history of back pain. He is well known to his GP as a frequent consulter with minor illnesses. His current episode has lasted three weeks and he has been off work for eight days. Having self-certified his absence he consults his GP for advice and further certification.

---

### Analysis of case study 1 with respect to the six domains of Being a GP

#### DOMAIN 1: PRIMARY CARE MANAGEMENT

The GP uses his skills in *clinical management* to take a history and perform an examination. He concludes that Mr Hughes has simple mechanical back pain without radiation. It is not controlled by simple paracetamol and is causing impairment of his daily activities – he needs help to dress and is not able to take a bath. There are no clinical red flags. His GP prescribes better pain relief in line with NICE and SIGN guidelines (he is using *information management* to access the latest guidance on back pain).

#### DOMAINS 2 AND 3: PERSON-CENTRED CARE AND SPECIFIC PROBLEM-SOLVING SKILLS

The GP also explores his thoughts regarding his back pain, using his *specific problem-solving skills* and *person-centred care* to elicit any yellow, blue or black flags in the history. He already knows that Mr Hughes is a frequent attender and considers that this may not be a straightforward consultation.

#### DOMAIN 4: A COMPREHENSIVE APPROACH

Using a *comprehensive approach* to the problem, he considers other possible confounding features. Mr Hughes indicates that he is concerned about returning to work as his job involves shelf stacking and moving boxes of tins on and off pallets. He is concerned that he might suffer from increased pain and damage his back. He also works on the till and takes customer orders over the telephone, then making them up in the warehouse. He is exhibiting 'fear-avoidance behaviour'. His GP explains the positive benefits of remaining active,' busts' the myth that pain means damage, uses his *communication skills* to educate Mr Hughes and reassure him about the lack of pathology, and advises on symptom control. He also mentions that with better pain control he could do parts of his job, but not all, and asks Mr Hughes to think about what he could do, not what he cannot, and to speak to his employer. The GP is aware that Mr Hughes's firm has an occupational health service (*working with colleagues in teams*) and suggests that Mr Hughes could speak to them for advice about his workplace and duties. He also provides Mr Hughes with simple, easy to understand literature about back pain and self-help (*IMT and person-centred care*); the leaflet contains some basic exercises for Mr Hughes to perform to reduce pain and increase his back movements. (Examples can be found at www.arthritisresearchuk.org/.)

**DOMAIN 6: A HOLISTIC APPROACH**

He gives a medical statement stating that he is not fit for work and arranges to see Mr Hughes again. Mr Hughes returns after one week with better pain relief and is able to dress himself. He has discussed his job with his employer and thinks he can do the till work, answer the telephone and make up orders, as he can move at his own pace. His employer is happy to have him back on limited duties. His GP explains the importance of avoiding lifting, twisting and repeated bending. The GP issues a medical statement advising that Mr Hughes may be fit for work with that advice and ticks the box on 'amended duties' on a two-week note. Mr Hughes is happy to return to work. As part of a *holistic approach*, Mr Hughes's GP offers a follow-up consultation in three weeks if the problem has not settled and suggests that Mr Hughes should start taking more regular exercise to build up his muscle strength and core stability, to reduce further back problems.

---

Box 20.4 ○ *Case study 2*

---

Mr Campbell is a 58-year-old data entry operator who works full time for the local council as a forklift truck driver. He has had severe neck pain, diagnosed as cervical spondylosis, for the last two weeks but is bored at home and wants to return to work. His employers are not happy about him returning to work because of Health and Safety concerns about his driving and being able to turn his head to check for obstacles.

## DOMAINS 1 AND 3: PRIMARY CARE MANAGEMENT AND SPECIFIC PROBLEM-SOLVING SKILLS

He consults his GP who uses skills in *clinical management* and *specific problem-solving skills* to take a history and examine the patient. He concludes that Mr Campbell has some restriction in neck movement, but can function as a driver. He refers Mr Campbell to the practice physiotherapist (*working with colleagues and in teams*) for manual therapy to improve the range of movement in Mr Campbell's cervical spine. There are no signs of radiculopathy, so this is a mechanical restriction. It should improve with manual therapy. An X-ray of Mr Campbell's neck, taken last year, was normal for his age, and the GP finds a record of the report in Mr Campbell's notes (*primary care administration and IMT*).

## DOMAINS 4 AND 6: A COMPREHENSIVE APPROACH AND A HOLISTIC APPROACH

With Mr Campbell's permission (the patient does not like using the telephone and feels intimidated by people in authority) (*holistic care*), the GP telephones Mr Campbell's employers and speaks to the OHP (*working with colleagues and in teams*), to discuss their concerns about Mr Campbell being at work as a driver. An appointment is arranged for the patient to be assessed by the OHP. In the mean time, the GP issues a Statement of Fitness for Work advising that he may be fit for work and ticks the box for amended duties, so that Mr Campbell can work on the factory floor until the OHP has assessed him. Mr Campbell's GP is aware that the patient suffers from depression and lives alone. Being off work will exacerbate Mr Campbell's mental health problem (*holistic care*) and his GP is very keen to get him back to work as soon as possible. Mr Campbell manages to return to his job as a forklift truck driver two weeks later. His physiotherapy continues for two months (*holistic care*) and he returns for a follow-up consultation with his GP six weeks later. His GP offers support in the future if required (*a comprehensive approach*).

### *Resources for GPs and patients*

▶ ACAS – for advice on disagreements with employers, **www.acas.org.uk**.
▶ Disability Discrimination Act 1995 and 2005, **www.equalityhumanrights.com**.
▶ Health and Safety Executive, **www.hse.gov.uk**.

▶ NHS Choices – back pain site,
**www.nhs.uk/conditions/Back-pain/Pages/Introduction.aspx.**
▶ Patient UK – information on non-specific low-back pain in adults,
**www.patient.co.uk/health/Back-Pain.htm.**

### Resources for employers

▶ 'Working Joints and Muscles' – a toolkit for employers that provides
practical advice and case studies of companies who have managed MSD,
**www.bitc.org.uk/resources/publications/working_jointsmuscl.html**
▶ 'Assessment of Repetitive Tasks' – a tool produced by the HSE to help
employers assess and reduce the risks of MSD,
**www.hse.gov.uk/msd/art-tool.htm.**
▶ ACAS – advice for employers managing conflict at work,
**www.acas.org.uk.**

**References**

1 • Arthritis Research UK, www.arthritisresearchuk.org/ [accessed October 2011].

2 • Smedley J, Dick F, Sadhra S. *Oxford Handbook of Occupational Health* Oxford: Oxford University Press. 2009.

3 • Jones J R, Huxtable C S, Hodgson J T. *Self-Reported Work-Related Illness in 2003/04: results from the Labour Force Survey* Sudbury: HSE Books.

4 • Department for Work and Pensions. Personal communication, 2009.

5 • Office for National Statistics. *Statistical Bulletin: national population projections, 2008-based* Newport: ONS, 2009, www.ons.gov.uk/ons/rel/npp/national-population-projections/2008-based-projections/index.html [accessed October 2011].

6 • Waddell G, Burton A K. *Is Work Good for Your Health and Well-being?* London: The Stationery Office, 2006.

7 • Black C. *Working for a Healthier Tomorrow* London. The Stationery Office. 2008.

8 • CBI/AXA Absence Survey 2008, www.cbi.org.uk [accessed October 2011].

9 • Health and Safety Executive, 1999, www.hse.gov.uk [accessed October 2011].

10 • Bevan S, Passmore E, Mahdon M. *Fit for Work: musculoskeletal disorders and labour market participation* London: The Work Foundation, 2008.

11 • Health and Safety Executive. *Ill-Health Costs Introduction*, www.hse.gov.uk [accessed October 2011].

12 • *Social Security (Prescribed Diseases) Regulations 1995* London: The Stationery Office.

13 • *Health and Safety at Work etc. Act 1974* London: The Stationery Office.

14 • National Institute for Health and Clinical Excellence. *Clinical Guideline 88, Low Back Pain: early management of persistent non-specific low back pain* London: NICE, 2009, www.nice.org.uk/CG88 [accessed October 2011].

15 • National Institute for Health and Clinical Excellence. *Managing Long-Term Sickness Absence and Incapacity for Work* London: NICE, 2009, www.nice.org.uk/PH19 [accessed October 2011].

16 • Waddell G, Burton A K, Kendall N A S. *Vocational Rehabilitation: what works, for whom and when?* London: The Stationery Office, 2008.

17 • Kendall N, Burton K, Main C, *et al. Tackling Musculoskeletal Problems: a guide for the clinic and workplace* London: The Stationery Office, 2009.

18 • Schultz I Z, Stowell A W, Feuerstein M, *et al.* Models of return to work for musculoskeletal disorders *Journal of Occupational Rehabilitation* 2007; **17(2)**: 327–52.

19 • de Croon E M, Sluiter J K, Nijssen T F, *et al.* Predictive factors of work disability in rheumatoid arthritis: a systematic literature review *Annals of the Rheumatic Diseases* 2004; **63(11)**: 1362–7.

20 • Department for Work and Pensions. *Statement of Fitness for Work* London: DWP, 2010, www.dwp.gov.uk/docs/fitnote-gp-guide.pdf [accessed October 2011].

Figure 1.1 ○ *The intervertebral disc*

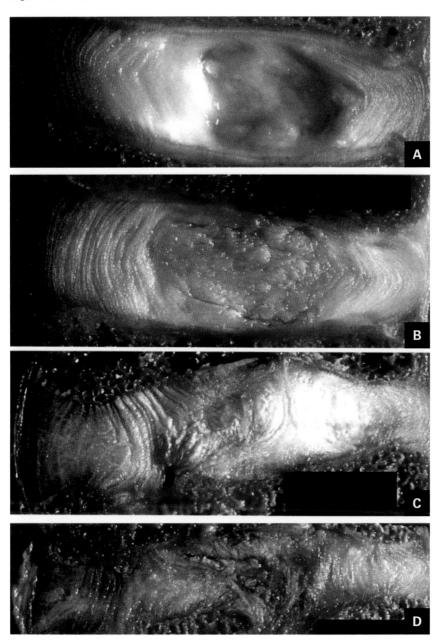

*Source*: M. Adams. *The Biomechanics of Back Pain* Edinburgh: Churchill Livingstone.
Copyright © Elsevier (2006).

Figure 6.3 ○ *A severely pronated 'flat' foot associated with systemic joint hypermobility*

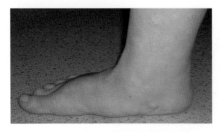

*Note*: this patient had a Beighton–Carter–Wilkinson score of 9/9.

Figure 6.4 ○ *A frank pes cavus, in this case associated with inherited peripheral neuropathy (HMSA type 1)*

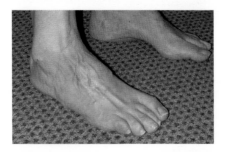

Figure 6.5 ○ *Severe localised OA of the midfoot*

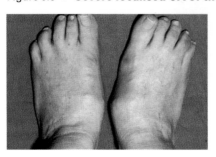

*Source*: published in Redmond AC, Helliwell PS. Musculoskeletal disorders. In: P Frowen, M O'Donnell, JG Burrow, *et al.* (eds). *Neale's Disorders of the Foot* (8th edn) Edinburgh: Churchill Livingstone, 2010.[18] Copyright © Elsevier (2010).

Figure 6.9 ○ *Grade 3 ankle sprain with syndesmosis injury (high sprain) presenting in primary care one week after the initial injury*

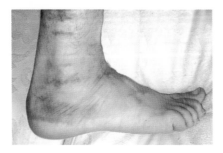

Figure 6.10 ○ *Typical ultrasound finding of a chronically degenerative Achilles tendon*

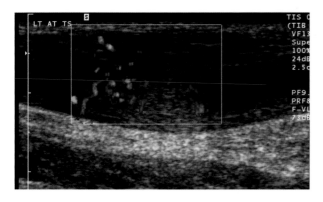

*Note*: the fusiform swelling indicates derangement of the normal fibrillar structure and the Doppler signal (orange overlay) indicates local inflammation.

Figure 6.12 ○ *Functional foot orthoses*

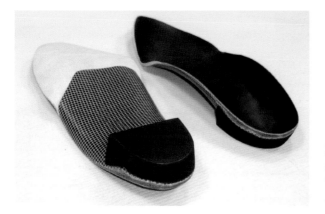

*Note*: made from carbon fibre, these orthoses alter foot joint function selectively and may be helpful in some overuse type conditions.

Figure 8.1 ○ *OA hands with Heberden's and prominent Bouchard's nodes*

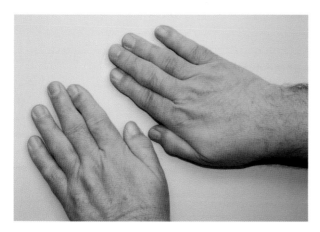

Figure 13.1 ○ **Psoriasis of the natal cleft**

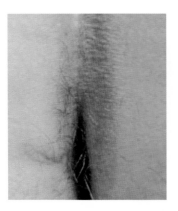

*Source*: Mease P, Helliwell P (eds). *Atlas of Psoriatic Arthritis* London: Springer-Verlag, 2007. Copyright© Springer-Verlag 2007.

Figure 13.2 ○ **Psoriatic arthritis affecting the metacarpophalangeal and proximal interphalangeal joints, hence mimicking rheumatoid arthritis**

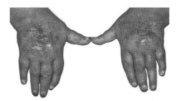

*Source*: Mease P, Helliwell P (eds). *Atlas of Psoriatic Arthritis* London: Springer-Verlag, 2007. Copyright© Springer-Verlag 2007.

Figure 13.3 ○ **There may be very few joints affected in psoriatic arthritis**

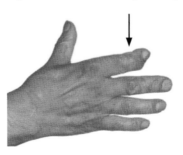

*Source*: Mease P, Helliwell P (eds). *Atlas of Psoriatic Arthritis* London: Springer-Verlag, 2007. Copyright© Springer-Verlag 2007.

Figure 13.4 ○ **Enthesitis of the Achilles tendon**

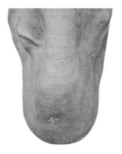

*Source*: Mease P, Helliwell P (eds). *Atlas of Psoriatic Arthritis* London: Springer-Verlag, 2007. Copyright© Springer-Verlag 2007.

Figure 13.5 ○ **Dactylitis of the second and third toes**

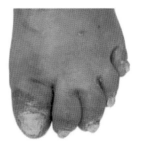

*Source*: Helliwell P. Psoriatic arthritis: its presentation and management in primary care. Reports on the Rheumatic Diseases (Series 6), *Hands On* 3. Copyright© Arthritis Research UK. Used with permission.

Figure 13.6 ○ **Distal interphalangeal disease with nail involvement, the latter cleverly (partly) concealed by nail varnish**

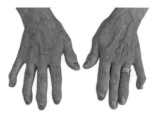

*Source*: Helliwell P. Psoriatic arthritis: its presentation and management in primary care. Reports on the Rheumatic Diseases (Series 6), *Hands On* 3. Copyright© Arthritis Research UK. Used with permission.

Figure 13.8 ○ **Severe mutilation in psoriatic arthritis**

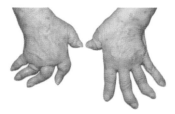

*Source*: Mease P, Helliwell P (eds). *Atlas of Psoriatic Arthritis* London: Springer-Verlag, 2007. Copyright© Springer-Verlag 2007.

Figure 13.10 ○ **Keratoderma blennorrhagica**

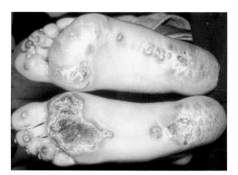

Figure 13.11 ○ *Circinate balanitis*

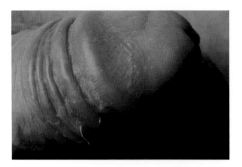

Figure 14.1 ○ *Raynaud's colour changes*

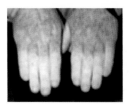
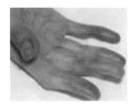

Initial white stages

Secondary blue
discoloration; this is
followed by redness

Figure 14.2 ○ *The various effects of SLE on the body*

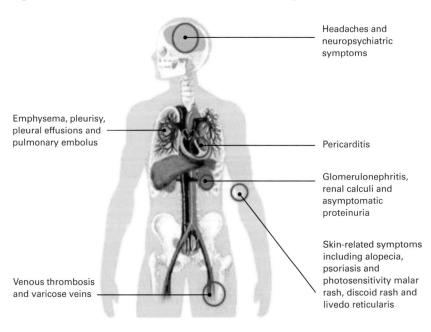

Headaches and
neuropsychiatric
symptoms

Emphysema, pleurisy,
pleural effusions and
pulmonary embolus

Pericarditis

Glomerulonephritis,
renal calculi and
asymptomatic
proteinuria

Skin-related symptoms
including alopecia,
psoriasis and
photosensitivity malar
rash, discoid rash and
livedo reticularis

Venous thrombosis
and varicose veins

Figure 14.3 ○ *Typical malar rash of SLE*

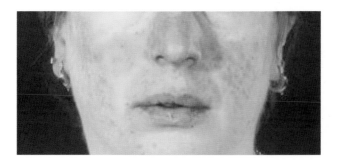

Figure 14.4 ○ *Jaccoud's arthritis*

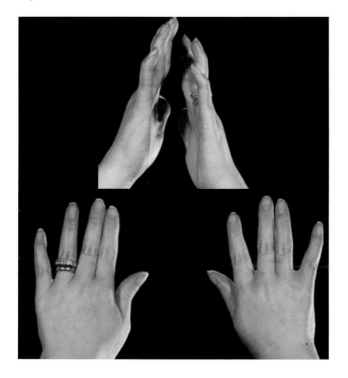

Figure 14.5 ○ *Subcutaneous calcified nodules in CREST syndrome*

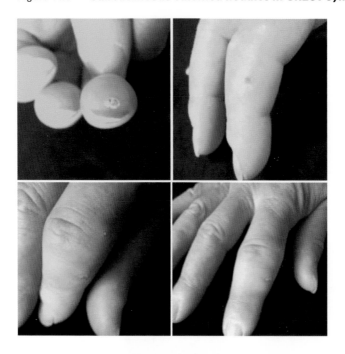

Figure 14.6 ○ *X-ray of subcutaneous skin nodules in CREST syndrome*

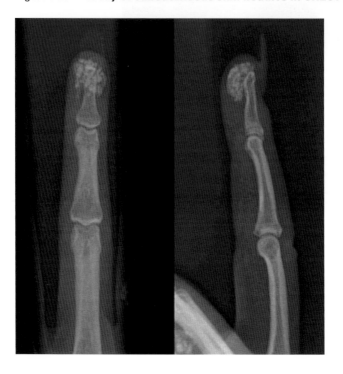

Figure 14.7 ○ *Schirmer's test*

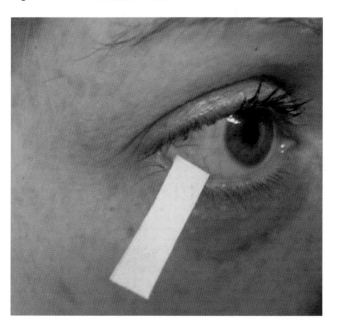

Figure 18.3 ○ *Burn of variable depth*

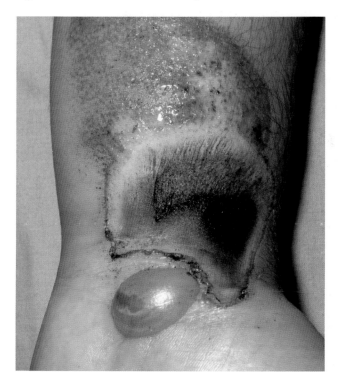

Figure 18.4 ○ *Superficial partial-thickness burn*

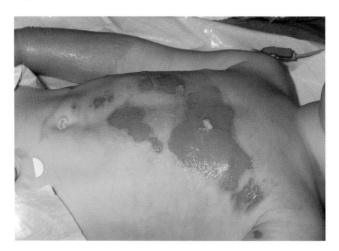

Figure 18.5 ○ *Deep dermal burn*

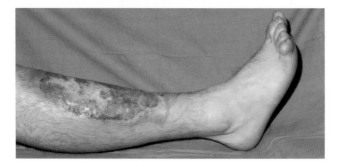

Figure 18.6 ○ *Full-thickness burn*

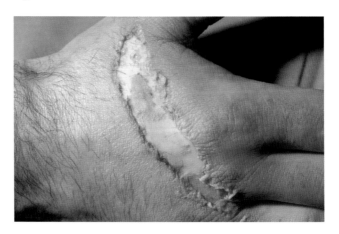

Figure 18.7 ○ *Paediatric scald*

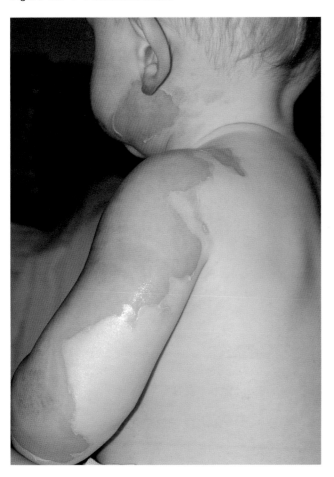

Figure 18.8 ○ *Contact burn*

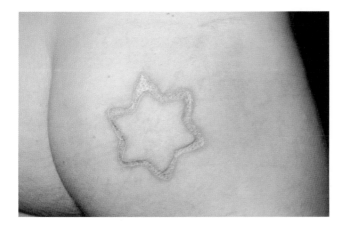

Figure 18.9 ○ *Full-thickness burn in an elderly patient who collapsed against a radiator*

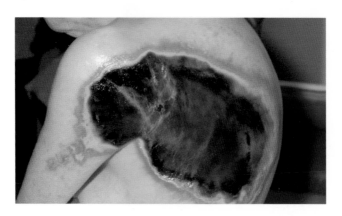

Figure 18.10 ○ *Full-thickness cement burn*

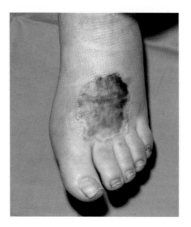

Figure 18.11 ○ *Electrical burn*

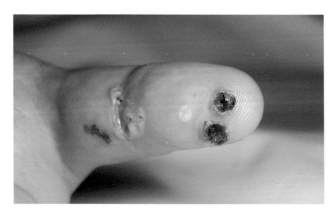

Figure 18.12 ○ *Superficial partial-thickness burn treated by excision of non-viable blister skin*

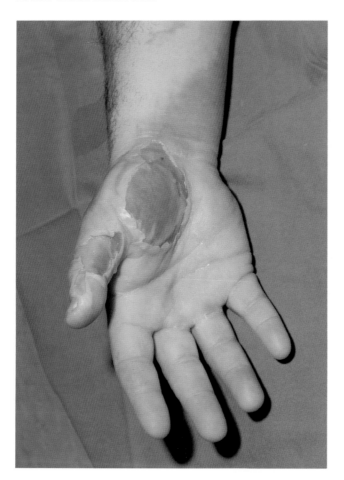

Figure 18.13 ○ *Hypertrophic scarring post-burn*

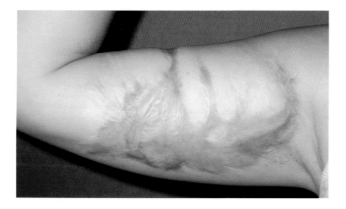

Figure 18.14 ○ *Contracted scarring post-burn*

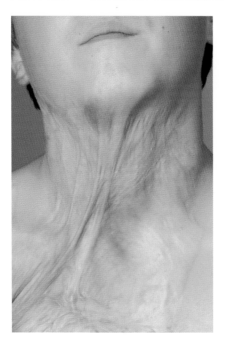

Figure 18.15 ○ *Keloid scarring post-burn*

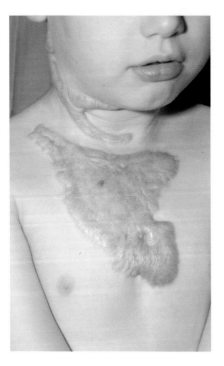

Figure 18.16 ○ *Infected burn*

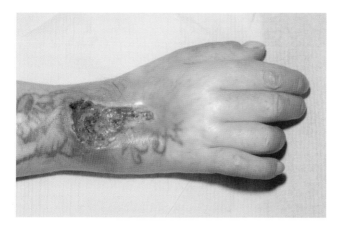

Figure 19.2 ○ *Tophaceous gout affecting the finger interphalangeal joint*

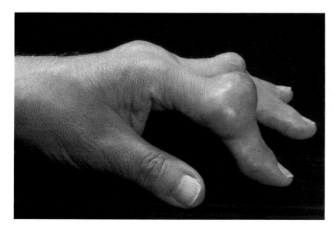

*Note*: the asymmetrical nodular swelling has overlying erythema.

# Index

Achilles bursitis 157
Achilles enthesitis 175, 315–16, 320
Achilles tendonopathy 154, 175
  case study 176
  treatment algorithm 155
  *see also* tendonopathy
acromioclavicular disorders 95
  treatment 99
acromioclavicular joint, anatomy 87
acupuncture 74
  in osteoarthritis 203
acute arthropathies 263
  in connective tissue disorders 339
  monoarthropathy
    case study 264, 280
    differential diagnosis 264
    gout 266–8
    haemophilia 272
    inflammatory arthritis 268–70
    investigations 265
    osteoarthritis 270–2
    red flags 266
    septic arthritis 265–6
    traumatic 272
  polyarthropathy
    case study 272, 281
    connective tissue disorders 277–8
    fibromylagia 278–9
    gout 279
    hypermobility 276–7
    osteoarthritis 275–6
    possible causes 272–3
    rheumatoid arthritis 273–5
    vitamin D deficiency 279
acute inflammation, classic signs 264
adalimumab 293–4
  in inflammatory bowel disease 332
adhesive capsulitis 94–5
  case study 103–5
  treatment 99
airway maintenance 413
alcohol consumption, risk of gout 441
alendronate
  in osteoporosis 222, 223, 225, 226
  in Paget's disease 232
Alexander Technique 70, 365

alkaline phosphatase
  in osteomalacia 232, 233
  in Paget's disease 231
allodynia 250
allopurinol 439–40, 444
  and acute gout 268
  dose 445
  drug interactions 445
  initiation of therapy 446
  side effects 445
allopurinol desensitisation 447
alphacalcidol 228
American College of Rheumatology, classification criteria for osteoarthritis 187–8
amitriptyline
  in acute back pain 17
  in chronic back pain 50–1
  in chronic musculoskeletal pain 256
  in fibromyalgia 246, 247
anaemia 398
  in connective tissue disorders 350–1
analgesia
  in acute back pain 17
  in cervical disc prolapse 26
  in chronic back pain 50–1
  in chronic musculoskeletal pain 255–6
  in fibromyalgia 247
  in foot pain 161–2
  in hypermobility 365
  in osteoarthritis 200–1, 206
  in osteoporosis 228
  in rheumatoid arthritis 286
  in shoulder pain 96
  in tendonopathy 173–4
ankle injuries 421–3
  sprains 152–3
ankle joint
  anatomy 421
  instability 153
  osteoarthritis 144–5
ankle pain
  Achilles tendonopathy 154, 155
  tibialis posterior dysfunction 154–6
ankylosing spondylitis 270, 308
  associated conditions 310

BASDAI 313
case study 311
clinical features 309–10
diagnosis 311–12
diagnostic triage 16
foot involvement 147
natural history and prognosis 310–11
pathogenesis 308–9
patient education 314
prevalence 1, 309
referral 312
treatment 312–14
treatment guidelines 314
see also inflammatory bowel disease (IBD)-associated arthritis
antalgic gait 18
anterior cruciate ligament (ACL) 110
assessment 114
rupture 420
anterior drawer test 114
anterior knee pain 112
case study 119–20
children 396–7
anterior springing of spine 22
anti-CCP antibodies 275, 284, 285
anticentromere antibodies 347
antidepressants, for chronic back pain 50–1
antinuclear antibodies (ANAs) 245, 340, 347, 350, 351
children 399
antiphospholipid syndrome (APS) 341, 345
anti-TNF therapy 293–4
in ankylosing spondylitis 313–14
in inflammatory bowel disease 331–2
in psoriatic arthritis 320
in reactive arthritis 326
anxiety 31
association with fibromyalgia 243
arch supports 162–3
Arthritis Care 204
arthroplasty referral 204
arthroscopy referral 204–5
aspirin therapy, low-dose
interaction with NSAIDs 201
in SLE 340
ataxic gait 18
atrophic bone response 191
audit 6
AVPU mnemonic, neurological

assessment 416
axial neck pain 27
azathioprine
in inflammatory bowel disease 331
in psoriatic arthritis 319
in reactive arthritis 326
steroid-sparing 375

B27 transgenic mouse 309
back pain
absence from work 10, 453–4, 459
acute
age-related incidence 11
analgesia 17
case study 24, 30
common sites of degenerative changes 11
communication of findings 16–17
costs 2, 9
CSAG guidelines 14
diagnosis and management 9
diagnostic triage 15–16
domains of care 30–1
dysfunction 12
explanation of symptoms 10–11
nocebo effect 11–12
outcomes 37
patients' beliefs and expectations 10
physical examination 18–23
importance of 16
prevalence 1, 9
psychological factors 12–13
red flags 14, 15
referrals 17
role of GP 13
sickness absence 10
surgical management 9–10
in ankylosing spondylitis 310
in children 397–8
case study 405–7
chronic 35
assessment tools 47–8, 49
case study 58–9
clinical assessment 39
definition 35–6
distress 36
distress assessment 42–4
ethnic and cultural factors 39
flag system 253
history taking 42–4
CERTIFICATE questions 47

injection therapy 51
investigations 41, 45
key points 59–60
key priorities 52
management 48, 50, 56–7
manual therapy 77
occupational aspects 54–6
outcomes 37
pain management programmes 54
pharmacotherapy 50–1
physical examination 44–5
physiotherapy referral 53–4
population-based measures 51–2
positive messages 57
predisposing factors 37–8
signs of serious disease 40–1
surgery 51
exercise therapy 68–9
facet joint osteoarthritis, prevalence 190
in hypermobility 362
massage 78
occupational issues, case study 467–8
physiotherapy 53–4, 74
prevalence 36, 37, 453
psychosocial intervention 48
risk factors for chronicity 13, 46
work-related 457
Baker's cyst 110, 112, 120, 194
management 117
balicatib 230
balneotherapy 247
Bath Ankylosing Spondylitis Disease Activity Index (BASDAI) 313
bazedoxifene 230
behavioural problems, children 385
Beighton score, hypermobility 360–1, 368
benzbromarone 446
biological therapies 292–4
in ankylosing spondylitis 313–14
in inflammatory bowel disease 331–2
in juvenile idiopathic arthritis 400
in psoriatic arthritis 320
in reactive arthritis 326
biopsychosocial approach 239
in fibromyalgia 246
bisphosphonates
in osteoporosis 222, 223, 226
in Paget's disease 231
black flags 55, 462

blood pressure, relationship to palpable pulses 415
blue flags 55, 462
bone marrow lesions, osteoarthritis 186–7
bone mineral density (BMD)
DXA 220
treatment thresholds 218
bone-sparing therapy 225–7
adherence and persistence 228–9
case studies 234–7
new drugs 229–30
bone stress reactions, foot 149–50
bone tumours 397
botulinum toxin A injections, in chronic neck pain 52
bow legs, children 392
braces 76
in osteoarthritis 202
brachalgia
nerve root block injections 51
physical treatments 53
breastfed babies, vitamin D supplements 233
breathing assessment 414
Brighton diagnostic criteria for hypermobility 277, 360, 361, 368
bruising, children 386
bunions 158–9
burns 423
assessment 425–6
complications 430
first aid 428
key points 432
long-term follow-up 431
management in primary care 428–9
mechanisms of injury 426–7
non-accidental injury 427
pathophysiology 424–5
psychosocial problems 431
referral, indications for 427–8, 429
role of primary care 424
zones of injury 425
bursae, knee joint 110
bursitis
association with tendonopathy 173, 174
heel 157
knee joint 112, 117
'butterfly' rash, SLE 339
buttock clench testing 22

C-reactive protein (CRP) 350
calcinosis, distinction from gouty tophi 346
calcitriol 228
calcium pyrophosphate crystals 196–7, 270
calcium supplements, in osteoporosis 226
callus removal, feet 160
Cam deformity, hip joint 127
*Campylobacter* infection, reactive arthritis 324
capsaicin, in osteoarthritis 200
cardiovascular disease risk
    in gout 439, 444
    from NSAIDs 96
    in psoriatic arthritis 318
    in rheumatoid arthritis 297
    in SLE 339–40
carpal tunnel syndrome
    causes 457
    Industrial Injuries Disablement Benefit 457
    ultrasound therapy 73
case studies 279
    Achilles tendonopathy 176
    adhesive capsulitis 103–5
    ankylosing spondylitis 311
    back pain
        acute 24, 30
        children 405–7
        chronic 58–9
    gout 447–8
    growing pains 402–4
    hip OA, physiotherapy 77–8
    hypermobility 366–7
    inflammatory bowel disease (IBD)-associated arthritis 329–30
    knee pain 3–6
        anterior 119–20
        Osgood–Schlatter's disease 122
        osteoarthritis 120–1
    lateral elbow pain 179
    meniscal tear 121
    monoarthropathy, acute 264–72, 280
    neck pain, acute 28, 31–3
    occupational issues 181–2, 467–9
    osteoarthritis 77–8, 120–1, 205–7
    osteoporosis 234–7
    polyarthropathy, acute 272–9, 281
    polymyalgia rheumatica 377–8

Raynaud's phenomenon 336
reactive arthritis 324–5
rheumatoid arthritis 3–6
    early disease 299–302
    established disease 302–4
    rotator cuff disorder 101–2
    soft-tissue injuries 75–6
    systemic lupus erythematosus 342–4
    work-related upper-limb disorder 181–2
cauda equina syndrome, diagnosis 16, 21
cavus/cavoid feet 140, 143–4
cerebral lupus 339
CERTIFICATE questions, back pain 47
certolizumab 293–4
cervical collars 53
cervical spine
    fractures 417–18
    rheumatoid arthritis 298–9
    *see also* neck pain
cervical spine control, emergency situations 413–14
chemical injuries 427
    *see also* burns
chest pain, non-cardiac 243
    *see also* medically unexplained symptoms
chickenpox exposure, immunosuppressed patients 297
children 381–2
    ankylosing spondylitis 309
    back pain 11, 17, 397–8
        case study 405–7
        red flags, 397
    cavoid foot postures 144
    clinical assessment 382–3
        history taking 384–5, 387–8
        pGALS screen 388–90
        physical examination 385–6, 388, 389
        suspected JIA 387
    complex regional pain syndrome 398–9
    development, normal variants 391
    distinguishing mechanical from inflammatory presentations 386
    'flat feet' 142–3
    gait and leg alignment, normal variants 392
    growing pains 393–4

case study 402–4
hip pain 122–3, 396
holistic approach 404
hypermobility 390–1
investigations 399–400
juvenile idiopathic arthritis (JIA),
    primary care management 400–2
knee pain 112, 396–7
    Osgood–Schlatter's disease 122
    red flags 113
Legg–Calvé–Perthes disease 396
limping 394, 396
    significant causes 383
neck pain 24–5
non-accidental injury 427
red flags 113, 387, 397
referral, indications for 392
sepsis 394, 396
systemic disease 398
transient synovitis (irritable hip) 396
chondrocalcinosis 195
chondroitin, in osteoarthritis 201–2
chronic back pain see back pain,
    chronic
chronic fatigue syndrome (CFS) 243,
    245
    see also medically unexplained
    symptoms
chronic health conditions, legal
    protection 463–4
chronic neck pain see neck pain,
    chronic
chronic pain
    assessment 249–50
    explanation to the patient 251–2
    flag system 252–3
    holistic approach 252
    management toolkit 251
    manner of description 43
    multidisciplinary approach 256, 257
    musculoskeletal causes 250
    occupational issues 256
    pharmacotherapy 255–6
    predictors of psychiatric co-morbidity
    255
    prevalence 249
    prognostic factors 252
    psychosocial factors 252
    referral options 257
    see also back pain, chronic; neck pain,
    chronic

chronic pain management programmes
    54
ciclosporin
    in inflammatory bowel disease 331
    in psoriatic arthritis 319
circinate balanitis 323
citrullinated peptides, antibodies see
    anti-CCP antibodies
Clarke's test 115
clawing of toes 159–60
'clumsiness', children 384
cognitive behavioural therapy
    in chronic pain 54
    in fibromyalgia 247, 248
colchicine 268, 439, 443
collateral ligaments, knee joint 110
    assessment 114
communication see information
    provision
community-oriented care, case study
    of rheumatoid arthritis 5
compensation claims 182
    neck injuries, prognostic significance
    26, 39
complex regional pain syndrome 180–1
    case study 181–2
    children 398–9
comprehensive approach, case study of
    rheumatoid arthritis 5
computed tomography (CT), foot 139
connective tissue disorders (CTDs)
    277–8, 335
    acute hot joints 339
    antiphospholipid syndrome 345
    common presentations 336
    investigations 350–2
    key points 355–6
    malignancy risk 349
    polymyositis and dermatomyositis
    347
    Raynaud's phenomenon 336–8
    Sjögren's syndrome 348
    treatment
        immunisations 353
        immunosuppressive therapy 353
        non-steroidal anti-inflammatory
        drugs (NSAIDs) 352–3
        steroids 353
    see also systemic lupus erythematosus;
    systemic sclerosis/scleroderma
core competences 2–3

case study of rheumatoid arthritis 3–6
costs of musculoskeletal disease 2
COT template 253–4
COX-2 inhibitors
    in acute gout 443
    in inflammatory bowel disease 331
    in osteoarthritis 200–1
    see also non-steroidal anti-
    inflammatory drugs (NSAIDs)
creatine kinase 347
CREST (calcinosis, Raynaud's,
  oesophageal dysmotility, sclerodactyly
  and telangiectasia) syndrome 278,
  345–6
Crohn's disease see inflammatory bowel
  disease (IBD)-associated arthritis
crooked toes, children 392
cruciate ligaments 110
cryotherapy 74–5
cultural factors, in chronic pain 39
cyclophosphamide, in juvenile
  idiopathic arthritis 400

dactylitis
    in psoriatic arthritis 316, 320
    in reactive arthritis 323
DAMASK trial 116
demographic trends 454–6
denosumab 223, 227, 229–30
depression
    in fibromyalgia 243
    in osteoarthritis 193
    in systemic sclerosis 346
depression screening 120
dermatomyositis 278, 347
    juvenile 398
    malignancy risk 349
developmental assessment, children
  384, 387
    motor milestones 391
    normal variants 391
diabetes, adhesive capsulitis 103
diagnostic labels, 'number needed to
  offend' 243
diclofenac 96
dietary modification, in gout 444
disability 2
Disability Discrimination Act (DDA)
  1995 463, 464
disc prolapse
    cervical 26

diagnostic features 23
surgical management 9–10
    see also back pain
discectomy 51
discitis, children 397
disease, distinction from illness 13
disease activity score (DAS),
  rheumatoid arthritis 287–8, 302
disease-modifying anti-rheumatic drugs
  (DMARDs) 289–90, 320
    biological therapies 292–4
    cautions 321, 327
    hydroxychloroquine 292
    in inflammatory bowel disease 331–2
    in juvenile idiopathic arthritis 400
    leflunomide 292
    malignancy risk 349
    methotrexate 290–1
    monitoring therapy 295–6
    in reactive arthritis 326
    sulfasalazine 291
dislocation of the shoulder 89
Display Screen Equipment Regulations
  458
distress, assessment in chronic pain
  42–4
diuretics, risk of gout 444
drop arm test 92
dry-eye syndrome 348, 349
duck walking test 113
duloxetine, in fibromyalgia 246, 247
DXA (dual energy X-ray
  absorptiometry) 219
dysaesthesia 250
dysfunction 12
dysmenorrhoea 243
dyspnoea, in rheumatoid arthritis 299

Early Arthritis Clinics 270, 275
effusions, knee joint 112
    differential diagnosis 123
    management 118
    physical examination 114
Ehlers–Danlos syndrome 357
elbows
    common pathology in hypermobility
    363
    see also lateral elbow pain
electrical injuries 427
    see also burns
electrotherapy 71

interferential therapy 72
low-level laser therapy 72–3
short-wave diathermy 73
in tendonopathy 174
transcutaneous electrical nerve
stimulation 71–2
ultrasound 73
emergency situations
airway maintenance 413
ankle injuries 421–3
breathing assessment 414
casualty safety 410–11
catastrophic haemorrhage 413
cervical spine control 413–14
circulation assessment 414–15
equipment for pre-hospital care
434–7
exposure 416
fractures
cervical spine 417–18
scaphoid 418–19
information relay 412
knee injuries 420–1
management template 412
neurological assessment 416
personal safety 409–10
primary survey 413
scene safety 410
treatment 415–16
triage sieve 411, 412
see also burns
emotional response to symptoms 2
enteropathic arthritis see inflammatory
bowel disease (IBD)-associated
arthritis
enthesitis
in inflammatory bowel disease 330
in psoriatic arthritis 315–16, 320
in reactive arthritis 323
enthesitis-related arthritis 398
entrapment neuropathies
in the foot 150–1
in rheumatoid arthritis 299
see also carpal tunnel syndrome
epicondylar clasps 180
epicondylopathy 179–80
Equality Act 2010 463–4
erector spinae muscles, physical
examination 22
erythema infectiosum, reactive arthritis
322

ESR (erythrocyte sedimentation rate)
350, 352
in polymyalgia rheumatica 375
etanercept 293–4
in juvenile idiopathic arthritis 400
ethnic factors, in chronic pain 39
etidronate 222, 223, 225, 226
etoricoxib
in acute gout 443
in ankylosing spondylitis 312
see also COX-2 inhibitors; non-
steroidal anti-inflammatory drugs
(NSAIDs)
European League Against Rheumatism
(EULAR), guideline for fibromyalgia
246, 247
Exercise on Prescription 199–200
exercise therapy 68, 69–70
Alexander Technique 70
in ankylosing spondylitis 313
in chronic neck pain 53
in fibromyalgia 247
hydrotherapy 70
in hypermobility 364
in low-back pain 69
maintenance 70
in osteoarthritis 69, 198–200
in osteoporosis 225
in upper-limb conditions 69–70
extractable nuclear antigens (ENAs)
340, 347, 351

FABER (Flexion ABduction and
External Rotation) test, hip joint 125
facet joint injections 51
facet joint osteoarthritis, prevalence 190
febuxostat 446, 447
femoral head, avascular necrosis 396
femoral neck fractures 124
femoral nerve stretch 22
femoro-acetabular impingement (FAI)
122, 127–8
causes 123–4
symptoms 124
fend-off position 410
fenofibrate, urate-lowering function
446–7
'fever WARMS' questions 40
fibromyalgia 239, 278–9, 372
baseline investigations 245
biopsychosocial assessment 246

diagnosis 241
   ACR criteria 240
   impact of diagnostic label 243
differential diagnosis 245
differentiation from polymyalgia
rheumatica 373
disability assessment 248
holistic approach 248
information provision 243
massage 78
over-investigation 244
overlap with allied disorders 243–4
   similarities to Sjögren's syndrome
   348
pathophysiology 242
patient-centred care 242, 246, 248
prevalence 239–40
prognosis 242–3
referral 248
self-assessment questions 257–9
self-help 248
symptoms 241
treatment 246–8
first metatarsophalangeal (MTP) joint
   gout 266–7
   osteoarthritis 190
   see also hallux limitus; hallux rigidus;
   hallux valgus
first-response equipment 435–7
fitness for work 465–7
   Fit Note 466
flag systems 252–3
flares, rheumatoid arthritis 298
'flat feet'
   asymptomatic 142–3
   children 392
   definition 140
   heel raise test 140, 142
   symptomatic 143
   tibialis posterior dysfunction 154–6
fluid resuscitation 415–16
fluoroquinolones, association with
  tendon pain 180
fluoxetine, in fibromyalgia 247
folic acid, administration with
  methotrexate 290
foot
   alignment in hypermobility 364
   assessment 134–5
   common pathology in hypermobility
   362

'flat feet' 140, 142–3
   normal ranges of movement 139
foot injuries, indications for X-rays 422
foot pain 133
   bone stress reactions and stress
   fractures 149–50
   bunions 158–9
   cavus / cavoid feet 143–4
   'flat feet' 143
   gout 148–9
   history taking 136
   impingement syndromes 151–2
   investigations
      high-resolution ultrasound 139
      MRI / CT 139
      X-rays 138–9
   lesser toe deformities 159–60
   metatarsalgia 157–8
   nerve entrapments 150–1
   observation 136–7
   orthoses 162–3
   osteoarthritis 144–5
   pharmacotherapy 161–2
   physical examination 138
   physical therapies 162
   rheumatoid arthritis 146–7
   self-management 160
   seronegative inflammatory arthritides
   147–8
   systemic sclerosis/scleroderma 148
   weightbearing versus non-
   weightbearing assessment 137
   see also ankle pain; ankle injuries,
   sprains; heel pain
Foot Posture Index 140, 141, 143
footwear 161
   in osteoarthritis 202
foraminal closing test 28
forefoot pain 157–8
Fracture Liaison Services 229
fracture risk, patient education 217
fractures
   ankle 422–3
   cervical spine 417–18
   epidemiology 216
   neck of femur 124
   scaphoid 418–19
   see also osteoporosis
fragility fractures
   investigations 220
   see also osteoporosis

FRAX calculator 223–4
FREEDOM trial 229
'frozen shoulder' 94–5
    case study 103–5
    treatment 99
functional orthoses 163
functional somatic disorders 243–4
    predictors of psychiatric co-morbidity
    255
    *see also* chronic pain; fibromyalgia

gabapentin
    in chronic musculoskeletal pain 256
    in radiculopathy 50
gait assessment 18
    children, normal variants 392
    in foot pain 136–7
    Trendelenburg's sign 125–6
GALS (gait, arms, legs and spine) screen
    134
gelling, in osteoarthritis 193
genu valgus/varus, children 392
giant cell arteritis 371
    diagnostic criteria 372–3
    differential diagnosis 374
    epidemiology 372
    ESR 350
    investigations 373
    treatment 376
giving way
    ankles 153
    knee joint 111
    in osteoarthritis 193
glenohumeral joint, anatomy 87
glenohumeral joint disorders 94–5
    treatment 99
glucosamine, in osteoarthritis 201–2
gluteal tendonopathy 127, 177
golimumab 293–4
Gottron's papules 347
gout 148–9, 266–7, 448–9
    acute management 442–3
    case study 447–8
    classification 440–2
    clinical features 440
    distribution of affected joints 441
    hyperuricaemia 440
    initial management 267–8
    investigations 117
    key points 439–40
    knee joint 111

long-term management 443–4
    co-morbidity and risk factor
    assessment 444
    urate-lowering therapies 444–7
    polyarthropathy 272
    prevalence 1, 440
    primary and secondary, comparison
    of features 442
    risk factors 441, 442
gouty tophi 440
    distinction from calcinosis 346
'greater trochanteric pain syndrome'
    126–7
grinding, in osteoarthritis 193
groin pain 178
growing pains 393
    case study 402–4
    examination 385
    history taking 384, 385
    information leaflet 395
    referral, indications for 394
growth, children 386, 388

haemarthroses 272
haemorrhage, fluid resuscitation 415–16
Haglund's bumps, heel pain 157
hallux limitus 145, 159
hallux rigidus 145, 159
hallux valgus 145, 158–9
hands
    common pathology in hypermobility
    363
    osteoarthritis 194
        classification criteria 187
        prevalence 189–90
        radiographic appearance 196
headaches 243
    *see also* medically unexplained
    symptoms
Health and Safety at Work Act 1974
    457–8
Health and Safety Executive (HSE) 458
'heartsink' feelings 242
Heberden's nodes, familial incidence
    191
heel pain
    bursitis 157
    Haglund's bumps 157
    plantar 156–7
heel raise test 140, 142
heel spurs 156

hepatitis B / C, reactive arthritis 323
high-resolution ultrasound (HRUS), of foot 139
high-stepping gait 18
hip adductor tendonopathy 178
hip joint
  anatomy 123–4
  arthroplasty 204
  developmental dysplasia 396
  movements 124
  physical examination 125–6
    children 394
hip pain 122–3
  femoro-acetabular impingement 127–8
  history taking 124
  in hypermobility 362
  lateral 126–7
  Legg–Calvé–Perthes disease 396
  osteoarthritis 126, 195
    classification criteria 188
    exercise 199
    manual therapy 77–8
    prevalence 190
    risk and prognostic factors 191
  referral from spine 124
  transient synovitis (irritable hip) 396
  traumatic 124
HLA-B27 genotype 269, 308–9
  in classification of reactive arthritis 322
  enthesitis-related arthritis 398
HLA-B27 testing, in diagnosis of ankylosing spondylitis 311–12
holistic approach
  children 404
  in chronic pain 252
  in fibromyalgia 248
  in osteoarthritis 193, 207
  in rheumatoid arthritis 5–6
  in SLE 340–1
hosiery 161
housemaid's knee 112
Hughes syndrome see antiphospholipid syndrome
hyaluronan injections, in osteoarthritis 201
hydrotherapy 70
hydroxychloroquine, in rheumatoid arthritis 292
hyperalgesia 250

hyperlipidaemia, as risk factor for rheumatoid arthritis 285
hypermobility 276–7, 357
  Brighton diagnostic criteria 277
  case study 366–7
  children 390–1, 394
  diagnosis 359–60
  investigations 363
  joint hypermobility syndrome 358–9
  management principles 363
  overuse/malalignment 358
  pain management 366
  presentation of joint problems 362–3
  prognosis 366
  scoring systems 360–1, 368
  symptoms 357–8
  treatment
    alignment check/correction 364
    pharmacotherapy 365
    physiotherapy 364–5
    rest 363
hypertension, in systemic sclerosis 346
hyperuricaemia 441
  see also gout
hypothyroidism 398
hypovolaemic shock 415–16

ibandronate, in osteoporosis 225, 226
ibuprofen 96
  in ankylosing spondylitis 312
  see also non-steroidal anti-inflammatory drugs (NSAIDs)
ICE (ideas, concerns and expectations) 254
idiopathic pain syndromes see complex regional pain syndrome
iliotibial band, anatomy 124
iliotibial band friction syndrome 113
  management 118
illness, distinction from disease 13
immunisations
  in connective tissue disorders 353
  immunosuppressed patients 297, 401
immunosuppressed patients
  children 400–1
  immunisations 297, 401
  malignancy risk 349
impingement syndromes, foot 151–2
Independent Care and Treatment Service (ICATS) 9, 17
indometacin

in acute gout 443
in reactive arthritis 326
*see also* non-steroidal anti-
inflammatory drugs (NSAIDs)
Industrial Injuries Disablement Benefit
(IIDB) 457
qualifying conditions 458
infection risk
anti-TNF therapy 293
burns 430
inflammatory arthritis 268
characteristics 273
spondyloarthropathy 269, 270
*see also* ankylosing spondylitis;
inflammatory bowel disease
(IBD)-associated arthritis; psoriatic
arthritis; reactive arthritis
inflammatory bowel disease (IBD)-
associated arthritis 269, 270, 327–8
case study 329–30
clinical features 328
diagnosis 330
natural history and prognosis 330–1
referral 331
treatment 331–2
inflammatory disorders, back pain 16
inflammatory markers 350
infliximab 293–4
in inflammatory bowel disease 332
information provision 67
in ankylosing spondylitis 314
in fibromyalgia 243, 248
in osteoarthritis 197–8
in osteoporosis 217
in rheumatoid arthritis 287
information sources 7, 104
insertional tendonopathy, Achilles
tendon 175
insoles 162–3
insufficiency stress fractures
foot 150
*see also* osteoporosis
interferential therapy (IFT) 72
intermetatarsal bursitis (IMB) 158
International Classification of
Functioning (ICF) 65
intervertebral discs, structure 11
in-toeing, children 392
irritable bladder 243
irritable bowel syndrome
association with fibromyalgia 243

*see also* medically unexplained
symptoms
irritable hip 396

Jaccoud's arthritis 341
joint aspiration 351
cloudy aspirates 266
in gout 267, 443
knee 116–17, 118
joint hypermobility syndrome (JHS)
358–9
juvenile idiopathic arthritis (JIA) 381
education 400
enthesitis-related arthritis 398
immunosuppression 400–1
impact of disease and treatment
401–2
investigations 399–400
limping 394
pharmacotherapy 400
presentation 397

Keele STarT Back Screening Tool 47–8,
49
keloid scars, burns 430
keratoconjunctivitis sicca 348, 349
keratoderma blenorrhagica 323
knee joint
arthroplasty 204
bursae 110
ligaments 110
locking 204–5
patella 111
physical examination
Clarke's test 115
inspection 113
menisci assessment 114–15
palpation 114
range of movement 113
stability assessment 114
stability 110
swelling 111
knee pain 110
anterior 112
case study 119–20
associated effusions 123
case study 3–6
children 396–7
differential diagnosis 123
history taking 111
in hypermobility 362

investigations
blood tests 117
joint aspiration 116–17
MRI 116
ultrasound scanning 115–16
X-rays 115
lateral 113
management
bursitis 117
effusions 118
iliotibial band friction syndrome 118
non-traumatic ligamentous pain 118
non-traumatic meniscal problems 118
osteoarthritis 117
medial 112
obesity 119–20
Osgood–Schlatter's disease, case study 122
osteoarthritis 194
case study 120–1, 205–7
classification criteria 188
management 117
massage 78
prevalence 190
radiographic appearance 197
risk and prognostic factors 192
Oxford knee score 130–2
red flags 113
referral from hip 115
trauma 420–1
meniscal tears, case study 121
knock knees, children 392
Kummel's signs 45

laryngeal mask airways (LMAs) 413
lasofoxifene 230
lateral collateral ligament, knee joint 110
lateral elbow pain 179
case study 179–80, 181–2
see also tendonopathy
lateral hip tendonopathy 177
Leeds foot assessment protocol 134, 135
leflunomide 290
cautions 321, 327
in psoriatic arthritis 320
in rheumatoid arthritis 292
leg alignment, children, normal variants 392
leg length differences 19, 20–1

children 386
Legg–Calvé–Perthes disease 396
leukaemia 398
lifestyle modification
in gout 444, 448
in osteoporosis 225
limping
children 383, 394, 396
see also gait assessment
locking, knee joint 111, 118, 121, 204–5
Looser's zones 233
losartan, urate-lowering function 446–7
low-back pain see back pain
low-level laser therapy (LLLT) 72–3
lumbar root entrapment, diagnostic features 23
lung cancer, pancoast tumours 27–8
Lyme disease, reactive arthritis 323
lymphoma risk, rheumatoid arthritis 297

magnetic resonance imaging (MRI)
in ankylosing spondylitis 311–12
foot 139
knee joint 116
in osteoarthritis 186, 195
malalignment of joints 358
malignancy
bone tumours, children 397
differentiation from polymyalgia rheumatica 373
risk in connective tissue disorders 347, 349
manipulation of joints 76–7
manipulation under anaesthetic (MUA), adhesive capsulitis 99
Manual Handling Operations Regulations 458
manual therapy 76–7
in osteoarthritis 202
'march fractures' 150
Marfanoid syndromes 390–1
massage 78
McKenzie Method 29, 68
McMurray's test 114
mechanical joint pain, characteristics 271, 276
medial collateral ligament, knee joint 110
medial epicondylitis see tendonopathy

medically unexplained symptoms
(MUPS) 10, 244
  prevalence 249
  *see also* chronic pain
meniscal cysts 113
meniscal injury
  case study 121
  children 396
  MRI 116
meniscectomy, subsequent knee pain
112
menisci, assessment 114–15
menopause, bone loss 216
mesalazine, in inflammatory bowel
  disease 331
metabolic syndrome 441, 444
  association with gout 267
  association with psoriatic arthritis 318
metatarsalgia 157–8
METHANE mnemonic, emergency
  situations 412
methotrexate 354–5
  cautions 321, 327
  in connective tissue disorders 353
  in juvenile idiopathic arthritis 400
  in psoriatic arthritis 319
  in reactive arthritis 326
  in rheumatoid arthritis 290–1
    combination with biological agents
    293–4
  steroid-sparing 375
microdiscectomy 9
midfoot pain 157–8
'milking' knee joint 114
milnacipran, in fibromyalgia 247
mobilisation of joints 76–7
moclobemide, in fibromyalgia 247
monoarthropathy
  case study 264
  differential diagnosis 264
  gout 266–8
  haemophilia 272
  inflammatory arthritis 268–70
  investigations 265
  osteoarthritis 270–2
  red flags 266
  septic arthritis 265–6
  traumatic 272
Morton's neuroma 151
motor milestones 391
movie-goer's knee 112

Multidisciplinary Interface Clinics 79
multidisciplinary working 78–9
  in rheumatoid arthritis 4, 287
muscle relaxants
  for acute back pain 17
  for chronic back pain 50
muscle strength testing 21
musculoskeletal disease
  costs 2
  prevalence 1
musculoskeletal interface services 104
Musculoskeletal Services Framework
  (MSF) 79
myalgic encephalitis (ME) *see* chronic
  fatigue syndrome (CFS)
myofascial pain syndrome 241

naproxen 96
  in ankylosing spondylitis 312
  in reactive arthritis 326
  *see also* non-steroidal anti-
    inflammatory drugs (NSAIDs)
navicular, stress fractures 149–50
neck examination, TWELVE mnemonic
  414
neck injuries, indications for X-rays
  417–18
neck pain
  acute
    case study 29, 31–3
    in children between ten and
    sixteen 25
    in children under five years 25
    diagnosis and management 9
    disc prolapse 26
    domains of care 32–3
    physical examination 28
    postural 26
    prevalence 9, 24
    red flags 27
    traumatic 25–6
    in young adults 25
  chronic 35
    clinical assessment 39
    distress 42–4
    drug therapy 52
    ethnic and cultural factors 39
    history taking 42–4
    investigations 41, 45
    key points 59–60
    management strategy 56–7

occupational aspects 54–6
physical examination 44–5
physical treatments 53
positive messages 57
predisposing factors 38–9
signs of serious disease 40–1
in hypermobility 362
manipulation and mobilisation 76–7
occupational issues, case study 468–9
prevalence 37
referral to shoulder 95
in rheumatoid arthritis 298–9
see also back pain
neovascularisation, tendonopathy 170
imaging 173
nerve entrapments see carpal tunnel
syndrome; entrapment neuropathies
nerve root blocks 51
nerve root pain, diagnostic triage 15
neurogenic cavoid feet 144–5
neurological assessment, emergency
situations 416
neurological symptoms, in rheumatoid
arthritis 298–9
neuropathic pain 250, 256
neuropathy
drugs as cause 40
investigations to consider 41
NICE guidelines
for ankylosing spondylitis 314
for osteoarthritis 198, 199
for osteoporosis 221–2, 223
for psoriatic arthritis 319
nifedipine, in Raynaud's phenomenon
337
nocebo effect 11–12
nociceptive pain 249–50
NOGG (National Osteoporosis Guideline
Group) guideline 221, 223–4
non-accidental injury, burns 427
non-steroidal anti-inflammatory drugs
(NSAIDs)
in acute gout 268, 439, 442–3
in ankylosing spondylitis 312–13
in back pain 50
in connective tissue disorders 352–3
in inflammatory bowel disease 331
in osteoarthritis 200–1, 271–2
in reactive arthritis 326
in rheumatoid arthritis 286
in shoulder pain 96

side effects 339, 354
'number needed to offend' (NNO),
diagnostic labelling 243

obesity, as risk factor for knee pain
119–20
occupational health physicians 461
occupational issues 453–4
benefits of work 456
case studies 467–9
chronic health problems 459
legal protection 463–4
chronic pain 256
back and neck pain 54–6, 58
demographic trends in workforce
454–6
fitness for work 465–7
key points 453
prevention of work-related
musculoskeletal ill health 457–8
rheumatoid arthritis 296–7
shoulder pain 96–7, 102, 104
vocational rehabilitation 459–60
key components of medical
consultation 462
messages for employees 460–1
messages for employers 460
messages for primary care health
professionals 461
psychosocial flags 462
stepped care approach 462
work as a cause of ill health 457
Working for a Healthier Tomorrow 465
working-age ill health 456
see also work-related upper-limb
disorder (WRULD)
odanacatib 230
old-age support ratio, projected trends
455
opioids
in acute back pain 17
in chronic back pain 50
in chronic musculoskeletal pain 255
in osteoarthritis 201
in shoulder pain 96
orthoses 76, 162–3
for anterior knee pain 119
for tendonopathy 174
Osgood–Schlatter's disease 112, 396
case study 122
osteoarthritis 185, 208

acromioclavicular 95
acute exacerbations 270–1
  investigations 271
  management 271–2
American College of Rheumatology
classification criteria 187–8
assessment
  history taking 194
  holistic approach 193
  physical examination 194–5
case study 205–7
everyday activity impairment 193
exercise therapy 69
of the foot and ankle 144–5
frequently affected joints 189–90
of the hip
  management 126
  manual therapy 77–8
  symptoms 124
investigations
  blood tests 196
  magnetic resonance imaging 195
  radiography 195, 196, 197
  synovial fluid analysis 196–7
  ultrasound scanning 196
joints commonly involved 271
of the knee 112, 113
  case study 120–1
  management 117
  massage 78
  X-rays 115
management 198
  acupuncture 203
  aids and devices 202
  analgesia 200–1
  corticosteroid injections 201
  education 197–8
  exercise 198–200
  glucosamine and chondroitin 201–2
  hyaluronan injections 201
  manual therapy 202
  thermotherapy 203
  transcutaneous electrical nerve
  stimulation (TENS) 71
  treatment guidelines 198, 199
  weight reduction 200
NICE guidelines 146
pathogenesis 186–7
polyarthropathy 275–6
prevalence 1
prevention 191

prognostic factors 190–1, 192
quality of life impairment 193
radiographic 189
referral 204–5
risk factors 190–1, 192, 271
role of primary care 185–6
self-help strategies 203–4
of the shoulder 94
symptomatic 189
symptoms 192–3
Osteoarthritis Research Society
 International (OARSI) guideline 198
osteochondritis dissecans 396
osteoid osteoma 397
osteomalacia 232, 279, 398
  investigations 233
  risk factors 233
  treatment 233
osteomyelitis, children 394, 396
osteonecrosis of the jaw, risk from
 bisphosphonates 227
osteopenia, T-score 219
osteoporosis 215, 230
  adherence and persistence with
  therapy 228–9
  AKT questions 233–4
  analgesia 228
  case studies 234–7
  commonly used codes 218
  diagnosis 219
  epidemiology 216
  FRAX calculator 223–4
  guidance 221
    NICE TA 160 and 161 221–2, 223
    NICE TA 204 223
    NOGG guideline 223–4
  high-risk patients, identification
  217–18
  investigations 220
  key learning points 214–15
  management
    drug treatment 225–7
    lifestyle advice 225
    new drugs 229–30
  management chart 224
  pathogenesis 216
  patient-centred care 217
  prevalence 1
  prevention in steroid therapy 374
  primary care roles and responsibilities
  215–16

referral 228
risk factors 217
steroid-induced 218–19, 344
osteotomy 204
Ottawa Ankle Rules 152, 422
Ottawa Foot Rules 422
Ottawa Knee Rules 420
over-investigation 244
oxygenation, trauma patients 414

Paget's disease 231–2
pain 2
in fibromyalgia 240
in osteoarthritis 192
*see also* analgesia; back pain; chronic pain; neck pain
pain management programmes 54
'painful arc', shoulder 92
painful heel drops regime 174
palindromic disease, rheumatoid arthritis 285
pancoast tumours 27
paracetamol, in osteoarthritis 200
parvovirus, as cause of arthritis 322
patella 111
patellar tendonopathy 112, 177
patellofemoral joint maltracking 112
case study 119–20
patellofemoral pain
Clarke's test 115
exercise therapy 69
patient education
in ankylosing spondylitis 314
in fibromyalgia 248
in osteoarthritis 197–8
in osteoporosis 217
in rheumatoid arthritis 287
peak bone mass 216
peek-a-boo heel sign 144
pelvis, common pathology in hypermobility 362
perimenopausal women, polyarthropathy 276
person-centred care, case study of rheumatoid arthritis 4
pes anserine bursitis 112
management 117
pes cavus 143–4
PEST screening questionnaire, psoriatic arthritis 317
pGALS screen 385, 389–90

practical tips 388
when to perform it 389
photobioactivation 73
photosensitivity 354
in SLE 339
Physio Direct 66
physiotherapy 79
acupuncture 74
in acute soft-tissue injury 75, 76
aims 65
in ankle instability 153
in ankylosing spondylitis 313
in anterior knee pain 119
in chronic back pain 53–4
in chronic neck pain 53
clinical assessment 66
cryotherapy 74–5
electrotherapy 71
interferential therapy 72
low-level laser therapy 72–3
short-wave diathermy 73
transcutaneous electrical nerve stimulation (TENS) 71–2
ultrasound 73
evidence-based practice 66
exercise therapy 68
Alexander Technique 70
hydrotherapy 70
in low-back pain 69
maintenance 70
in osteoarthritis 69
in upper-limb conditions 69–70
in foot pain 162
in hypermobility 364–5
information and advice provision 67
in low-back pain 74
manual therapy 76–7
massage 78
in osteoarthritis 202–3
progressive eccentric loading 174–5
referral, indications for
service delivery 66
in shoulder problems 97
adhesive capsulitis 99
rotator cuff disorders 97
splints, strapping, bracing and orthoses 76
in tendonopathy 174
therabands 180
thermotherapy 74
Pincer deformity, hip joint 127

pirlindole, in fibromyalgia 247
Pittsburgh Decision Rules, knee injuries 420
placebo effects, manual therapy 77, 78
plantar heel pain / plantar fasciitis 156–7
pleurisy, in SLE 342–4
pneumonitis, as side effect of methotrexate 291
podagra 266–7
podiatry 160, 162, 205
polyarthropathy
    connective tissue disorders 277–8
    fibromyalgia 278–9
    gout 279
    hypermobility 276–7
    osteoarthritis 275–6
    possible causes 272–3
    rheumatoid arthritis 273–5
    vitamin D deficiency 279
polymyalgia rheumatica 371
    bone-sparing therapy 236–7
    case study 377–8
    diagnosis 89, 372
    differential diagnosis 374
    distinction from polymyositis 347
    epidemiology 372
    investigations 373
    prevalence 1
    problem situations 375–6
    referral guidelines 376
    treatment 374–5
polymyositis 278, 347
Poncet's disease 323
popliteal cysts *see* Baker's cyst
posterior cruciate ligament (PCL) 110
    assessment 114
posture
    in hypermobility 365
    neck pain 26, 27–8
post-viral reactive arthritis 322
    *see also* reactive arthritis
pramipexole, in fibromyalgia 247
prazosin, in Raynaud's phenomenon 337
prednisolone
    in acute gout 443
    in giant cell arteritis 376
    in polymyalgia rheumatica 374–5, 377–8
    *see also* steroids

pregabalin
    in chronic musculoskeletal pain 256
    in fibromyalgia 247
    in radiculopathy 50
premenstrual syndrome 243
pre-patellar bursitis 112
prevalence of musculoskeletal disease 1
primary gout 440–1, 442
probenecid 446
progressive eccentric loading 174–5
proprioception training 364
prosthetic joints, septic arthritis 266
proton pump inhibitors (PPIs), prescription with NSAIDs 201
pseudogout 148, 197, 270
psoriasis, 'hidden' areas 315, 332
psoriatic arthritis 269, 270
    clinical features 315–16
    diagnosis 316–17
    foot involvement 147–8
    monitoring 321
    natural history and prognosis 318
    PEST screening questionnaire 317
    prevalence 315
    referral 318
    treatment 318–20
psychosocial history taking 253
psychosocial intervention, back pain 48
PTPN22 285
public health campaigns, back pain 52
pulsed electromagnetic energy (PEME) 73
pulsed short-wave diathermy (PSWD) 73
pump bumps (Haglund's bumps) 157

Quality and Outcomes Framework (QoF) 6
Quebec Task Force guidelines, whiplash-associated disorders 25–6

radiography
    in ankle injuries 152, 422
    children 400
    in chronic back pain 45
    foot 138–9
    knee joint 115
        in knee injuries 420–1
    in neck injuries 417–18
    in osteoarthritis 189, 195
    in osteomalacia 233

in osteoporosis 220
in psoriatic arthritis 321
in tendonopathy 173
raloxifene, in osteoporosis 221, 223, 225, 227
RANKL 229
rashes, SLE 339
Raynaud's phenomenon 336–7, 354, 355
  case study 336
  foot involvement 148
  self-assessment questions 338
  systemic sclerosis 346
reactive arthritis 269–70, 321–2
  case study 324–5
  classification 322
  clinical features 322–3
  diagnosis 323–4
  foot involvement 148
  knee pain 113
  monitoring 327
  natural history and prognosis 325
  prevalence 322
  referral 326
  treatment 326
reasonable adjustments, Disability Discrimination Act (DDA) 1995 463, 464
red flags
  back pain 14, 15
    children 397
    thoracic spine 36
  children 113, 387, 397
  knee pain 113
  neck pain 27–8
  shoulder pain 89
referred pain 95, 182
reflex sympathetic dystrophy see work-related upper-limb disorder (WRULD)
Reiter's syndrome 269
  see also reactive arthritis
REMS (Regional Examination of the Musculoskeletal System) screen 134, 135
repetitive pain symptoms 26–7
repetitive strain injury see work-related upper-limb disorder (WRULD)
resources 7
rheumatoid arthritis 283
  case studies
    early disease 299–302

established disease 302–4
multidisciplinary working 3–6
clinical expression 285
co-morbidities 297
constitutional symptoms 274
disease activity assessment 287–8
disease-modifying drugs 289–90
  biological therapies 292–4
  hydroxychloroquine 292
  leflunomide 292
  methotrexate 290–1
  monitoring therapy 295–6
  sulfasalazine 291
early treatment, importance 273
emergency situations
  dyspnoea 299
  flares 298
  joint sepsis 298
  new-onset neurological symptoms 298–9
emotional impact 296
epidemiology 284
family history 274
foot involvement 146–7
immunisations 297
information provision 287
initial management 286
investigations 275
low-level laser therapy 73
lymphoma risk 297
manual therapy 77
multidisciplinary working 287
NICE guidelines 275
occupational issues 296–7
pattern of joints affected 273–4
physical examination 274
prevalence 1
prognosis 288
public awareness campaign 147
referral 146, 286–7
risk factors 284–5
shared care 294
  communication between primary and secondary care teams 289
  primary care responsibilities 294–5
  secondary care responsibilities 295
similarities to polymyalgia rheumatica 374
transcutaneous electrical nerve stimulation (TENS) 71
treatment principles 286

rheumatoid factor 284, 351
  children 399–400
rheumatology referral 205
rickets 279
rickety rosary 233
risedronate
  in osteoporosis 222, 223, 226
  in Paget's disease 232
rituximab 294
rotation provocation test 23
rotator cuff disorders 178
  case study 101–2
  investigations 95
  referral 98
  tears 89
    clinical features 92, 93–4
  tendonopathy 93
  treatment 97–8
  see also tendonopathy
rubella, reactive arthritis 323
runners, iliotibial band friction
  syndrome 113, 118

S4 predictors of psychiatric co-
  morbidity 255
saddle area anaesthesia/paraesthesiae
  16, 21
safety considerations, emergency
  situations 409–11
    protective equipment 434
sag sign, knee joint 114
scalds 423, 426
  see also burns
scaphoid fractures 418–19
scarring, burns 430
Schirmer's test 348
Schober's test 18–19
Schuermann's disease 398
scleroderma
  prevalence 1
  see also systemic sclerosis/scleroderma
scleroderma crisis 346
secondary gout 442
self-help strategies
  in fibromyalgia 248
  in osteoarthritis 203–4
sensory limb symptoms, investigations
  to consider 41
septic arthritis 265–6
  children 394, 396
  in rheumatoid arthritis 298

shared epitope 284
Shigella infection, reactive arthritis 322
short-wave diathermy (SWD) therapy
  73
shoulder joint
  instability 100
  structure and function 86–7
shoulder pain
  acromioclavicular disorders 95
  analgesia 96
  assessment 88
    clinical assessment algorithm 93
    history taking 90–1
    physical examination 91–2
  calcific tendonitis, ultrasound therapy
  73
  case studies 100–5
  causes 90
  diagnosis 92
  glenohumeral disorders 94–5
  in hypermobility 363
  investigations 95–6
  occupational and lifestyle issues 96–7
  orthopaedic referral 100
  outcomes 86
  prevalence 85
  prognostic factors 88
  red flags 89
  referral pointers 100
  referred mechanical neck pain 95
  rheumatology referral 100
  risk factors 87–8
  rotator cuff disorders 93–4, 97–8, 178
  treatment 96
    acromioclavicular disorders 99
    glenohumeral disorders 99
    physiotherapy 97
    rotator cuff disorders 97–8
shoulder-tip pain, malignant disease
  349
sicca syndrome 348, 349
Sjögren's syndrome 278, 341, 348
  ESR 350
  malignancy risk 349
  treatment 354
  see also connective tissue disorders
  (CTDs)
SLE see systemic lupus erythematosus
sleep disturbance 120, 121
  children 385
  management 256

slipped epiphysis, upper femoral 396
slump test 19–20
smoking
  and ankylosing spondylitis 311
  and rheumatoid arthritis 285, 297
soft-tissue injuries, physiotherapy 75, 76
somatisation 244
spinal fusion surgery 51
spinal joint dysfunction, diagnostic
 features 23
spinal stenosis 11
  X stop 10
spine
  common pathology in hypermobility
  362
  common sites of degenerative
  changes 11
  facet joint osteoarthritis, prevalence 190
  see also back pain; cervical spine;
  neck pain
splints 76
  in osteoarthritis 202
spondylitis
  in inflammatory bowel disease 328
  in psoriatic arthritis 316
  in reactive arthritis 323
  see also ankylosing spondylitis
spondyloarthropathies 269, 270, 307–8
  reactive arthritis 269–70
  self-assessment questions 332–3
  see also ankylosing spondylitis;
  inflammatory bowel disease (IBD)-
  associated arthritis; psoriatic arthritis;
  reactive arthritis
spondylolisthesis 23
  children 398, 406–7
spondylolysis, children 398
spondylosis 11
sports injuries
  knee pain 113
    meniscal tear 121
  physiotherapy 75, 76
  tendonopathy 171, 172, 176
sports massage 78
statins
  association with tendon pain 180
  in SLE 340
stepped-care approach, vocational
 rehabilitation 462
steroid-induced osteoporosis 218–19,
 344

prevention 237, 374
steroid injections
  in acromioclavicular disorders 99
  in acute gout 443
  in adhesive capsulitis 99
  in hypermobility 365
  in osteoarthritis 201
  in rotator cuff disorders 98
  in tendonopathy 173–4
steroids
  in acute gout 268, 443
  in connective tissue disorders 353
  in giant cell arteritis 373, 376
  in inflammatory bowel disease 331
  in juvenile idiopathic arthritis 400
  in polymyalgia rheumatica 373,
  374–5, 377–8
  in reactive arthritis 326
  in rheumatoid arthritis 289
stiffness, in osteoarthritis 192
straight-leg raise 20
strapping 76
stress fractures, foot 149–50
stretching, in hypermobility 364
strontium ranelate, in osteoporosis 222,
 223, 225, 227
subacromial impingement syndrome
 69–70
subchondral bone turnover, in
 osteoarthritis 187
sulfasalazine
  in inflammatory bowel disease 331
  in reactive arthritis 326
  in rheumatoid arthritis 291
sulfinpyrazone 446
sunburn 426
  see also burns
supra-patellar bursitis 112
supraspinatus tendinitis 178
supraspinatus muscle, anatomy 87
swimming, value in osteoarthritis 199
synovial fluid analysis 196–7
synovial fluid aspiration see joint
 aspiration
synovitis
  in osteoarthritis 186, 187
  in rheumatoid arthritis 285
systemic illness, 'fever WARMS'
 questions 40
systemic lupus erythematosus (SLE)
 278, 338–9, 355

acute hot joints 339
  case study 342–4
  cerebral lupus 339
  children 398, 399–400
  clinical features 346
  diagnosis 340
  full blood count 350
  holistic care 340–1
  pleurisy 342–4
  premature coronary artery disease
  339–40
  presentation 341
  prevalence 1
  renal function monitoring 340, 341
  self-assessment questions 342
  statin therapy 340
  see also connective tissue disorders
  (CTDs)
systemic sclerosis/scleroderma 341,
  345–6
  diagnosis 347
  foot involvement 148
  malignancy risk 349
  treatment 347
  see also connective tissue disorders
  (CTDs)

T-scores, DXA 218, 219
tarsal tunnel syndrome 151
temperomandibular joint, common
  pathology in hypermobility 363
temperomandibular joint syndrome 243
  see also medically unexplained
  symptoms
temporal artery biopsy 373
tendon pain, drug-associated 180
tendon tears 172
  imaging 173
  treatment 174
tendonopathy 182
  Achilles tendonopathy 175–7
  assessment
    history taking 172
    imaging 173
    physical examination 172–3
  causes 170–2
  frequently affected sites 169
  hip adductor tendonopathy 178
  lateral elbow pain 179–80
  lateral hip tendonopathy 177
  old and new thinking 170

patella tendonopathy 177
  pathological changes 169–70
  presentation 172
  rotator cuff disorders 178
  tibialis posterior tendonopathy 177
  treatment 173–4
    novel treatments 175
    progressive eccentric loading 174–5
  work-related upper-limb disorder
  (WRULD) 180–2
  see also Achilles tendonopathy;
  rotator cuff disorders
tennis elbow 179
  case study 179–80
  see also tendonopathy
tenosynovitis 180
teriparatide 223, 225, 227
therabands 180
thermal burns 426–7
  see also burns
thermotherapy 74–5
  in osteoarthritis 203
Thessaly's test 114, 115
thoracic spine pain 36
  investigations to consider 41
thyroid disease 398
tibialis posterior dysfunction (TPD) 151,
  154–5
  classification 156
tibialis posterior tendonopathy 177
Tinel's sign 151
tocilizumab 294
toe deformities 159–60
  see also hallux valgus
toe walking, children 392
toxic shock syndrome, risk from burns
  430
tramadol
  in acute back pain 17
  in chronic musculoskeletal pain 256
  in fibromyalgia 247
transcutaneous electrical nerve
  stimulation (TENS) 71–2
  in osteoarthritis 202–3
transient synovitis 396
trauma 272, 311
  in ankylosing spondylitis 311–12
  see also emergency situations
Trendelenburg gait 18, 125–6
triage sieve 411, 412
triage systems, physiotherapy 66

trigger point injections 256
  in chronic neck pain 52
trochanteric bursa 124
trochanteric bursitis 126, 177
  symptoms 124
tropisetron, in fibromyalgia 247
tuberculosis, reactive arthritis 323
tumour necrosis factor-alpha (TNF),
  role in rheumatoid arthritis 292
TWELVE mnemonic, neck examination
  414

ulcerative colitis *see* inflammatory
  bowel disease (IBD)-associated
  arthritis
ultrasound scanning
  foot 139
  knee joint 115–16
  in osteoarthritis 196
  in polymyalgia rheumatica and giant
  cell arteritis 373
  in tendonopathy 173
ultrasound therapy 73
urate-lowering therapies
  allopurinol 444, 445–6
  in allopurinol intolerance 446–7
  indications 444–5
  target urate levels 445
uric acid crystals 267
urinalysis 351
uveitis, chronic anterior, in JIA 397

varicella zoster prophylaxis,
  immunosuppressed patients 297, 401
vitamin D deficiency 43, 279
  breastfed babies 233
  osteomalacia 232–3
vitamin D metabolism 233
vitamin D supplementation
  in osteomalacia 233
  in osteoporosis 226
vocational rehabilitation 453, 459–60
  key components of medical
  consultation 462
  messages for employees 460–1
  messages for employers 460
  messages for primary care health
  professionals 461
  psychosocial flags 462
  stepped-care approach 462

Waddell's signs 44–5
walking aids, in osteoarthritis 202
warfarin, interaction with leflunomide
  292
'wear and tear' 186
weight reduction
  in foot disorders 160
  in osteoarthritis 200
whiplash-associated disorders (WAD)
  25–6, 37
  physical treatments 53
  prognostic factors 38–9
'window of opportunity', rheumatoid
  arthritis 289
work
  benefits of 456
  *see also* occupational issues
workforce, demographic trends 454–6
*Working for a Healthier Tomorrow* 248,
  256, 465
working-age ill health 456
  work as a cause 457
work-related musculoskeletal ill health,
  prevention 457–8
work-related upper-limb disorder
  (WRULD) 171, 172, 180–1, 454
  case study 181–2
Wright, Verna 307–8

X stop 10

yellow flags 12, 55, 253, 462

zoledronate
  in osteoporosis 225, 226
  in Paget's disease 232

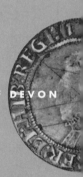

THE CONCISE HISTORIES OF **DEVON**

# ELIZABETHAN
# DEVON

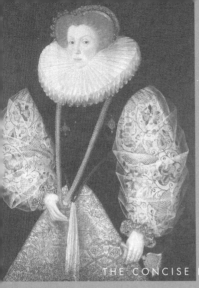

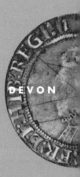

THE CONCISE HISTORIES OF **DEVON**

# ELIZABETHAN
# DEVON

TODD GRAY

First published in Great Britain by The Mint Press, 2001

© Todd Gray & The Mint Press 2001

The right of Todd Gray to be identified as author of this work has been asserted by him in accordance with the Copyright, Designs & Patents Act 1988.

ISBN 1-903356-12-1

Cataloguing in Publication Data
CIP record for this title is available from the British Library


The Mint Press
18 The Mint
Exeter, Devon
England EX4 3BL

Cover and text design by Delphine Jones

Main cover illustration: portrait of Mary Cornwallis, Countess of Bath, by George Gower (courtesy of Manchester City Art Galleries).

Coin: Silver shilling struck in 1601, found in the East Worlington hoard (by courtesy of Exeter Museums Service.)

Printed and bound in Great Britain
by Short Run Press Ltd, Exeter.

# CONTENTS

| | |
|---|---|
| Introduction | 7 |
| The People | 11 |
| Industries | 21 |
| *Tin Mining* | 21 |
| *Agriculture* | 24 |
| *Cloth-making* | 31 |
| *Maritime enterprize* | 35 |
| The Sea Dogs | 53 |
| Exploration and colonies | 77 |
| Religion | 83 |
| The Legacy of the Elizabethan Age | 89 |

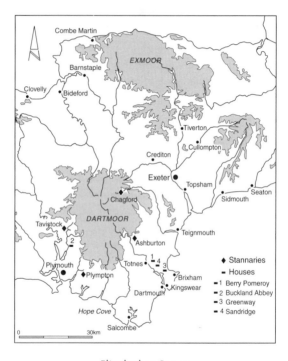

Elizabethan Devon

# INTRODUCTION

Elizabethan Devon's geographical distance from London placed it at a disadvantage with many other counties. Not once, from 1557 to her death in 1603, did the queen visit the county: there were no great country houses of the calibre needed to host her which other parts of the country could boast. Its distance helped ensure this paucity of building. The Duke of Somerset's grand refurbishment of Berry Pomeroy

Castle in the 1540s and 1550s was unusual and probably seemed eccentric even to Devonians: land communications were notoriously poor and inhibited the county's attraction as a location for country seats. As late as the 1680s a visitor from Sussex wryly commented that the devil himself would not purchase a Devon home because of the travel difficulties: one Elizabethan wrote that strangers only needed one journey to forbear ever travelling in Devon again.

And yet there were discrepancies, the county's mariners, particularly its fishermen, were well-travelled. Many seamen who lived in coastal parishes were familiar with parts of Ireland, Iceland, Newfoundland and the North Sea whereas it is unlikely they ever visited Dartmoor.

Devon's mariners were also becoming acquainted with Africa, North and South America, the West Indies and the Far East. It would be easy to think that Sir Francis Drake circumnavigated the globe on his own: historians largely ignore the presence of his crew. But the tales they had of the strange world outside England were no doubt highly sought-after and for years listened to and then repeated, even if not believed, in private and public houses throughout Devon.

Irrespective of their insights into the New World, the majority of the population of Devon were not well-travelled but were born and brought up within relatively short distances.

In spite of this general isolation, the

county was at the forefront of national affairs: its courtiers were regarded by the queen as exceptional in their number and quality, Devon was one of the most prosperous counties in the country, for technological and strategic reasons it became important that the navy retained a presence in the county, particularly Plymouth, and Devon's gentlemen and merchants were premier in many of the country's overseas maritime enterprises. The county remained of special interest and importance to the queen throughout her long reign.

# THE
# PEOPLE

At the end of the sixteenth century John Hooker, Devon's first historian and Exeter's first archivist, gathered together documents with an intention of writing the county's first history. He copied a number of original sources but managed to finish only part of his *Synopsis Chorographical* of Devonshire which, while incomplete and unpublished, has been tremendously influential in our interpretation of Devon's past. The historians who followed in the seventeenth and eighteenth centuries heavily 'borrowed' from his manuscript in their own writings and this continued to a great degree in the nineteenth and twentieth centuries.

Hooker described the class system then prevalent in Devon, as it was elsewhere in England, by noting that men could be grouped into four 'sorts and degrees'. At the top were the nobility and the gentry. There were very few noblemen resident in Devon although for a short while 'Princess Katherine, Countess of Devon, daughter, sister and aunt of kings' resided in the county: the daughter of Edward IV, sister of Edward V and aunt of Henry VIII lived in exile, or at least safety, at Tiverton Castle from about 1512 to her death in 1527. It was partly due to her marriage into the Courtenay family, and the political machinations in London, which resulted in their loss of the title earls of Devon; her son, the senior member of the family, the marquis of Exeter, was executed for treason in 1538 and the last male of his line died in Italian exile the year before Elizabeth came to the throne.

The one resident nobleman was William, fourth Earl of Bath, who lived at Tawstock near Barnstaple. A portrait of his first wife, the ill-fated Mary Cornwallis, Countess of Bath, is featured on this book's cover. To modern eyes she is easily confused with Queen Elizabeth. In 1577, at the age of twenty, the earl married Mary Cornwallis in circumstances which led to an annulment: it was later claimed that the young man met his bride-to-be at a country house party in Suffolk, given excessive amounts of alcohol, placed in bed with the slightly older woman and then found to the supposed shock of the household. The resulting marriage took place in the early hours of the morning and was legally disputed for years. The bride's family claimed that the earl had been in love with her. Irrespectively, the earl's mother secured an annulment and at Exeter in 1582 the earl married Lady Elizabeth, daughter of Francis Russell, second Earl of Bedford. Bedford was Lord Lieutenant and Devon's other aristocrat with large land holdings. Bedford kept only a nominal residence in Devon but the marriage brought together the county's two noble families. Notwithstanding, up to her death in 1627 Mary Cornwallis still considered herself the Countess of Bath.

In contrast to the number of resident aristocracy, Devon had a great number of gentry. There were possibly as many as four hundred families. Even so, they tried to emulate the nobility by aspiring to live in London at least part of the year so the county was, to a certain degree, also denuded of its gentlemen and ladies. Hooker, the son of a gentleman, praised the high moral fibre of Devon's gentry; he wrote they were extraordinarily well-behaved and never tempted by 'disorders and filthiness as be found in the courts of

Bachus and the palaces of Venus'. Nevertheless, four times a year those members of the gentry who were county justices, as well as many others, flocked to Exeter for the quarter sessions. Exeter was the religious, economic and political centre of the region and the focus for county society. One of the largest landowners was Sir William Petre whose son John was created Baron Petre of Writtle on the accession of James I. The gentry's houses were mainly on old sites, built for shelter of local materials: the fashion for views came later. The making of brick did not come to Devon until the 1590s and even then was confined to East Devon. Local quarries provided the building stone for larger houses and Dartmoor granite was found on the surface.

The second class were men Hooker described as merchants. Not surprisingly William Harrison, a colleague of Hooker's, distinguished society into similar groupings in his *Description of England* but referred to merchants firstly as citizens and burgesses. Neither term made it into Hooker's description of merchants. Harrison, the son of one such man, wrote with more approval than Hooker who dismissively noted that merchants aspired to be gentlemen by buying land 'and by little and little they do creep and seek to be gentlemen'. However, he was impressed by the international aspect of their trade which had greatly expanded in the latter part of the sixteenth century.

Below them were the yeomen, a term of

status rather than occupation, which signified free men who lived off their land and held it in their own right or rented it at a sufficiently high level. Even they, considered Hooker, were not satisfied with their station as they had previously been accustomed but "every man is now of an aspiring mind and not contented with their own estate, do like better of another's".

One unusual manuscript is that of the late Elizabethan account book of William Honeywell, a yeoman of Ashton. In it he records the day-to-day life of a farmer in planting and reaping corn, the buying and selling of livestock, his hiring of servants and the shearing of his sheep. He was a prosperous yeoman but his lifestyle would probably have been disapproved of by

Hooker: he bought fine clothes, was fond of playing cards and bowls and visited London.

The lowest in the social scale were workers for daily wages. Hooker wrote there were two sorts, the first were the artificers who lived in towns and the second were labourers employed in husbandry or other rural trades. They did most of the work in specialised areas such as the cobblers, chimney sweeps, bakers and butchers. Women too were employed in such roles as laundresses and midwives and some earned additional income by weeding the fields. In coastal parishes they were engaged in the shore fisheries. Although these men and women made up the majority of the population, they received the least attention by Hooker and there are few records left by them, unlike those in the other three social groups, which can provide glimpses of society from their perspectives.

Hooker thought men should accept the position they were born into and he ignored women altogether in his considerations. These social distinctions had legal implications and privileges even if the four divisions were not universally accepted; one Elizabethan Devonian in Hooker's lowest group was overheard claiming that if his blood was mixed in a bowl with that of a nobleman it would be impossible to tell the difference between the two.

# INDUSTRIES

In John Hooker's estimation there were four principal industries in Elizabethan Devon comprising farming, cloth-making, tin-extraction and maritime enterprises. Each of these four contributed commodities that could be exported.

## Tin-mining

In the medieval period, if not in many of the generations before, Devon had been best known for its mining activities. There was some gold and silver found in the county, notably silver at Combe Martin under the guidance of Adrian Gilbert of Greenway near Dartmouth, but overwhelmingly the main interest was in tin extraction on Dartmoor. During the Elizabethan period most production came from streaming: like the gold prospectors of nineteenth-century California, deposits were found on the surface, the ore washed and then later smelted. Shaft mining took place later.

The production of tin peaked in the early 1500s and then declined by the end of the century to the level of the late 1400s. In contrast, the amount of Cornish tin continued to increase in value and relative importance and later outstripped Devon's production. Even so, during the Elizabethan period great profits were still being made in Devon.

The industry was overseen in most of Elizabeth's reign by the second Earl of Bedford through the office of Lord Warden of the Stannaries until 1585 when Sir Walter Raleigh was appointed. Tinners enjoyed special privileges as members of the Stannary including the right to be tried for legal offences outside the legal system and within their own Stannary court. They were also exempt from royal taxation and from service in the county militia.

The county was divided into four Stannaries. These areas of administrative jurisdiction, centred on Ashburton, Chagford, Plympton and Tavistock, required that the tin was assayed and taxed in the Stannary in which it was mined. Of the four Plympton was the least important in the sixteenth century while Tavistock had the largest share of production. It not only maintained its dominance in the early seventeenth century but increased it. Ashburton declined through Elizabeth's reign while Chagford slightly gained in the late sixteenth century and nearly continued at the same level up to the start of the Civil War.

## Agriculture

Farming was, in Hooker's opinion, not only more important than tin mining but

the most significant industry of all. This is
hardly surprising given the
overwhelmingly rural nature of the
county which is, at best, seven days'
travel from London. Small farms that
practised mixed farming were more the
rule than the exception. The degree to
which stock was raised as opposed to crops
planted was mostly dependent upon local
soil and climate conditions. There were a
handful of open fields left but on the
whole Devon had already been enclosed.

A county as large as Devon inevitably
has wide variations in farming conditions
and the Exe valley, East Devon and the
South Hams were more profitable for the
Elizabethan farmer than the soils of Mid-
Devon or Dartmoor. Wheat, barley, oats

and rye were all grown as well as peas, beans and occasionally flax and hemp. Hops were raised in north Devon in the early seventeenth century but, even if it were an Elizabethan crop in Devon, most supplies came from the south east of England. Potatoes, if they were familiar to any but the ships' companies of the Elizabethan adventurers, are not known to have been grown in Elizabethan Devon although it is possible experimental plantings were made by Sir Francis Drake at Buckland Abbey.

Many householders, not only farmers, kept herb gardens in which they grew plants for ornament, medicine and cooking including rosemary, thyme, sage, oregano, parsley, hyssop, rue, several types of roses, lettuce, cabbages, onions, leeks, carrots, parsnips and garlic. In the early seventeenth century there were also melons and *pompions*, that is pumpkins, but it is unclear whether these were raised in the sixteenth century. Soft fruit, notably strawberries and raspberries, were also grown and not surprisingly many other useful plants were easily found in hedgerows. Every household in Elizabethan Devon was within an easy walk of the countryside.

In orchards there were apples, pears, cherries, mazards (the black cherry known best in north Devon), plums, medlars, and exotic trees such as quinces and mulberries were planted in gentry gardens. All were grown as table fruit but apples had a further use in the making of cider for which the county became known. It was not complimented for the quality of its beer or ale although local March Ale, so called because it was ready in the spring, was claimed by Sir Walter Raleigh to have the ability to make men dumb and cats speak.

Cattle, sheep and pigs were the most common farm animals although meat was unlikely to have been a frequent part of the general diet. When meat was consumed it could include parts of the animals, such as pigs' feet and even cows' udders, which would be rarely eaten today. Geese, ducks and chickens were also raised with geese being the most predominant because they could be raised cheaply on grass. Wild birds, including rooks, blackbirds and even seagulls, were also eaten.

The county excelled in the making of clotted cream, less so in butter, and produced two types of cheese that were distinguished by the fat content. Imported sugar was still too expensive for mass use and many farmers kept bee-hives to supply the continuing demand for honey.

Even with all this apparent plenty, Elizabethan Devon did not have the ability to feed itself. Harvest failure was problematic in the 1590s but was a continual dilemma. In the 1580s and 1590s Adam Wyott, town clerk of Barnstaple, continually noted in his 'Book of Matters carried on about the town of Barnstaple' the high prices of grain brought about by floods, drought or other extreme weather conditions. The general diet was based on bread and pulses, not yet supplemented by potatoes or rice, and there were dire consequences for the poor when these were expensive or not available. In some years the city of Exeter and some towns purchased grain from France or Poland to supplement local supplies with the hope that prices would be lowered and the poor could afford to buy grain. The more serious problem was when stores ran out. Wyott was particularly concerned in 1596 and 1597: he wrote that 'such snatching and catching for that little and such a cry that the like was never heard'. Some £1,200 was raised in Barnstaple to acquire a full ship's load of grain. Shortages continued into the early seventeenth century.

## Cloth-making

The high number of sheep raised in the county was due to the importance of the local manufacture of woollen cloth. Devon had progressed from having a wool trade to one based on the manufacture of cloth. By the Elizabethan period, the county could not produce enough wool and it was brought in from Cornwall and Ireland.

The cloth industry complemented farming by offering, for many men, women and children, a useful by-employment; they could be employed during spare hours in one of the jobs needed to produce cloth. Once the wool was shorn from the sheep it was washed and carded or combed, and then spun into yarn. The yarn was woven on looms and then fulled, a process for cleansing of grease by the use of water and an alkali, either fuller's earth or soap, or even stale urine. The cloth was also hammered so that, together with the cleaning, it shrunk and had a closer texture. At this point the cloth was stretched on racks, burled (searched for rough imperfections), dubbed (the nap raised), sheared, and finally, pressed and folded for sale. The cloth received its colour either as dyed yarn or afterwards as cloth.

A great number and range of individuals were involved in the different processes. Exeter was the main centre for finishing and selling cloth but it, together with the small market towns in the county, were dependent upon cloth being produced in its various stages in small villages and isolated farmhouses and cottages. There were as yet no large factories in which great numbers of workers gathered as they later did in the eighteenth and nineteenth centuries. Hooker wrote that 'where-so-ever any man doth travel you shall find at the hall door (as they do name the fore door of the house) he shall, I say, find the wife, their children and their servants at the turn spinning or at their cards carding, and by which commodity the common people do live'.

Devon specialised in kerseys, a lighter and coarser material than that produced in some other parts of the country, and made it in lengths of twelve yards. On this account they were known as 'Devonshire Dozens'. Shortly after the death of Elizabeth the county began producing a more hard-wearing and heavier cloth, serge, for which it became even more well-known. Much of the Elizabethan cloth was sold to the London market or sent directly overseas.

Of much less importance was the making of bone-lace, an activity which later became solely identified with East Devon and in particular with Honiton.

There is some evidence which indicates men were involved making lace.

## Maritime Enterprise

Hooker's final industry was somewhat ill-defined in that it encompassed all the maritime trades. The brevity of his account may have been due to his unfamiliarity with coastal life but he appreciated that Elizabethan trade had increased in importance. In the 1540s John Leland, the topographical surveyor, noted a number of coastal towns and villages, including Bideford, Dartmouth, Kingswear, Brixham and Topsham, as being 'pretty'. Leland was not complimenting them for their picturesque qualities but rather commenting on their considerable size and was suggesting an economic vitality. Each of these places, as well as all the other Devon ports, had different patterns of trade.

Devon's two coastlines provide a variety of different types of harbours. In the sixteenth century many of them were already inaccessible, to some degree, to ocean-going vessels through years of silting. The rivers Otter, Sid and Axe were fully crossed at their mouths by banks of gravel while ports such as Salcombe, Teignmouth, Barnstaple and Bideford also had sandbars which made navigation difficult. Efforts were made to emulate the success of Lyme Regis by creating artificial harbours at both 'Ottermouth' and at Seaton. In 1574 a national public 'brief', otherwise known as an appeal for funds, brought money in from around the country to execute what was a very ambitious plan for a quay at Seaton. Churchwardens' account books for parishes around the country recorded donations made to create this new economic centre. The enterprise failed possibly because of storm damage and East Devon continued to dwindle into insignificance as an area for any vessels other than small boats.

The great success story in artificial harbours was not on the south coast but in North Devon. In the 1580s the Cary family at Clovelly constructed a fishing port out of what was virtually a barren stretch of coastline. The great stone quay still stands, more than four hundred years later, as do some of the ancillary buildings. The arrival of herring on the north coast in that decade ensured the financial success of the enterprise but it was helped by the lack of a sufficient number of good harbours along the north Cornish and Devon coasts.

Another engineering feat was achieved at Exeter. For more than 150 years the city was inaccessible to ocean-going vessels. Controversial river restrictions, over which Exeter had no control, hindered the movement of goods to the sea. However in 1564 the city began work on what became the country's first pound lock waterway and it was finished by the end of 1566. Ships still had to unload at Topsham, from whence goods travelled by lighters or via land, but their movement was easier. The city continued to extend and modify the canal into the nineteenth century.

Devon's trade was dominated by cloth export particularly at Exeter. The city's merchants were dependent on the hinterland not just for the production of cloth but Exeter was also important because merchants in many inland towns, such as Crediton, Cullompton, Taunton and Tiverton, used it as the means of exporting their goods. Trade from Exeter, as with other South Devon ports, was of long-standing significance with northern France because of the close proximity but the city's merchants were also actively involved with western France as well as with many ports in Spain and Portugal. However, the steady course of Exeter's trade was not easy: a trade depression in the first years of Elizabeth's reign and trade embargoes with the Spanish in the 1560s, 1570s and from the mid 1580s through to the death of Elizabeth in 1603 seriously hampered the pursuit of legitimate trade.

To a certain degree this was compensated by increased activity with France and also through trade with the Channel Islands. Goods arrived there from Spain and Portugal with whom it became illegal for the English to directly trade.

A greater amount of tin was exported

from Dartmouth and Plymouth than at Exeter because of the easier access to Dartmoor. Plymouth had the additional advantage of its proximity to supplies of Cornish tin. The military uses for tin in the making of armour and weaponry made it a strategic commodity during an era in which there was war in the Netherlands, between England and Spain, and with the Spanish conquering a considerable part of the Americas.

The main imports from the continent were wine, salt, canvas and rope, exotic foodstuffs (including spices, prunes, figs, raisins, almonds, oranges), paper, sugar and many finished goods. Spanish iron was particularly important to a country that was not able to meet its own needs.

There were also a great deal of smaller and more incidental items, such as playing cards and plaster of Paris, which were brought in but not always recorded individually in customs accounts.

The majority of shipping in Devon, as with the rest of the country, is thought to have been jointly owned by a number of individuals, mostly merchants. Some gentlemen owned vessels but most ships were commercial enterprises in which the potential risks of loss were shared between men engaged in maritime trade. Several surveys were made of ships and seafarers in Elizabethan Devon which are very detailed but unfortunately provide contradictory and somewhat misleading information. The details were needed by government to assess resources for potential war use. In 1572 there were 131 vessels recorded for Devon (including 30 from the Exe estuary, 40 from Dartmouth and Teignmouth, 30 from Plymouth and Salcombe, and 24 in North Devon) while in 1582 the figure had dropped to 124 (including 37 which were from the Exe, 12 from the Dart river and Teignmouth, 21 from Plymouth and Salcombe, and 38 in North Devon). The greatly varying numbers of ships between the surveys was partly caused by inaccurate reporting, neither Dartmouth or Plymouth were recorded fully in 1582, or possibly even partially by loss through shipwreck. In spite of the unreliable nature of the details, it is clear there were four main centres of shipping in Plymouth, Dartmouth, Exeter and in the north Devon communities of Barnstaple, Bideford and Northam.

The number of seamen in the county were also surveyed: in 1560 there were 1,268 mariners while in 1570 there were 1,580, or in another survey of that year, 1,675, and finally, in 1582 there were 2,166 seamen. Few of these men would have been full-time mariners but rather men engaged in seafaring on a part-time and occasional basis. Fishing in particular attracted men who were otherwise employed outside of the season. There are no statistics on how many men lost their lives at sea so it is impossible to gauge how quickly they were supplemented by unexperienced men known then as 'green' men.

John Hooker's fourth industry also included fishing. In addition to increasing the number of ships and training men in seafaring, a particular strategic interest of Queen Elizabeth, it was important as a means of supplementing food supplies and in providing a valuable export.

Devon's two coastlines were abundant with fish and along certain stretches there were mussels, oysters and other shellfish. Two fish stocks were particularly important. On the north coast, during the autumn months, herring was significant to local and other fishermen. The fish suddenly reappeared in the 1580s and provided a short seasonal activity which supplemented food supplies and offered employment. On the south coast a pilchard fishery stretched from Cornwall to Dorset and could last many weeks in late summer and early autumn. The fish, and the extracted oil, were valuable commodities for both internal and external sale. Fresh fish was sold but much of it was cured either by salting ('White Herring') or smoking ('Red Herring' or *fumadoes*). The fish were caught in seine nets generally along sand or shingle stretches of coastline and processed in 'Pilchard Palaces' most notably at Hope Cove, Slapton, Teignmouth and Dawlish but in many other coastal villages as well.

There were other types of fish caught but these two fisheries employed the greatest number of men and women in Elizabethan Devon. Men sailed their boats considerable distances from one coast to another to engage in the fisheries and could spend several weeks away from their homes. As impressive as this may have been, the Devon men had considerable experience, by the beginning of Elizabeth's reign, in many other fisheries. For generations Ireland and Wales had been popular destinations for Devon fishermen. There they caught herring, cod, salmon and a great deal of other fish. For example, Thomas Beaple of Barnstaple was one fisherman who fished at Aberdyfi in 1567. In the fifteenth century men from Dartmouth and Plymouth, and probably many other places as well, had fished off the Icelandic coast for cod and this continued into the sixteenth century although it appears to have been curtailed during Elizabeth's reign.

Another medieval fishing ground was to the east of Devon: fishermen from along the south coast of the county sailed along the English Channel to Sussex and Kent where they fished for a number of stocks. They could stay for several weeks and rented huts along the shore. These men also sailed into the North Sea where among the places they visited were Great Yarmouth, Lowestoft and Scarborough. The East Coast activity died away in the seventeenth century only to be taken up again generations later.

The greatest fishery for Devon was of

course Newfoundland. It is uncertain how long it took for English fishermen to regularly fish there after John Cabot discovered the island for Bristol in 1497. Some were there within the next few years but the first reference to Devon men at Newfoundland is in the 1540s. In the following forty years it had grown large enough for Sir Walter Raleigh to then claim it was the 'stay of the west countries'. The fishery employed during Elizabeth's reign many hundreds of local men and engaged scores of vessels. The ships left Devon in early spring and then, after a voyage of a month or so crossing the three thousand miles of the Atlantic, they spent the summer fishing mostly for cod. The fish was cured, mostly salted, and then sold in either

England or on the Continent. As with the pilchard fishery, there was an additional incentive to catch Newfoundland cod because they were particularly oily: the by-product, 'train-oil' now known as cod-liver oil, was highly commercial.

The Devonians interest in fishing, and in developing new fisheries which could supplement the existing ones, led them to the northern shores of the region that later became known as New England. It has generally been thought that the Devon men, under the guidance of the Gilberts, of Greenway near Dartmouth on the river Dart, began exploring that coast in the last year of Elizabeth's reign. However, one document from the collection of the borough of Dartmouth claims that a ship of Dartmouth explored the New England coast in 1597, fully five years before a voyage is known to have been undertaken. Shortly afterwards the Devon men began another fishery in the Gulf of Maine and continued to fish there until the outbreak of the Civil War some forty years later.

In all of these fisheries the interest was a migratory one: the mariners defined Devon as home and perceived the long-distance fisheries merely as short-term employment. Each had its own seasons and dangers. In both Newfoundland and New England there were recurring problems with the native populations and Newfoundland had the added danger of icebergs. The life of an overseas fisherman was not easy.

Although Devon had this network of fisheries, the participation by its fishermen was not universal. As with other maritime endeavours, the topography of the coastline determined not only which stock of fish was available but also the ability of villagers to engage in long-distance fishing: the men of Sidmouth could send ships to Ireland but their limited anchorage meant their ships were too small to cross the Atlantic. Mariners from Dartmouth however had no such restrictions and engaged in all the fisheries. Indeed, a later mayor claimed that it was the town's only asset and therefore the townspeople concentrated their endeavours on the fisheries.

# THE
## 'SEA DOGS'

The Devon men who ventured to sea against the Spanish, including Sir John Hawkins, Sir Walter Raleigh and, most notably of all, Sir Francis Drake, made the greatest impact on the popular imagination: moreover, it could be claimed with some justification that their actions defined the Elizabethan Age. The term 'Sea Dog' was used as early as the seventeenth century to describe both

English and Dutch sailors who engaged in private or public warfare against the Spanish. Throughout the seventeenth century these men were used as symbols of the cause of Protestant England against Catholicism and in the middle of the nineteenth century they were reinterpreted to boost patriotism and underpin Britain's legitimacy for imperial expansion. Finally, during the second world war Drake was revamped by Hollywood. One leading studio presented their activities as a struggle against the Spanish oppression of innocent people in the New World and equated them with the RAF and the Battle of Britain: the message was that just as the Sea Dogs had implored Elizabeth to give them ships to fight the Spanish, so too did modern England need American planes, and vessels, to fight the Nazis. Romanticising has overlooked some of the hard questions regarding their original motivation.

In the first half of the sixteenth century England mostly acted as a spectator to the overseas drama that Spain and Portugal performed in carving out empires for themselves in the New World. Catholic England was constrained by the papal edict which effectively restricted European involvement to the Iberians. But the coronation of the young queen, and the prospect it held out of a long Protestant rule of England, particularly after the Catholic hiatus of her sister

Mary, emboldened a number of gentlemen in the 1560s to seek a personal share of New World wealth. There could be no moral impediment to the English involving themselves in the West Indies and South America as they no longer recognised the authority of Rome. The only obstacles were practical ones; they needed to gauge what activities Elizabeth and the Spanish would permit.

There were some exceptions to England's inactive role in the New World. In 1497 John Cabot sailed from Bristol and discovered Newfoundland after the Europeans had forgotten its existence since the Viking settlements were established some four centuries earlier. The voyage eventually had considerable commercial consequences in that it established English primacy to the island. A second initiative came a generation later in 1530: William Hawkins sailed from Plymouth to Africa, traded English commodities for local goods, voyaged to the West Indies and finally continued trading before returning to England. He entertained the Court in presenting a Brazilian to Henry VIII and symbolised the commercial possibilities of participation in American trade. Hawkins returned to South America two years later.

It was nearly another generation later, in 1562, that his son John was ready to follow in his father's wake. The family had one of the greatest merchant fleets in the West Country but the Spanish and

Portuguese had not relaxed their prohibitions on foreigners trading in their overseas territories and this carried considerable risks both at home and abroad: what could be claimed by the English as peaceful trans-oceanic enterprises could equally be interpreted by the Spanish as commercial warfare.

In the 1560s Hawkins undertook three voyages to the West Indies which proved highly momentous to Elizabethan England and have remained just as notable today. His initiative lay in carrying not merely traditional trading goods to the New World but in introducing slaves from Africa. Hawkins accurately assessed the Spanish need for cheap labour and began a practice which lasted for nearly three hundred years. The consequence of Hawkins' voyages was transforming not only the New World but Africa and Europe.

Hawkins' third voyage in 1568 ended in controversy not over the ethics of the selling of human beings as slaves, although there were existing concerns of the treatment of indigenous Americans, but regarding the Spanish treatment of him and his crew. Although the English were, somewhat, welcome to those Spaniards who were resident in the West Indies, there was considerable pressure from the Spanish government not to deal with the armed and insistent English. The ensuing attack, after Hawkins was assured of his safety, enraged public opinion.

English eagerness to share in the New World wealth was masked with a moral superiority claimed by them over the Spanish Catholic. It was with this justification that the English later attacked the Spanish: it was argued that by removing the Spanish and their Catholicism from the Americas the English were saving many millions of native Americans from eternal damnation.

Two points are often overlooked when considering the implications of Hawkins' actions. First, it should not be assumed that the slave trade was only trans-Atlantic and secondly, it was not only Africans who were made slaves.

Africans were not just being brought

to the West Indies but also transported to Devon. One of the first, if not the earliest, reference to an African in Devon is 'Anthony, a blackmore' who was baptised in Barnstaple on 18 June 1565. It is possible his presence in Devon resulted from one of Hawkins' voyages. Some thirty years later in 1596, also in Barnstaple, there were two Africans noted as Negro or 'neiger' servants. Both 'Grace' and 'Peter Mingus' were baptised and brought to different households in Barnstaple because of Richard Dodderidge, a leading local merchant and member of the English Guinea Company which had exclusive trading rights on the Senegal and Gambia. It is unclear whether they were considered personal property or paid as servants. Within a few years of Elizabeth's death yet another African was living in Barnstaple: Elizabeth, a 'Negro servant', gave birth in 1605 and 1606 to illegitimate daughters who were named Mary and Susannah. The identity of the father and his race was not recorded.

Other races were 'kidnapped'. A Native American from Virginia was baptised with the name Raleigh and lived in nearby Bideford in 1589. Another was 'Adrian the Indian' who in 1599 visited, if not lived in, the parish of Stoke Gabriel near Dartmouth. Both individuals were in those places through local men associated with the New World: Raleigh was in Bideford because of Sir Richard Grenville, who lived nearby and was active in Virginia, and Adrian could have been in the household of the Gilberts of nearby Greenway, who were leading explorers of the American coastline, and probably that of Adrian Gilbert himself. Most likely there were other Africans and Native Americans in Devon who were not noted in the county's documents. In the early seventeenth century there were more, the most famous of them was Pocahontas. Although the Elizabethan numbers were probably small, the movement is not without its significance.

Within only a few years' of Elizabeth's death, but with precedents going back generations, English men and women were also enslaved by Africans. Initially the numbers were small but by 1620 many hundreds of English mariners were being held captive and kept as slaves in North African ports along the Barbary Coast. The movement was partly religiously inspired but largely dominated by commercial incentives. By the outbreak of the Civil War the number of English slaves was comparable to those taken from Africa.

The news of John Hawkins' ill-treatment in the West Indies in 1568 coincided with an event which provoked a crisis for Elizabeth and her Councillors. In the closing months of that year Hawkins' news reached England just as a fleet of Spanish ships sailed into Plymouth, Fowey and Southampton in an attempt to avoid pursuing Dutch and French privateers. The ships carried bullion destined for the Spanish troops fighting in the Netherlands.

Technically the coinage belonged to a group of Genoese bankers from whom Philip of Spain had arranged to borrow the money. The Hawkins family laid claim to the bullion as compensation for the Caribbean losses but Elizabeth impounded the bullion for her own use. In retaliation the Spanish seized all English goods and residents in the Low Countries. Elizabeth raised the stakes by arresting all Spaniards and their property in England as well as ordering the capture of Spanish ships at sea. In 1570 the Spanish preparations for a large fleet to sail through the Channel bringing Anne of Austria to Spain prompted fears of an invasion and Elizabeth ordered the survey of English ships and seamen noted above.

Devon ships were among those which set sail against the Spanish. Francis Drake, who had been with Hawkins on the voyage of 1568, led expeditions from Plymouth in 1570 and 1571. However it was his voyage in 1573 which was extraordinarily effective and made his name. The expedition was a financial success because of a daring raid on the treasure train in Panama and when, as a longstanding story is told, Drake returned home unexpectedly on a Sunday in August, the people of Plymouth left church in the midst of a sermon.

Emboldened with confidence and enabled by his new wealth, Drake began organising what would be the most illustrious of his endeavours. In 1574 state relations between England and Spain eased but anti-Spanish feelings remained, particularly among those men who wanted a portion of the American wealth. One option was for legitimate trade through Spain opening her overseas territories to English merchants, which the Spanish were reluctant to do. The second lay in continuing hostile operations against Spanish interests.

In November of 1577 Drake set sail from Plymouth aboard the *Pelican* under the guise of a voyage to Tripoli, Alexandria and Constantinople. His actual destination was South America. Historians have questioned Drake's motivations: he was certainly intent on raiding and may well have planned trading outside of Spain's territories. But less plausible are various theories that he hoped to establish trade with the Far East or was acting as an unofficial agent of the crown in trying to provoke Spain into a declaration of war.

Reports slowly reached England, via Spain, of some of Drake's activities: a series of attacks on Spanish interests along both the Atlantic and Pacific coasts of South America were viewed with alarm in Spain and expectation in England. Drake then disappeared across the Pacific and his successful circumnavigation of the globe became apparent several years later when, in the autumn of 1580, the *Pelican*, renamed the *Golden Hind*, returned to Plymouth.

Those who invested in the voyage, including the queen, were significantly wealthier but the full financial details were not released. Drake himself had sufficient wealth to buy Buckland Abbey. The son of a poor cleric had become one of the richest and most influential men in Devon.

Elizabeth did not punish Drake in spite of Spain's protests for what clearly were a series of illegal attacks on Spanish property; to the contrary, the queen knighted the man who had become a popular hero. Tensions between the two countries once again increased. In 1585 English ships were confiscated in Spain which prompted Elizabeth to openly support the Dutch Protestants in their struggle against the Spanish. She also unleashed Drake after many months of indecision on another plan of his: Devon remained at the forefront of national affairs when in September he sailed with a large fleet from Plymouth for a voyage to the Spanish coast. Open warfare between England and Spain looked more certain.

Drake's priority was to release the English vessels and their crews and in this the voyage theoretically looked after national interests but at the same time it offered a profit incentive for private investors. The Spanish were humiliated when Drake surprised the town of Vigo in north-west Spain and secured supplies on his own terms but he did not achieve the release of English ships and men. The fleet then sailed to the West Indies where it caused great destruction. The voyage was not the commercial success many of the investors had hoped but in strategic terms it was clear that Spain could not protect its empire from a well-armed English fleet.

Drake returned in 1586 and in that year a plot was discovered to kill the queen and it implicated Mary Queen of Scots. Her trial and execution in February of 1587 was quickly followed by an attempt to head off a Spanish invasion of England. In April Drake's fleet sailed from

Plymouth and arrived at Cadiz where they destroyed as many as thirty-nine vessels. The 'Singeing of the King of Spain's Beard' was followed by the loss of many more vessels at St Vincent and an attempt to blockade Lisbon. Once again, private interests were served when Drake abandoned Lisbon and headed for the Azores where he captured a rich East Indies prize. The voyage was both a commercial and strategic success. It was hoped that the loss of ships and supplies would impede the building of a Spanish invasion fleet, which in part it did, but it was clear that within the year the ships would attack England.

Devon remained at the forefront of national affairs when, in the spring of

1588, Drake, Vice Admiral of the Fleet, waited at Plymouth for the Spanish Armada. In the third week of July the Spaniards were reported nearby (prompting the enduring tale of Drake's nonchalant attitude while playing a game of bowls on the Hoe) and the theatre of operations quickly moved up channel as the English pursued the Spanish navy. The events of the next few days, particularly the role of the subsequent storm, has somewhat overshadowed the contemporary anxieties of the extent of the Spanish loss and the certainty of English victory: the full destruction of the Spanish fleet took several months longer as the ships rounded Scotland in an attempt to return to Spain.

One of those ships was the *San Pedro Mayor* which in late October went ashore in Hope Cove near Salcombe. This was not the only Armada vessel in Devon. Drake also brought in a prize, the *Nuestra Senora del Rosario*, in circumstances still questioned, to Torbay where the crew was initially imprisoned in what has since been known as 'The Spanish Barn'.

The loss of the Armada was followed by other attempts in the 1590s to attack England, most notably when a small Spanish force attacked Mount's Bay in Cornwall. This was a decade of intensive action by the English against the Spanish. On the day after Christmas in 1590 the town clerk of Barnstaple looked on with disbelief and wonder of the arrival of the

*Prudence* with its prize ship carrying four chests of gold worth more than £16,000. He wrote 'such a value as the like prize hath not before this time been brought into this port' but in the following years he grew accustomed to such prize ships.

The greatest prize was the *Madre de Dios*, brought into Dartmouth in 1592. The amount of precious jewels and musk was staggering to onlookers including the London official sent to salvage the government's share of the spoils. It was widely alleged, and acknowledged, that 'the common sort', the actual crew who captured the ship, were the chief beneficiaries.

It can be claimed that in the late 1580s and through the 1590s the English were justified in their attacks on the Spanish in that they were legally sanctioned. But many of the early seizures of Spanish ships and property were not made by privateers, those with an official government license, but by pirates. Moreover, the English established a form of undeclared war which was taken up by other nations and became as great a problem for Elizabeth's successor as it had been for Philip of Spain.

The 1590s brought the death of Sir Richard Grenville from a Spanish onslaught on the *Revenge* and, less illustriously, that of Drake from dysentery in the West Indies. However, the late 1590s continued to bring in enormous wealth and Plymouth was the busy centre of the privateers' world.

# EXPLORATION
## AND
# COLONIES

E xploration, trade, colonisation, privateering and piracy were often linked-components of Elizabethan voyages. While some men were motivated by scientific curiosity, all voyages needed to make a financial return for the men who had invested in them. The greatest exploration prize, in terms of fame and wealth, lay in the search for a northern passage to the Far East; the consequences of such a route would open Asia to English merchants and end the Spanish monopoly. John Davis, who lived at Sandridge on the river Dart near the Gilbert family, made three voyages in search of a North-West passage in the three years immediately before the Armada. The Spanish war interrupted his search which yielded the most comprehensive details of that region.

Other Devonians made less well-known voyages and many, such as John Chudleigh of Ashton who voyaged through the Magellan Straits en route to Peru in 1589, never returned.

In 1582 Sir Humphrey Gilbert, half-brother to Sir Walter Raleigh, sailed to Newfoundland and formally claimed the island as the first colony for England. The queen had given Gilbert exclusive rights to settle English colonies in North America. Unfortunately Gilbert was drowned on his return voyage to England; the last he was heard to utter was that at sea he was as close to heaven as on land. The choice of Newfoundland was of particular interest and relevance for Devon's fishermen and it accelerated a process of attempting the forced exclusion from that fishery of other European mariners. However, the permanent settlement of the island by the English would not be commercially successful for several more generations.

In 1584 Sir Walter Raleigh obtained his half-brother Humphrey's license to

North American exploration and settlement. That year he sent two vessels, led by two Devonians, to discover the most appropriate site for a colony; his motivations were part mercantile and strategic, a colony would be a useful base for English privateers. The following year an expedition left Devon to establish a settlement at Roanoke in 'Virginia', named after the Virgin Queen, situated in what is now North Carolina. Only a year later deteriorating relations with the native population prompted the colonists to leave with Sir Francis Drake's fleet which had unexpectedly arrived on its return voyage to England. A few weeks later Sir Richard Grenville landed at Roanoke and upon finding the colony deserted left a number of his crew there in an attempt to continue the settlement. The men were never seen again. Notwithstanding, the two enterprises, Devon-led and inspired, were symbolically important and had long-term consequences.

Of more immediate importance was Ireland, which has been argued as England's first colony. A number of the leading players were Devonians: not only Drake, Raleigh and Gilbert were concerned with establishing Protestant settlements there but others gave considerable financial backing, notably the Champernowne family of Modbury. From the start the enterprise was violent, and the profits uncertain, but Devon men, and later women, remained keenly involved for the following two centuries. As with the American colonial plans, the prospect of obtaining extensive grants of land, a commodity in short supply at home, was a powerful incentive to the Devon gentleman with ready cash.

# RELIGION

With Elizabeth's coming to the throne the county of Devon, like the rest of the country, returned to its Protestant state. Only eight years previously the Prayer Book Rebellion (or the 'Western Rebellion') had torn through Devon and it is likely, after the swift lurches in religion under the previous three monarchs, that it took many years before ordinary Devonians were assured that the country would stay Protestant.

It is a matter of conjecture as to how closely the new religion was taken to heart in Devon as well as to how many remained allied to the old one: there are no reliable figures of Catholics during Elizabeth's reign. Those that were faced heavy fines but a list was made in the last year of her reign: it noted only 35 Catholics in the county. Other records show the list to be incomplete but it is interesting that it was of a few dozen individuals only.

There are also only occasional references to individuals termed 'Puritans', a name which many used in a derogatory manner, but this markedly increases in early seventeenth-century records. Those places with which Puritanism was associated can often be linked to the introduction of 'godly' men by patrons such as Sir John Chichester who placed two such men in the churches at Shirwell and Pilton. In 1586 Adam Wyott at Barnstaple made a cryptic note in his journal that in two neighbouring villages men and women gathered to hear a trental of sermons, that is a set of thirty lectures, which they called an 'Exercise' or 'Holy Fast'. He compared it to a pilgrimage because they made offerings but noted it was 'to the admiration of all Protestants'. The two villages were Shirwell and Pilton.

Of the great figures in the county

more can be found but it is a mixed message. Raleigh can himself hardly be held up as a strong believer in Protestantism, in fact it was whispered he was an atheist. Some Devon families long remained Catholic, such as the Courtenays. Drake's religious convictions were well known and his choice of the converted former Catholic Buckland Abbey for his home was a highly symbolic act. Even so, Drake's widow chose a member of the Catholic Courtenay family for her next husband. The first wife of the earl of Bath was from a prominently Catholic family who were supporters of Queen Mary and yet his second wife was the daughter of the earl of Bedford, a staunch Protestant who suppressed the Prayer Book Rebellion.

As for Devon's merchants, they were if anything pragmatic in that they were prepared, at least, to suspend their beliefs in the furtherance of their profession. Throughout Elizabeth's reign their main foreign trading partners were not fellow Protestants but Catholics. While it is true they learned to rob from the Spanish, and excelled at it, they embraced trade once peace was declared after the accession of James I. One of the greatest commodities was fish and it had a strong market in Catholic Europe because the diets there were determined by religious beliefs. While in church Devonians may have complimented themselves on their righteousness, the wine they celebrated communion with was produced by Catholic hands and the prosperity of Devon was based on the sale of goods to those they may have scorned privately, or publicly, as idolaters.

# THE
# LEGACY
## OF THE
# ELIZABETHAN
# AGE

The final appraisal on Elizabeth Devon could belong to John Hooker. He wrote without, he claimed, any vanity that 'England may better live of itself without another nation than any other nation without it. And even so also this little corner of this land can live better of itself without the rest of the land, than all the residue can live without it'. At the close of the sixteenth century, John Hooker was an elderly man and perhaps had not appreciated the sweeping changes in his native Devon. Exploration and colonies little figured in his assessment of the county's history. It is probably true that Devon could survive on it's own but it could not prosper. As much as Devon had thrived in the years before Elizabeth's reign, it was the subsequent gain of maritime expertise in navigation and in the knowledge of other lands that brought it great wealth. Perhaps one particular room in Buckland Abbey most ably symbolizes this 'sea change' in Devon: in Sir Richard Grenville's Great Hall are the faces, created in plaster, of peoples from a mixture of often ill-defined races. The Elizabethan Devonian was beginning to understand the complexities and extent of the wider world and in so doing he was defining himself.

The disposable wealth taken during the long Spanish war was the result not of activity conducted within the county but outside of it, and at the expense of others. In the years immediately following Elizabeth's death Devon men utilised their knowledge of new horizons to expand trade and establish lasting colonies. The Elizabethan legacy lay with the successful integration of Devon with the Old and New Worlds.

ELIZABETHAN DEVON

# FURTHER READING

The best general study of late sixteenth-century Devon is Joyce Youings, *Ralegh's Country* (North Carolina, 1986). The two studies of particular relevance in Todd Gray, Margery Rowe and Audrey Erskine (eds), *Tudor and Stuart Devon: The Common Estate and Government* (Exeter, 1992) are Tom Greeves, 'Four Devon Stannaries: A Comparative Study of Tinworking in the Sixteenth Century', and Alison Grant, 'Breaking the Mould: North Devon Maritime Enterprise, 1560-1640'. There are also several relevant articles in *The New Maritime History of Devon* (London, 1992), notably Ronald Pollitt, 'Devon and the French and Spanish Wars', 108-114 and Joyce Youings with Peter W. Cornford, 'Seafaring and Maritime Trade in Sixteenth-Century

Devon', 98-107. The only edition, to date, of Hooker's partial history is William J. Blake, 'Hooker's Synopsis Chorographical of Devonshire', *Devonshire Association Transactions,* xlvii (1915), 334-48, and for the diary of Adam Wyott see Todd Gray (ed.), *The Lost Chronicle of Barnstaple* (Exeter, 1998). Two recent biographies of Drake are John Sugden, *Sir Francis Drake* (London, 1990) and the less well-written Harry Kelsey, *Sir Francis Drake; The Queen's Pirate* (New Haven, 1998).

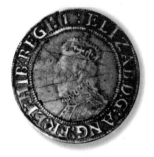

*Silver shilling struck in 1601, found in the*
*East Worlington hoard*

(by courtesy of Exeter Museums Service)

**Also available in the Concise Histories of Devon
Series**

| | |
|---|---|
| *Roman Devon* | Malcolm Todd |
| *The Vikings and Devon* | Derek Gore |
| *Devon and the Civil War* | Mark Stoyle |

*Also by* **The Mint Press**

**The Devon Engraved Series**

> *Exeter Engraved: The Secular City* (2000)
>
> *Exeter Engraved: The Cathedral,
> Churches, Chapels and Priories* (2001)
>
> *Devon Country Houses and Gardens
> Engraved* (2001)
>
> *Dartmoor Engraved* (2001)

**The Travellers' Tales Series**

> *Exeter* (2000)
>
> *East Devon* (2000)
>
> *Cornwall* (2000)